Mental Health Practitioner's Guide to HIV/AIDS

Sana Loue
Editor

Mental Health Practitioner's Guide to HIV/AIDS

Springer

Editor
Sana Loue
Department of Epidemiology and Biostatistics
Case Western Reserve University
Cleveland, OH
USA

ISBN 978-1-4614-5282-9 ISBN 978-1-4614-5283-6 (eBook)
DOI 10.1007/978-1-4614-5283-6
Springer New York Heidelberg Dordrecht London

Library of Congress Control Number: 2012953263

Printed on acid-free paper

Springer is part of Springer Science+Business Media (www.springer.com)

Preface

Although significant progress has been made in the development and implementation of HIV prevention strategies and HIV treatments, new infections continue to occur, particularly among those who are most vulnerable due to poverty, marginalization, isolation, and violence. Too often, individuals with mental illness may fall within one or more of these groups. Researchers have identified HIV prevention strategies that are effective in preventing HIV transmission among those with mental illness. Nevertheless, many individuals do not have access to either the information or the skills development programs that would help them prevent HIV transmission, often due to lack of access to care, the unavailability of such programs within their communities, language or cultural barriers, or logistical issues such as transportation difficulties and lack of child care.

Additionally, individuals who become infected with HIV/AIDS often experience depression, anxiety, and the mental health consequences of the disease. Mental health care providers may or may not have received training related to the wide variety of issues that may arise in this context.

This volume is intended to provide mental health care providers, such as psychiatrists, social workers, psychologists, and marriage and family therapists, with the information necessary to address both HIV-related issues with individuals with a preexisting mental illness diagnosis and with HIV-positive individuals who experience mental illness or the mental health consequences of HIV infection. The volume commences with two in-depth chapters. The first, authored by Busby, Lytle, and Sajatovic, provides an overview of the biology of HIV and mental illness, mental health issues that may arise when working with HIV-positive clients, and the management of co-occurring mental illness and HIV infection. The second chapter, authored by Johnson and Henderson-Newlin, examines the legal issues relevant to the HIV-infected client, many of which are also relevant to HIV-negative clients; many of these legal issues may impact the provision of mental health care at varying stages of HIV infection.

These two in-depth chapters are followed by brief entries arranged in alphabetical order. These entries, authored by 46 different authors with training in diverse disciplines and experience in HIV research, prevention, or care, cover a multitude of topics related to HIV and mental health and illness. As an example, topics range from antiretroviral medication to social support to cognitive impairment to case management to sex toys. Each entry is followed by a listing of suggested references and/or Web-based resources that will enable the reader to access the most current literature.

Mental health care providers represent a critical link in the promotion and maintenance of well-being among those with mental illness, whether HIV-negative or HIV-positive. This volume is intended to assist them in fulfilling that role.

Cleveland, OH, USA Sana Loue, J.D., Ph.D., M.P.H., M.S.S.A., MA., LISW
April 2012

Contents

D

E/F

G/H

List of Contributors

David Arute Wheaton College, Wheaton, IL, USA

Domniţa Oana Bădărău Institute for Biomedical Ethics, University of Basel, Basel, Switzerland

Ana Gabriela Benghiac Department of Bioethics, Case Western Reserve University, Cleveland, OH, USA

David Bruckman Cleveland Department of Public Health, Cleveland, OH, USA

Katherine Kovalski Busby Department of Psychiatry, University Hospitals-Case Medical Center, Cleveland, OH, USA

Cristina Chinole Cazacu Center for Ethics and Public Policies, Bucharest and Iasi, Romania

Aiswarya Lekshmi Pillai Chandran Pillai Department of Epidemiology and Biostatistics, School of Medicine, Case Western Reserve University, Cleveland, OH, USA

Simona Irina Damian University of Medicine and Pharmacy Gr. T. Popa, Iasi, Romania

Brittany Daugherty-Brownrigg John Carroll University, South Euclid, OH, USA

Nicole Deming Department of Bioethics, Case Western Reserve University, Cleveland, OH, USA

Diana Diaconu Department of Dermatology, University of Medicine and Pharmacy "Gr. T. Popa", Iasi, Romania

Beth Faiman Cleveland Clinic Taussig Cancer Institute, Cleveland, OH, USA

Vanessa Forro Neurological Outcomes Center, Case Western Reserve University, Cleveland, OH, USA

Oscar Grusky Department of Sociology, University of California Los Angeles, Los Angeles, CA, USA

Susan Hatters-Friedman Department of Psychiatry, School of Medicine, Case Western Reserve University, Cleveland, OH, USA

Lisa M. Henderson-Newlin McAnany, Van Cleave & Phillips, P.A., St. Louis, MO, USA

Beatrice Gabriela Ioan Legal Medicine, Medical Deontology and Bioethics Department, University of Medicine and Pharmacy "Gr. T. Popa", Iasi, Romania

Abishek Jain Cleveland, OH, USA

Zane Jennings Mandel School of Applied Social Sciences, Case Western Reserve University, Cleveland, OH, USA

Brandy L. Johnson Rynearson, Suess, Schnurbusch & Champion, L.L.C, St. Louis, MO, USA

Cabrina Kang Wellesley College, Wellesley, MA, USA

Ezer Kang Department of Psychology, Wheaton College, Wheaton, IL, USA

Anton Knieling University of Medicine and Pharmacy Gr. T. Popa, Iasi, Romania

Helen Land School of Social Work, University of Southern California, Los Angeles, CA, USA

Kristen Limbach School of Medicine, Case Western Reserve University, Cleveland, OH, USA

Sana Loue Department of Epidemiology and Biostatistics, Case Western Reserve University, Cleveland, OH, USA

Sarah Lytle Department of Psychiatry, University Hospitals-Case Medical Center, Cleveland, OH, USA

Lisa Norman Ponce School of Medicine, Ponce, Puerto Rico

Daniel J. O'Shea Public Health Service, County of San Diego, San Diego, CA, USA

Stefani Parrisbalogun Department of Psychiatry, University Hospitals Case Medical Center, Cleveland, OH, USA

Bettina Rausa Salk Institute for Biological Studies, La Jolla, CA, USA

Eric Rice School of Social Work, University of Southern California, Los Angeles, CA, USA

Martha Sajatovic Department of Psychiatry, University Hospitals-Case Medical Center, Cleveland, OH, USA

Nicholas Schiltz Department of Epidemiology and Biostatistics, School of Medicine, Case Western Reserve University, Cleveland, OH, USA

Kristen Shirey Departments of Psychiatry and Behavioral Sciences and Medicine, Duke University Medical Center, Durham, NC, USA

Laura Solovastru Department of Dermatology, University of Medicine and Pharmacy "Gr. T. Popa", Iasi, Romania

Robert W. Stephens Rynearson, Suess, Schnurbusch & Champion, L.L.C., St. Louis, MO, USA

Bryan Taylor Cleveland, OH, USA

Dan Vata Department of Dermatology, University of Medicine and Pharmacy "Gr. T. Popa", Iasi, Romania

Mihaela Vicol Department of Bioethics, University of Medicine and Pharmacy "Gr. T. Popa", Iasi, Romania

Lucia Volk Middle East and Islamic Studies, San Francisco State University, San Francisco, CA, USA

Todd Wagner University Hospitals Case Medical Center, Cleveland, OH, USA

Margaret Winchester Department of Bioethics, School of Medicine, Case Western Reserve University, Cleveland, OH, USA

Hailey Winetrobe School of Social Work, University of Southern California, Los Angeles, CA, USA

Heather Wollin School of Social Work, University of Southern California, Los Angeles, CA, USA

Introduction

Sana Loue

The Beginning of the Epidemic

In 1981, five homosexual men were reported to have *Pneumocystis carinii* pneumonia (PCP) (Centers for Disease Control, 1981b). Kaposi sarcoma was detected in 26 others (Centers for Disease Control, 1981a). Both conditions were later found to be the result of an underlying immune deficiency (Gottlieb et al., 1981; Masur et al., 1981). First referred to as gay-related immune deficiency (GRID) and attributed to lifestyle choices (Centers for Disease Control, 1986), reports soon surfaced of its detection in nongay individuals, prompting the identification of "risk groups": homosexuals, heroin users, Haitians, and hemophiliacs (New York City Commission on Human Rights, 1986, 1987; Shilts, 1987). The identification of risk groups rather than risk behaviors and the emphasis on transmission through unprotected male–male sex and intravenous drug use severely hampered the detection of the illness in women and the prevention of the disease across populations (American Public Health Association, 1991; Mays & Cochran, 1987).

The underlying cause of the immune deficiency was identified in 1983–1984 as the human immunodeficiency virus (HIV), the causative agent of the acquired immunodeficiency syndrome (AIDS) (Barre-Sinoussi et al., 1983; Popovic, Sarngadharan, Read, & Gallo, 1984). There are four primary modes of HIV transmission: unprotected intercourse with an HIV-infected sexual partner, the use of HIV-contaminated injection and other medical paraphernalia, blood transfusion, and mother-to-child transmission. Sexual intercourse includes vaginal (Laga, Taelman, Van der Stuyft, & Bonneux, 1989; Peterman, Stoneburner, Allen, Jaffe, & Curran, 1988), anal (Darrow et al., 1987; Detels et al., 1989; Moss et al., 1987; Winkelstein et al., 1987), and oral intercourse (Lifson et al., 1990). Transmission

S. Loue (✉)
Department of Epidemiology and Biostatistics, Case Western Reserve University, Cleveland, OH, USA
e-mail: sana.loue@case.edu

S. Loue (ed.), *Mental Health Practitioner's Guide to HIV/AIDS*,
DOI 10.1007/978-1-4614-5283-6_1, © Springer Science+Business Media New York 2013

through injection drug use with contaminated injection equipment may occur as a result of using contaminated needles, syringes, cookers, and/or cotton (Hoffman, Larkin, & Samuel, 1989; Sasse, Salmaso, Conti, & First Drug User Multicenter Study Group, 1989; Schoenbaum et al., 1989). Transfusion with virus-contaminated blood or blood products may also lead to HIV infection. Mother-to-child transmission, also known as vertical transmission, may occur before birth, during delivery, or through breastfeeding. Vehicles for transmission include semen (Chiasson, Stoneburner, & Joseph, 1990; Ho, Schooley, Rota, Kaplan, & Flynn, 1984; Levy, 1989), vaginal and cervical secretions (Vogt et al., 1986; Wofsy et al., 1986), blood and blood products (Donegan et al., 1990), tissue and organs from HIV-infected donors (Centers for Disease Control, 1987, 1988; Kumar et al., 1987), and breast milk (Colebunders et al., 1988; Thiry et al., 1985; Ziegler, Cooper, Johnson, & Gold, 1985). HIV cannot be transmitted through casual and household contact (Friedland et al., 1990; Rogers et al., 1990), despite its presence in tears (Fujikawa et al., 1985) and saliva (Ho et al., 1985).

The risk of HIV transmission as a result of unprotected intercourse differs depending upon the nature of the sexual act. Receptive individuals are at increased risk of infection compared to the insertive partner. Unprotected anal intercourse carries a 1 in 50 chance of HIV transmission from the insertive to the receptive partner (Vittinghoff et al., 1999), whereas the risk of transmission associated with vaginal intercourse ranges from 1 in every 1,000 or 2,000 without a condom to 1 in 10,000 to 1 in 20,000 when a condom is used (Downs & De Vincenzi, 1996). Other activities, such as kissing and biting, that involve body fluids other than blood carry a negligible risk of transmission (Campo et al., 2006; Royce, Seña, Cates, & Cohen, 1997). The presence or absence of other factors, such as a sexually transmitted infection, circumcision of the male partner, the health of the uninfected partner, and the viral load of the infected partner, may serve to increase or decrease the risk of transmission (Fowler, Melnick, & Mathieson, 1997; Royce et al., 1997; Williams et al., 2006).

The Demographic Impact

The UNAIDS Report on the Global AIDS Epidemic 2010 estimated that worldwide, 30.8 million adults and 2.5 million children were living with HIV at the end of 2009 and approximately 16.6 million children under the age of 18 had lost one or both parents to HIV/AIDS. That same year, approximately 2.6 million individuals were newly infected with HIV and 1.8 million deaths from AIDS occurred. Approximately one-half of all HIV-infected individuals contract the infection before they have reached the age of 25 years. Worldwide, AIDS is the second most common cause of death among individuals between the ages of 20 and 24 years.

Sub-Saharan Africa, home to 10% of the world's population, continues to be the most highly impact geographic region, with 68% of all HIV-infected people living there. The HIV/AIDS epidemic is rapidly expanding in Eastern Europe and Central Asia. Unlike other regions of the world, there has been a significant increase in the number of adults and children living with HIV in the countries of North Africa and the Middle East.

The Centers for Disease Control and Prevention (2011) estimated that as of 2009, 1.2 million people in the United States were living with HIV. However, approximately 20% were unaware that they were infected. Although men who have sex with men are believed to comprise only 2% of the US population, they accounted for 61% of all new HIV infections in 2009. Unprotected heterosexual intercourse accounted for an additional 27% and injection drug use accounted for another 9%. Blacks and Latinos continue to be disproportionately impacted by HIVAIDS, as detailed further in the entries relating to African-Americans and Latinos (Centers for Disease Control and Prevention, 2006).

Mental Health and Illness and HIV

Individuals with mental illness and particularly those with severe mental illness have consistently been found to be at increased risk for HIV infection. Researchers have reported prevalence rates among individuals with severe mental illness ranging from 4 to 22%, although the prevalence has been found to vary by age, gender, ethnicity, and treatment setting (Cournos et al., 1991; Cournos, Horwath, Guido, McKinnon, & Hopkins, 1994; Empfield et al., 1993; Lee, Travin, & Bluestone, 1992; Meyer, Cournos, et al., 1993; Meyer, McKinnon, et al., 1993; Sacks, Dermatis, Looser-Ott, & Perry, 1992; Schwartz-Watts, Montgomery, & Morgan, 1995; Silberstein, Galanter, Marmor, Lisshutz, & Krasinski, 1994; Stewart, Zuckerman, & Ingle, 1994; Susser, Valencia, & Conover, 1993; Volavka et al., 1991). Nevertheless, this prevalence far exceeds the prevalence of 0.3–0.4% among the general population of the United States (McQuillan, Khare, Karon, Schable, & Vlahov, 1997; Steele, 1994). As many as 40% of individuals with severe mental illness have reported having more than one sexual partner during the preceding year (Hanson et al., 1992; Kelly et al., 1992), contrary to the often-held belief that individuals with severe mental illness due not engage in sexual activity (Carey, Carey, & Kalichman, 1997; Carey, Carey, Weinhardt, & Gordon, 1997). As many as 20–26% of severely mentally ill individuals have reported having had sexual intercourse with an injection drug user (Knox, Boaz, Friedrish, & Dow, 1994; Steiner, Lussier, & Rosenblatt, 1992), resulting in increased HIV risk. Further, as many as 27% or more of samples of SMI have reported trading sex for drugs (Kalichman, Kelly, Johnson, & Bulton, 1994; McKinnon, Cournos, Sugden, Guido, & Herman, 1996) Many individuals with severe mental illness may have relatively low levels of HIV knowledge of HIV risk and prevention and relatively low and/or inconsistent use of condoms (Aruffo, Cloverdale, Chacko, & Dworkin, 1990; Carey, Carey, Weinhardt, et al., 1997; Katz, Watts, & Santman, 1994; Kelly et al., 1992; Kelly et al., 1995; Knox et al., 1994; McDermott, Sautter, Winstead,

& Quirk, 1994; McKinnon et al., 1996; Otto-Salaj, Heckman, Stevenson, & Kelly, 1998; Sacks et al., 1992; Steiner et al., 1992).

Women with severe mental illness may be at particularly high risk of HIV infection (Katz et al., 1994). This increased risk of HIV may be due to (1) deficits in the ability to process information, resulting in difficulties in the identification and avoidance of risky situations and (2) deficits in social competence, resulting in a decreased ability to form lasting relationships, refuse unreasonable requests, solve problems effectively, and negotiate risky situations (Gearon & Bellack, 1999). Women with severe mental illness have also been found to be at increased risk of partner violence (Hatters-Friedman & Loue, 2007), which may place them at increased risk of HIV infection.

This text is designed as a desk reference for mental health professionals in providing services to both HIV-infected and HIV-negative individuals. The text begins with two full-length chapters, one that addresses in detail both the increased risk of HIV among individuals with mental illness and the increased likelihood that some HIV-positive individuals may experience mental health issues. Guidance is provided with respect to differential diagnosis, medication interactions, and other related issues. The chapter on legal issues provides information that will be helpful to both HIV-positive and HIV-negative individuals with mental health concerns in planning for their health care. These two chapters are followed by alphabetically organized shorter entries on topics relevant to mental health care and HIV prevention and treatment.

References

American Public Health Association. (1991). *Women and HIV disease: A report of the special initiative on AIDS of the American Public Health Association*. Washington, DC: Author.

Aruffo, J., Cloverdale, J. H., Chacko, R. C., & Dworkin, R. J. (1990). Knowledge about AIDS among women psychiatric outpatients. *Hospital and Community Psychiatry, 41*, 326–328.

Barre-Sinoussi, F., Cherman, J. C., Rey, F., Chamaret, S., Gruest, J., Dauguet, C., et al. (1983). Isolation of a T-lymphotropic retrovirus from a patient at risk for acquired immune deficiency syndrome (AIDS). *Science, 220*, 868–870.

Campo, J., Perea, M. A., de Romero, J., Cano, J., Hernando, V., & Bascones, A. (2006). Oral transmission of HIV, reality or fiction? *Oral Diseases, 12*, 219–228.

Carey, M. P., Carey, K. B., & Kalichman, S. C. (1997). Risk for human immunodeficiency virus (HIV) infection among persons with severe mental illnesses. *Clinical Psychology Review, 17*, 271–291.

Carey, M. P., Carey, K. B., Weinhardt, L. S., & Gordon, C. M. (1997). Behavioral risk for HIV infection among adults with a severe and persistent mental illness: Patterns and psychological antecedents. *Community Mental Health Journal, 33*, 133–142.

Centers for Disease Control. (1981a). Kaposi's sarcoma and Pneumocystis pneumonia among homosexual men—New York and California. *Morbidity and Mortality Weekly Report*, 30, 305–308.

Centers for Disease Control. (1981b). Pneumocystis pneumonia—Los Angeles. *Morbidity and Mortality Weekly Report*, 30, 250–252.

Centers for Disease Control. (1986). *Reports on AIDS published in the Morbidity and Mortality Weekly Report, June, 1981 through February, 1986*. Springfield, VA: National Technical Information Service.

Centers for Disease Control. (1987). Revision of the CDC surveillance case definition of acquired immunodeficiency syndrome. *Morbidity and Mortality Weekly Reports*, 36 (Suppl. 1S), 1S–3S.

Centers for Disease Control. (1988). Transmission of HIV through bone transplantation: Case report and public health recommendation. *Morbidity and Mortality Weekly Reports*, 37, 597–599.

Centers for Disease Control and Prevention. (2006). *HIV/AIDS among Hispanics*. Atlanta, GA: Author.

Centers for Disease Control and Prevention. (2011, November). *HIV in the United States*. Retrieved December 29, 2011 from http://www.cdc.gov/hiv/resources/factsheets/PDF/us.pdf

Chiasson, M. A., Stoneburner, R. L., & Joseph, S. C. (1990). Human immunodeficiency virus transmission through artificial insemination. *Journal of Acquired Immune Deficiency Syndromes, 3*, 69–72.

Colebunders, R., Kapita, B., Nekwei, W., Bahwe, Y., Lebughe, I., Oxtoby, M., et al. (1988). Breastfeeding and transmission of HIV. *Lancet, 2*, 1487.

Cournos, F., Empfield, M., Horwath, E., McKinnon, K., Meyer, I., Schrage, H., et al. (1991). HIV seroprevalence among patients admitted to two psychiatric hospitals. *American Journal of Psychiatry, 148*, 1225–1230.

Cournos, F., Horwath, E., Guido, J. R., McKinnon, K., & Hopkins, N. (1994). HIV-1 infection at two public psychiatric hospitals in New York City. *AIDS Care, 6*, 443–452.

Darrow, W. W., Echenberg, D. F., Jaffe, H. W., O'Malley, P. M., Byers, R. H., Getchell, J. P., et al. (1987). Risk factors for human immunodeficiency virus (HIV) infections in homosexual men. *American Journal of Public Health, 77*, 479–483.

Detels, R., English, P., Visscher, B. R., Jacobson, L., Kingsley, L. A., Chmiel, J. S., et al. (1989). Seroconversion, sexual activity and condom use among 2915 HIV seronegative men followed up to 2 years. *Journal of Acquired Immune Deficiency Syndromes, 2*, 77–83.

Donegan, E., Stuart, M., Niland, J. C., Saks, H. S., Azen, S. P., Dietrich, S. L., et al. (1990). Infection with human immunodeficiency virus type I (HIV) among recipients of antibody-positive blood donations. *Annals of Internal Medicine, 113*, 733–739.

Downs, A. M., & De Vincenzi, I. (1996). Probability of heterosexual transmission of HIV, relationship to the number of unprotected sexual contacts. *Journal of Acquired Immune Deficiency Syndromes, 11*, 388–395.

Empfield, M., Cournos, F., Meyer, I., McKinnon, K., Horwath, E., Silver, M., et al. (1993). HIV seroprevalence among homeless patients admitted to a psychiatric inpatient unit. *American Journal of Psychiatry, 150*, 47–52.

Fowler, M. G., Melnick, S. L., & Mathieson, B. J. (1997). Women and HIV: Epidemiology and global overview. *Obstetrics and Gynecology Clinics, 24*, 705–729.

Friedland, G., Kahl, P., Saltzman, B., Rogers, M., Feiner, C., Mayers, M., et al. (1990). Additional evidence for lack of transmission of HIV infection by close interpersonal (casual) contact. *AIDS, 4*, 639–644.

Fujikawa, L. S., Salahuddin, S. Z., Palestine, A. G., Nussenblatt, R. B., Salahuddin, S. Z., Masur, H., et al. (1985). Isolation of human T-lymphotropic virus type III from the tears of a patient with the acquired immunodeficiency syndrome. *Lancet, 2*, 529–530.

Gearon, J. S., & Bellack, A. S. (1999). Women with schizophrenia and co-occurring substance use disorders: An increased risk for violent victimization and HIV. *Community Mental Health, 35*, 401–419.

Gottlieb, M. S., Schroff, R., Schanker, H. M., Weisman, J. D., Peng, T. F., Wolf, R. A., et al. (1981). *Pneumocystis carinii* pneumonia and mucosal candidiasis in previously healthy homosexual men: Evidence of a newly acquired immunodeficiency. *New England Journal of Medicine, 305*, 1425–1431.

Hanson, M., Kramer, T. H., Gross, W., Quintana, J., Li, P., & Asher, R. (1992). AIDS awareness and risk behaviors among dually disordered adults. *AIDS Education and Prevention, 4*, 41–51.
Hatters-Friedman, S., & Loue, S. (2007). Incidence and prevalence of intimate partner violence by and against women with severe mental illness. *Journal of Women's Health, 16*(4), 471–480.
Ho, D., Byington, R.E, Schooley, R.T., Flynn, T., Rota, T.R., & Hirsch, M.S. (1985). Infrequency of isolation of HTLV-III virus from saliva in AIDS. *New England Journal of Medicine, 313*, 1606.
Ho, D. D., Schooley, R. T., Rota, T. R., Kaplan, J. C., & Flynn, T. (1984). HTLV-III in the semen and blood of healthy homosexual men. *Science, 226*, 451–453.
Hoffman, P. N., Larkin, D. P., & Samuel, D. (1989). Needlestick and needleshare—The difference. *Journal of Infectious Diseases, 160*, 545–546.
Kalichman, S. C., Kelly, J. A., Johnson, J. R., & Bulton, M. (1994). Factors associated with risk for HIV infection among chronically mentally ill adults. *American Journal of Psychiatry, 151*, 221–227.
Katz, R. C., Watts, C., & Santman, J. (1994). AIDS knowledge and high risk behaviors in the chronically mentally ill. *Community Mental Health Journal, 30*, 395–402.
Kelly, J. A., Murphy, D. A., Bahr, G. R., Brasfield, T. L., Davis, D. R., Hauth, H. C., et al. (1992). AIDS/HIV risk behavior among the chronically mentally ill. *American Journal of Psychiatry, 149*, 886–889.
Kelly, J. A., Murphy, D. A., Sikkema, K. J., Somlai, A. M., Mulry, G. W., Fernandez, M. I., et al. (1995). Predictors of high and low levels of HIV risk behavior among adults with chronic mental illness. *Psychiatric Services, 46*, 813–818.
Knox, M. D., Boaz, T. L., Friedrish, M. A., & Dow, M. D. (1994). HIV risk factors for persons with severe mental illness. *Community Mental Health Journal, 30*, 551–563.
Kumar, P., Pearson, J. E., Martin, D. H., Leech, S. H., Buisseret, P. D., Bezak, H. C., et al. (1987). Transmission of human immunodeficiency virus by transplantation of renal allograft, with development of acquired immunodeficiency syndrome. *Annals of Internal Medicine, 106*, 244–245.
Laga, M., Taelman, H., Van der Stuyft, P., & Bonneux, L. (1989). Advanced immunodeficiency as a risk factor for heterosexual transmission of HIV. *AIDS, 3*, 361–366.
Lee, H. K., Travin, S., & Bluestone, H. (1992). HIV-1 in inpatients. *Hospital and Community Psychiatry, 43*, 181–182.
Levy, J.A. (1989). Human immunodeficiency virus and the pathogenesis of AIDS. *Journal of the American Medical Association, 261*(20), 2997–3006.
Lifson, A. R., O'Malley, P. M., Hessol, N. A., Buchbiner, S. P., Cannon, L., & Rutherford, G. W. (1990). HIV seroconversion in two homosexual men after receptive oral intercourse with ejaculation: Implications for counseling concerning safe sexual practices. *American Journal of Public Health, 80*, 1509–1511.
Masur, H., Michelis, M. A., Greene, J. B., Onorato, I., Vande Stouwe, R. A., Holzman, R. S., et al. (1981). An outbreak of community-acquired *Pneumocystis carinii* pneumonia: Initial manifestations of cellular immune dysfunction. *New England Journal of Medicine, 305*, 1431–1438.
Mays, V. M., & Cochran, S. D. (1987). Acquired immunodeficiency syndrome and black Americans: Special psychosocial issues. *Public Health Reports, 102*, 224–231.
McDermott, B. E., Sautter, F. J., Jr., Winstead, D. K., & Quirk, T. (1994). Diagnosis, health beliefs, and risk of HIV infection in psychiatric patients. *Hospital and Community Psychiatry, 45*, 580–585.
McKinnon, K., Cournos, F., Sugden, R., Guido, J. R., & Herman, R. (1996). The relative contributions of psychiatric symptoms and AIDS knowledge to HIV risk behaviors among people with severe mental illness. *Journal of Clinical Psychiatry, 57*, 506–513.
McQuillan, G. M., Khare, M., Karon, J. M., Schable, C. A., & Vlahov, D. (1997). Update on the seroepidemiology of human immunodeficiency virus in the United States household

population: NHANES III, 1988–1994. *Journal of Acquired Immune Deficiency Syndromes and Human Retrovirology, 4*, 355–360.

Meyer, I., Cournos, F., Empfield, M., Schrage, H., Silver, M., Rubin, M., et al. (1993). HIV seroprevalence and clinical characteristics of the mentally ill homeless. *Journal of Social Distress and the Homeless, 2*, 103–116.

Meyer, I., McKinnon, K., Cournos, F., Empfield, M., Bavlis, S., Engel, D., et al. (1993). HIV seroprevalence among long-stay psychiatric patients. *Hospital and Community Psychiatry, 44*, 282–284.

Moss, A. R., Osmond, D., Bacchetti, P., Chermann, J. C., Barre-Sinoussi, F., & Carlson, J. (1987). Risk factors for AIDS and HIV seropositivity in homosexual men. *American Journal of Epidemiology, 125*, 1035–1047.

New York City Commission on Human Rights. (1986). *AIDS and people of color: The discriminatory impact*. New York, NY: Author.

New York City Commission on Human Rights. (1987). *AIDS discrimination and its implications for people of color and other minorities*. New York, NY: Author.

Otto-Salaj, L. L., Heckman, J. G., Stevenson, L. Y., & Kelly, J. A. (1998). Patterns, predictors and gender differences in HIV risk among severely mentally ill men and women. *Community Mental Health Journal, 34*, 175–190.

Peterman, T. A., Stoneburner, R. L., Allen, J. R., Jaffe, H. W., & Curran, J. W. (1988). Risk of human immunodeficiency virus transmission from heterosexual adults with transfusion-associated infections. *Journal of the American Medical Association, 259*, 55–58.

Popovic, M., Sarngadharan, M. G., Read, E., & Gallo, R. C. (1984). Detection, isolation, and continuous production of cytopathic retroviruses (HTLV-III) from patients with AIDS and pre-AIDS. *Science, 224*, 497–500.

Rogers, M. F., White, C. R., Sanders, R., Schable, C., Ksell, T. E., Wasserman, R. L., et al. (1990). Lack of transmission of human immunodeficiency virus from infected children to their household contacts. *Pediatrics, 85*, 210–214.

Royce, R. A., Seña, A., Cates, W., & Cohen, M. S. (1997). Sexual transmission of HIV. *New England Journal of Medicine, 336*, 1072–1078.

Sacks, M. H., Dermatis, H., Looser-Ott, S., & Perry, S. (1992). Seroprevalence of HIV and risk factors for AIDS in psychiatric inpatients. *Hospital and Community Psychiatry, 43*, 736–737.

Sasse, H., Salmaso, S., Conti, S., & First Drug User Multicenter Study Group. (1989). Risk behaviors for HIV-1 infection in Italian drug users: Report from a multicenter study. *Journal of Acquired Immune Deficiency Syndromes, 2*, 486–496.

Schoenbaum, E. E., Hartel, D., Selwyn, P. A., Klein, R. S., Darenny, K., Rogers, M., et al. (1989). Risk factors for human immunodeficiency virus in intravenous drug users. *New England Journal of Medicine, 321*, 874–879.

Schwartz-Watts, D., Montgomery, L. D., & Morgan, D. W. (1995). Seroprevalence of human immunodeficiency virus among inpatient pretrial detainees. *Bulletin of the American Academy of Psychiatry and Law, 23*, 285–288.

Shilts, R. (1987). *And the band played on: Politics, people, and the AIDS epidemic*. New York, NY: St. Martin's Press.

Silberstein, C., Galanter, M., Marmor, M., Lisshutz, H., & Krasinski, K. (1994). HIV-1 among inner city dually diagnosed inpatients. *American Journal of Drug and Alcohol Abuse, 20*, 101–131.

Steele, F. R. (1994). A moving target: CDC still trying to estimate HIV-1 prevalence. *Journal of NIH Research, 6*, 25–26.

Steiner, J., Lussier, R., & Rosenblatt, W. (1992). Knowledge about and risk factors for AIDS in a day hospital population. *Hospital and Community Psychiatry, 43*, 734–735.

Stewart, D. L., Zuckerman, C. J., & Ingle, J. M. (1994). HIV seroprevalence in a chronically mentally ill population. *Journal of the National Medical Association, 86*, 519–523.

Susser, E., Valencia, E., & Conover, S. (1993). Prevalence of HIV infection among psychiatric patients in a New York City men's shelter. *American Journal of Public Health, 83*, 568–570.

Thiry, L., Sprecher-Goldberger, S., Jonckheer, T., Levy, J., Van de Perre, P., Henrivaux, P., et al. (1985). Isolation of AIDS virus from cell-free breast milk of three healthy virus carriers. *Lancet, 2*, 891–892.

Vittinghoff, E., Douglas, J., Judon, F., McKiman, D., MacQueen, K., & Buchinder, S. P. (1999). Per-contact risk of human immunodeficiency virus transmission between sexual partners. *American Journal of Epidemiology, 150*, 306–311.

Vogt, M. W., Witt, D. J., Craven, D. E., Crawford, D. F., Witt, D. J., Byington, R., et al. (1986). Isolation of HTLV III/LAV from cervical secretions of women at risk for AIDS. *Lancet, 1*, 525–527.

Volavka, J., Convit, A., Czobor, P., Dwyer, R., O'Donnell, J., Jr., & Ventura, A. (1991). HIV seroprevalence and risk behaviors in psychiatric inpatients. *Psychiatry Research, 39*, 109–114.

Williams, B. G., Lloyd-Smith, J. O., Gouws, E., Hankins, C., Getz, W. M., Hargrove, J., et al. (2006). The potential impact of male circumcision on HIV in sub-Saharan Africa. *PLoS Medicine, 3*, 1032–1040.

Winkelstein, W., Lyman, D. M., Padian, N., Grant, R., Sameul, M., Wiley, J. A., et al. (1987). Sexual practices and risk of infection by the human immunodeficiency virus: The San Francisco Men's Health Study. *Journal of the American Medical Association, 257*, 321–325.

Wofsy, C., Cohen, J., Hauer, L., Michaelis, B. A., Cohen, J. B., Padian, N. S., et al. (1986). Isolation of AIDS-associated retrovirus from genital secretions of women with antibodies to the virus. *Lancet, 1*, 527–529.

Ziegler, J. B., Cooper, D. A., Johnson, R. O., & Gold, J. (1985). Postnatal transmission of AIDS-associated retrovirus from mother to infant. *Lancet, 1*, 896–898.

Mental Health Comorbidity and HIV/AIDS

Katherine Kovalski Busby, Sarah Lytle, and Martha Sajatovic

Introduction

New data on the incidence and prevalence of HIV both in the United States and throughout the world underscore the continuing magnitude of the AIDS epidemic clearly. There are now an estimated 1.2 million people in the United States and 34 million people in the world living with HIV, with 2.7 million new infections in the world in 2010, including an estimated 390,000 among children (UNAIDS, 2011). The UNAIDS report urgently calls for accelerated responses from countries in efforts to completely halt the spread of the disease and highlights the declining incidence and death rate from the disease. However, there are still no current cures or available vaccines. Although medications which are available to manage HIV have been helpful in decreasing the ravages of the disease and prolonging life, each has drawbacks. We in health care must be prepared to manage HIV and AIDS for decades to come.

Psychiatric comorbidity in persons living with HIV is relatively high, specifically for psychiatric diagnoses such as depression and substance use disorders, as well as certain anxiety disorders, psychotic disorders, and cognitive disorders. The reverse relationship also seems to be true, namely that in general psychiatric populations, the rates of HIV infection are elevated. Furthermore, persons living with HIV are specifically at risk for increased symptoms related to psychiatric disorders. In some of these conditions the relationship is bidirectional; for example, persons with substance use disorders have a higher likelihood of also having HIV. In this chapter, we discuss the relationships between mental health and HIV, including the role of mental health in HIV transmission and treatment, the role of HIV in psychiatric illness and its course, and current recommendations for assessment and treatment of mental health in persons living with HIV.

K.K. Busby • S. Lytle • M. Sajatovic (✉)
Department of Psychiatry, University Hospitals Case Medical Center, Cleveland, OH, USA
e-mail: Martha.Sajatovic@UHHospitals.org

S. Loue (ed.), *Mental Health Practitioner's Guide to HIV/AIDS*,
DOI 10.1007/978-1-4614-5283-6_2, © Springer Science+Business Media New York 2013

Sample Clinical Treatment Scenario

The following composite case from a clinical practice setting demonstrates some of the relevant issues for consideration in assessment and treatment of people with mental health and HIV comorbidity.

A 45-year-old man presented to a community mental health center for treatment of depression and difficulty with attention. He reported that his mood symptoms had been severe since his mid-20s, including persistent low mood and thoughts of death. Although he indicated that he had also had low moods and poor attention in childhood, these had not been severely disabling and he had obtained some higher education and was a talented musician. He had used street drugs heavily at times, most notably having developed a methamphetamine addiction which peaked in his 20s and 30s. However, he states he has not used methamphetamines in 10 years. He is not sure when he acquired HIV, but feels it was likely in his late 20s from sexual contact with men. He is being treated for HIV with several medications. He admits that the symptoms of depression and inattention have interfered with his ability to take his HIV medications; at times when he is particularly depressed, he may spend an entire day in bed and fail to eat or take medications. At other times, he may simply forget to take a dose. Because of the increased recent depressive symptoms, decreased levels of movement and activity, and general physical debility, he is no longer able to continue his work in music at the same level as he had previously.

His treatment course has been difficult due to refractory depression and complex comorbidities of attentional difficulties and substance abuse. On presentation to the community mental health center, he was being prescribed two antidepressants with different actions, a benzodiazepine, and a stimulant by his clinician with whom he had worked with for several years; cross-referencing through the state-wide pharmacy repository confirmed that he did not have multiple providers. Chart review and conference with the previous provider confirmed that the medications had been added individually to address symptoms, and attempts to wean him off of any of the medication classes had been unsuccessful. In fact, as all of the diseases progressed, and he developed tolerance to certain medications, he seemed to need higher doses. He had particular difficulty with fatigue, low motivation versus a lack of interest, and poor appetite. He has not recently been able to access individual or group therapy other than supportive therapy per his psychiatrist and social work support at the clinic that manages his HIV. However, he is agreeable to these, as well as medication management.

Relationship Between Mental Illness and HIV Transmission

Several clinically relevant relationships exist between mental illness and HIV status. Having a preexisting mental illness may influence the likelihood of both contracting HIV as well as progression to AIDS. Conversely, it also seems that having HIV or AIDS increases the likelihood of developing certain mental illnesses or disorders, as well as symptoms of mental illness that, although extremely troublesome to patients, may not reach the level of a disorder. Although more needs to be done, some research has begun to identify both illness and psychosocial factors that may be important in modulating these relationships. While it is important to keep in mind that many things about HIV may be changing (in particular, its prevalence in different demographics and associated psychosocial stressors, available treatments, prognosis), and care must be taken not to overgeneralize studies, we must rely on what may be available to understand the relationships between HIV and mental health.

Studies of persons who have mental illness or substitute measures that suggest mental illness, such as having an inpatient psychiatric hospitalization, have found that this population has had a higher rate of HIV infection in comparison with the general population. Studies done two decades ago found that the prevalence of HIV in a population of psychiatrically hospitalized patients was several times higher than that of the general population (Cournos, Horwath, Guido, McKinnon, & Hopkins, 1994; Gewirtz, Horwath, Cournos, & Empfield, 1988; Sacks, Dermatis, Looser-Ott, & Perry, 1992), particularly among patients who had multiple sexual partners, had traded sex for money or drugs, or had used injection drugs (Kalichman, Kelly, Johnson, & Bulto, 1994). Later studies have again shown that patients with a psychiatric diagnosis have a much higher rate of HIV, which has been estimated to be seven to eight times higher than control groups (Otto-Salaj, Heckman, Stevenson, & Kelly, 1998; Rosenberg et al., 2001; Vanable, Carey, Carey, & Maisto, 2007).

Several factors may explain why certain mental illnesses increase the risk of contracting HIV. Patients with serious mental illnesses such as schizophrenia, recurrent major depression, and certain anxiety disorders such as posttraumatic stress disorder (PTSD) may have increased risk-taking behavior or lowered use of risk-reduction strategies in regard to sexual contacts and/or drug abuse during exacerbations; they may have lower knowledge about how to protect themselves from becoming infected; and they may also have other sexually transmitted or blood-borne infections that may increase the likelihood of HIV infection (Blumberg & Dickey, 2003). Studies examining the correlation between mental illness and higher rates of HIV transmission to others have not found this to be true. However, there is likely a link between depression and unprotected sex in HIV-negative men who have sex with men that may increase the likelihood of contracting the virus; a link was not found between depression and unprotected sex in HIV-positive men who have sex with men (Houston, Sandfort, Dolezal, & Carballo-Dieguez, 2012).

Mental illnesses and symptoms of mental illnesses also likely have an effect on HIV treatment success, which may be mediated by treatment adherence, biological factors, or other factors. Patients who have both HIV and a mental illness are likely to have worse outcomes, including higher likelihood of progression to AIDS and death (Evans et al., 1997; Rothbard, Miller, Lee, & Blank, 2009). Patients with symptoms associated with depression, even without meeting full criteria for depression, have been shown to have higher rates of poor HIV-related outcomes, such as higher rates of treatment failure and death (Leserman, 2008). A recent study has similarly found that patients with HIV and co-occurring schizophrenia, bipolar disorder, and substance use disorders have higher rates of mortality, and that progression to AIDS was more likely in patients with substance use disorders (Nurutdinova et al., 2012).

Having HIV or AIDS also increases the likelihood of developing mental illness or sub-threshold symptoms of these disorders, or exacerbating preexisting mental illness.

Biology of HIV and Psychiatric Illness

The biological relationship between mental illness and HIV has received increasing attention in the past two decades. Knowing the common biological links between HIV and mental illness can inform clinical treatment decisions.

Depression may contribute to the progression of HIV by several direct and indirect mechanisms. The neurotransmitter serotonin has been studied as a direct mediator of the process, as it plays a role in both depression and immunity. In immune cells, serotonin is felt to regulate the cell's production of additional receptors and signaling molecules and enhance the body's production of the types of immune cells responsible for effectively containing the infection by killing infected cells. Serotonin has been found to decrease HIV replication within the infected cell (Fauci, Mavilio, & Kottilil, 2005). Recent research has found that medications used to alleviate depression by blocking reuptake and subsequent degradation of this neurotransmitter may also enhance the body's ability to suppress HIV through actions on key immune cells (Benton et al., 2010).

According to a recent review of the topic by Schuster and colleagues, direct mechanisms also involve depression-related increases in cortisol and other stress-related hormones, in turn causing poor immune function by blunting and dysregulating the response of immune cells and their infection-fighting products, as well as enhancing HIV replication (Schuster, Bornovalova, & Hunt, 2012). Additionally, biopsychosocial factors, including increased hopelessness, increased substance abuse, decreased social support, decreased medication adherence, and increased risk taking behaviors with likelihood of contracting additional sexually transmitted diseases, play an important role through some of the same central mediators. The resultant load of contributing factors, each triggering biologic pathways that affect the immune system, leads to measurably worse outcomes for patients, in particular increased disability, faster progression to AIDS, and decreased lifespan. It is important for the mental health provider to assess for these contributing factors, as each of them represents an area where intervention may be needed to achieve better immune outcome. Of note, it has been shown that improvement in depressive symptoms can improve not only cell counts and decrease viral load but also improve immune cell function (Cruess et al., 2005).

The relationship between psychosis and HIV likely has completely different biological mechanisms, although some mediators are likely shared. Studies of patients with HIV and new onset psychosis including hallucinations and delusions have suggested HIV encephalopathy (inflammation of the central nervous system), or the direct infection of the brain with HIV, with resultant changes in the brain due to the infection, as the cause (Sewell et al., 1994).

HIV and Mental Illness Comorbidity

Depression, Anxiety, and HIV

A 2001 meta-analysis of ten studies concluded that patients with HIV are at two-fold higher risk of depression than those without HIV; this effect appears to be independent of disease stage or sexual orientation (Ciesla & Roberts, 2001). The presence of depressive disorders has been estimated to approach 40% of patients with HIV (Bing et al., 2001). A substantial percentage of patients with a depressive disorder remain undiagnosed, and increased efforts should be made to improve detection. Differences in biological sex in this regard have also been studied in a large, prospective, cross-sectional study by Lopes et al. (2012). When compared with HIV-negative men, HIV-positive men were significantly more likely to have a mood disorder, major depressive disorder or dysthymia having the highest prevalence, followed by any anxiety disorder, and lastly any personality disorder. In contrast, HIV-positive women were not found to have an elevated prevalence of psychiatric disorders in general or in specific (Lopes et al., 2012). Of note, different studies of various demographic populations have also correlated female sex with depression or depressive symptoms as well. HIV has also been found to increase sub-threshold symptoms of depression and anxiety. The role that HIV plays in increasing depression may be partly mediated by the effects of social support and family functioning (Dyer, Stein, Rice, & Rotheram-Borus, 2012).

Certain aspects of mental health are particularly important to emphasize. In a study of patients who had attempted suicide after recent diagnosis of HIV, researchers found that HIV diagnosis increased the risk of suicide by approximately 16%, and that patients endorsed many comorbid stressors related to HIV as being present, particularly fear of negative impact on psychological, social, economic and health statuses due to HIV, lack of psychosocial and health support, and fear of being ostracized or victimized (Schlebusch & Vawda, 2010). The study also supported earlier findings that factors such as younger age, female sex, and mental health diagnoses further increased the risk of suicide.

Treatment of depression has been shown to improve not only the depressive symptoms, but also improve measures of the HIV infection, such as viral load and cell counts (Coleman, Blashill, Gandhi, Safren, & Freudenreich, 2012). Assessment of depression and anxiety at the primary point of contact for patients who have HIV can facilitate correct treatment referral, act to destigmatize mental illnesses for the patient, and serve to support the patient even if he or she does not meet criteria for a psychiatric disorder. Rating tools can be used to quickly screen for many disorders, and can be used by a broad array of clinical providers. Tools that have been studied specifically with patients who have HIV include the Zung rating scale (Lombardi, Mizuno, & Thornberry, 2010), the Beck Depressive Inventory (Levine, Aaron, & Criniti, 2008), the PHQ-2 and the PHQ9 (Monahan et al., 2009). Other scales may also be useful in clinical practice as well. Continued research is needed to determine the optimal rating scale. Diagnosis should then be made based on clinical interview that will be able to rule out conditions that may mimic depression or anxiety. Of particular importance in this regard is HIV-associated dementia, which shares many symptoms of depression and anxiety, bipolar spectrum disorders, medication-related mood disorders, substance use disorders, and various medical illnesses, all of which will affect treatment decisions.

Treatments that appear to have at least some evidence base for people with HIV and depression include psychotherapies and antidepressant medications (Kelly et al., 1993; Olatunji, Mimiaga, O'Cleirigh, & Safren, 2006; Psaros, Israel, O'Cleirigh, Bedoya, & Safren, 2011). Medication treatment choices for treatment of depression and anxiety in the HIV patient should take into account medication interactions and particularly bothersome versus clinically useful side effects. A recent review of medication treatment for psychiatric disorders in patients with HIV and AIDS notes that there is a relative lack of research done since the advent of currently used antiretroviral regimens; however, antidepressants and anxiolytics are widely used (Repetto & Petitto, 2008). As in the general population with depression, use of antidepressant medications side effect profile that minimizes possible exacerbation of physical complaints such as fatigue or insomnia should be considered before medication initiation. It is reported that antidepressant medications that may be useful in treating depression in people with HIV include imipramine, desipramine, nortriptyline, amitriptyline, fluoxetine, sertraline, paroxetine, citalopram, escitalopram, fluvoxamine, venlafaxaine, nefazodone, trazodone, bupropion, and mirtazapine (Mainie, McGurk, McClintock, & Robinson, 2001). Double-blind trials have been conducted with imipramine, fluoxetine, sertraline, and paroxetine (Ferrando, 2005). No single antidepressant drug appears to have evidence of superior efficacy (Yanofski & Croarkin, 2008).

Psychotherapeutic approaches that appear to be helpful include cognitive behavioral therapy and interpersonal therapy (Psaros et al., 2011). Important elements of psychotherapy for people with HIV/AIDS may include dealing with stigma, discrimination, punishment beliefs and addressing barriers to illness self-management for both HIV and for depression such as adherence with antiretroviral medication. One report noted that patients with HIV who are treated for depression with antidepressants appear to benefit from improved levels of adherence to their antiretroviral therapy as well (Dalessandro et al., 2007).

Psychosis and HIV

Psychotic disorders are characterized by delusions, hallucinations and impaired insight. HIV-infected individuals presenting with psychosis require a thorough clinical assessment to determine the underlying etiology of the psychotic state.

An increased risk of psychosis in HIV infected individuals has been found to be associated with a history of psychiatric illness (de Ronchi et al., 2000; Dew et al., 1997), psychosis caused by physical illness such as opportunistic infections of the central nervous system (Johannessen & Wilson, 1988; Sewell, 1996), a high lifetime prevalence of stimulant and sedative/hypnotic abuse (Sewell et al., 1994), as well as lower cognitive abilities (de Ronchi et al., 2000) and stressful life events (Sewell, 1996).

A psychiatric history to evaluate for a preexisting (primary) psychotic disorder such as schizophrenia or bipolar disorder should be obtained. Schizophrenia is more prevalent (approximately 5%) in individuals with HIV than in the general populations (about 1%) (Walkup, Crystal, & Sambamoorthi, 1999). Despite this, a study of people with schizophrenia in an inpatient population showed that only 17% had been tested for HIV within the last month (Walkup, McAlpine, Olfson, Boyer, & Hansell, 2000), suggesting that screening for HIV in this population could be improved. Individuals with schizophrenia may be at an increased risk of contracting HIV due to symptoms or effects of schizophrenia including poor impulse control, delusions (Psaros et al., 2011), impaired judgment, substance abuse including intravenous drug use, a high risk of trading sex for money or drugs (Cournos, Guido, et al., 1994; Kalichman et al., 1994; Kelly et al., 1992; McKinnon, Cournos, Sugden, Guido, & Herman, 1996), and lack of effective HIV education (Gottesman & Groome, 1997; Sewell, 1996). Despite being at high risk for contracting HIV, individuals with psychotic disorders are less likely to be tested for HIV than those with other severe mental illnesses or substance abuse, possibly due to cognitive or social deficits, lack of patient education, and lack of clinician knowledge about risk behaviors in this population (Meade & Sikkema, 2005). However, timely diagnosis and treatment is critical since people with comorbid schizophrenia and HIV are at a greater risk of morbidity and mortality due to impaired ability to comply with medical care, difficulty explaining symptoms to medical personnel, and possibly receiving less attention than those without psychosis as it relates to physical complaints (Sewell, 1996; Sewell et al., 1994).

The differential diagnosis of psychosis in HIV infected individuals also includes substance intoxication or withdrawal, HIV encephalopathy, delirium, dementia or side effects of medications (Table 1) (Brogan & Lux, 2009; Foster, Olajide, & Everall, 2003; Sewell et al., 1994). Between 0.2 and 15% of HIV-positive individuals have no prior history of a psychotic illness and experience secondary or new onset psychosis (Sewell, 1996). Psychosis in HIV-positive individuals may be clinically distinct from primary psychotic conditions with more paranoid, grandiose and somatic delusions than bizarre delusions, impairment in attention and concentration, more visual hallucinations, fewer affective symptoms and a greater

Table 1 Differential diagnosis of psychosis in individuals with HIV/AIDS

Primary psychotic disorders	Schizophrenia
	Bipolar disorder
	Other psychotic disorders, e.g., schizoaffective disorder, depression
Secondary psychotic disorders	HIV infection
	HIV-related infections/opportunistic infections
	HIV encephalopathy
	Secondary mania
	Substance intoxication or withdrawal
	Delirium
	HIV-associated dementia
	Medication side effects or interactions
	Medical disorders (i.e., electrolyte disturbances, sepsis, hypoglycemia)

likelihood of remission (De Ronchi et al., 2006; Harris, Jeste, Gleghorn, & Sewell, 1991).

A variety of drug interactions or side effects of medications may induce psychotic symptoms in HIV-infected individuals. Medications used to treat HIV and associated conditions have significant side effects and a medication list should be obtained, including an assessment of any temporal relationship between starting new medications and the onset of psychotic symptoms. In particular, psychosis has been observed in those treated with the HIV medication efavirenz (de la Garza, Paoletti-Duarte, Garcia-Martin, & Gutierrez-Casares, 2001; Lowenhaupt, Matson, Qureishi, Saitoh, & Pugatch, 2007) and another HIV medication, zidovudine, may induce mania (O'Dowd & McKegney, 1988). Other HIV medications including nevirapine (Wise, Mistry, & Reid, 2002) and abacavir (Foster et al., 2003) have also been implicated in causing transient psychosis. Other drugs, including ganciclovir and ethambutol, used in the treatment of HIV-related illnesses such as cytomegalovirus and mycobacterium avium complex have also been reported to cause psychosis (Hansen, Greenberg, & Richter, 1996; Martin & Bowden, 2007).

HIV and hepatitis C virus (HCV) have similar routes of transmission (i.e., intravenous drug use) and 30–50% of individuals with HIV are coinfected with HCV (Dodig & Tavill, 2001). Individuals infected with HIV alone or HIV and HCV together were found to have higher rates of bipolar disorder, schizophrenia and psychotic disorders than those without HIV (Baillargeon et al., 2008). Interferon alpha is a medication used in the treatment of HCV (Ferguson, 2011) that may cause psychiatric side effects including psychosis in HIV-positive individuals (Hoffman et al., 2003).

Adherence with treatment for both HIV antiretroviral drugs and antipsychotic medications may be adversely affected by psychosis (Bansil, Jamieson, Posner, & Kourtis, 2009), although one study suggested that adherence may be better in HIV-infected people with schizophrenia than HIV-infected people who do not have schizophrenia due to increased access to medical care (Walkup, Sambamoorthi, & Crystal, 2001). Since adherence with antiretrovirals may be an issue and since psychotic individuals may present a risk of harm to themselves or others, it is critical to treat psychotic symptoms in HIV positive individuals.

Newer atypical antipsychotics such as quetipaine, risperidone, olanzapine, and aripiprazole can be used for psychosis and for mood stabilization and are generally preferred over the older, typical antipsychotics, such as haloperidol and thorazine. Typical antipsychotics are known to cause more extrapyramidal symptoms (EPS) such as abnormal movements, dystonia, or parkinsonism. However, atypical antipsychotics carry a greater risk for metabolic syndrome and those with the higher risk should generally be avoided or closely monitored. Increased appetite, obesity, and abnormal triglycerides and cholesterol as a result of antipsychotic medication can lead to diabetes and cardiovascular events and switching to an antipsychotic with lower metabolic risks may be considered (Stahl, Mignon, & Meyer, 2009).

A consensus survey conducted by Freudenreich et al. (2010) showed that the atypical antipsychotics quetiapine, risperidone, and aripiprazole were most often used for treatment of psychosis. Risperidone has been shown to be efficacious in the treatment of HIV-related psychosis (Singh, Golledge, & Catalan, 1997) but has higher rates of EPS than other atypical antipsychotics, especially at higher doses; individuals with HIV may be more likely to develop EPS due to loss of dopaminergic neurons (Hriso, Kuhn, Masdeu, & Grundman, 1991). Clozapine, another atypical antipsychotic, is generally not recommended for the treatment of psychosis in HIV-infected people due to concerns for agranulocytosis (a dangerous decrease in white blood cell count), toxicity, and drug interactions (Cournos, McKinnon, & Sullivan, 2005).

General recommendations for treating HIV-positive individuals with antipsychotic medications include starting at lower doses than in individuals without HIV, up-titrating doses slowly, and closely monitoring for side effects (Cournos et al., 2005). Discontinuing antiretroviral treatment until remission of the psychotic symptoms occurs should be considered (Arendt, de Nocker, von Giesen, & Nolting, 2007; Foster et al., 2003). Following stabilization of psychotic symptoms, individuals may benefit from psychotherapy, and psychosocial interventions for people with schizophrenia including skills training, cognitive therapies, education and HIV risk reduction programs. All of these approaches may improve self-care and overall functioning (Cournos et al., 2005; Heinssen, Liberman, & Kopelowicz, 2000).

Manic episodes in HIV-infected individuals may be due to a preexisting (primary) bipolar disorder which can be characterized by elevated mood, grandiosity, impulsivity, a decreased need for sleep, and/or pressured speech (American Psychiatric Association, 2000). First-episode (secondary) mania which is directly related to HIV infection in the brain or HIV-related infections may present differently with greater irritability, aggression, disruptive behaviors, decreased need for sleep, higher rates of psychotic symptoms, visual and auditory hallucinations, and cognitive impairment (Nakimuli-Mpungu, Musisi, Mpungu, & Katabira, 2006). Secondary mania, in contrast to primary mania, has been shown to develop later in the course of HIV/AIDS (Kieburtz, Zettelmaier, Ketonen, Tuite, & Caine, 1991; Lyketsos, Schwartz, Fishman, & Treisman, 1997) with a rate of 1.2% in

HIV-positive individuals and 4.3–8% in those with AIDS (Ellen, Judd, Mijch, & Cockram, 1999; Lyketsos et al., 1993). There is a limited amount of evidence suggesting that antiretroviral drugs that strongly penetrate the cerebrospinal fluid may decrease the likelihood of secondary mania (Mijch, Judd, Lyketsos, Ellen, & Cockram, 1999).

Secondary manias are most often treated with quetiapine, valproic acid and risperidone (Freudenreich et al., 2010). While the mood stabilizing drugs lithium and valproic acid both may be used in the treatment of secondary mania, they must be used cautiously in those with HIV and AIDS. Kidney disease and altered levels of critical electrolytes such as sodium and potassium are common in individuals with AIDS and increase the risk for lithium toxicity which can manifest as nausea, confusion, gait disturbances, kidney failure, seizures and coma (Freudenreich et al., 2010). Valproic acid undergoes metabolism in the liver and use may be affected in those with HIV due to comorbid HCV infection or drug interactions (Freudenreich et al., 2010; Romanelli, Jennings, Nath, Ryan, & Berger, 2000). The mood stabilizing medication carbamazepine, which is sometimes used in the treatment of bipolar mania, induces liver enzyme activity (cytochrome P450 CYP3A) and thus may lead to decreased efficacy of HIV medications (Romanelli et al., 2000).

Substance Use Disorders and HIV

Injection drug use (IDU) and non-injection drug use (NIDU) are risk factors for contracting HIV/AIDS (Koblin et al., 2006; Lampinen, Mattheis, Chan, & Hogg, 2007; Ostrow et al., 2009). In 2009, 8% of diagnosed HIV infection in males and 15% in females were due to injection drug use (Centers for Disease Control and Prevention, 2011). The use of contaminated injection equipment is a significant risk factor for HIV transmission; however, drug use via methods other than injection can also increase the risk of HIV transmission or exposure due to increased sexual risk-taking, multiple partners, sex trade, and decreased condom use (Meade, 2006). In addition, mother-to-child transmission of HIV may be increased in women who use drugs during their pregnancy (Purohit, Rapaka, & Shurtleff, 2010).

Alcohol and stimulant use is associated with an increased risk of HIV transmission among heterosexuals and men who have sex with men (MSM) (Morin et al., 2007). For example, amphetamine use increases high risk sexual behavior, thereby increasing the risk of HIV transmission (Plankey et al., 2007). Substance use is likely to continue after seroconversion, with 40% of HIV-infected individuals using illicit drugs other than marijuana and 12.5% screening positive for substance dependence (Bing et al., 2001). Substance abuse disorders (either active or in remission) among those with HIV/AIDS have been reported to be as high as 75% (Treisman & Angelino, 2007). Unfortunately, diagnosis of HIV may occur later in injection drug users than in others (Grigoryan, Hall, Durant, & Wei, 2009) and this population is less likely to have ever received Highly Active Antiretroviral Therapy (HAART), a combination of medications used in the treatment of HIV (Malta et al.,

2009; McGowan et al., 2011; Tegger et al., 2008) or may experience delayed initiation of antiretroviral therapy (Rodriguez-Arenas et al., 2006).

Decreased adherence to HIV medications has been associated with substance use, including alcohol dependence (Azar, Springer, Meyer, & Altice, 2010; Hendershot, Stoner, Pantalone, & Simoni, 2009; Hinkin et al., 2007; Sandelowski, Voils, Chang, & Lee, 2009). Less than maximal adherence can increase the likelihood of developing resistance to HIV therapies, thereby limiting treatment options (Colfax et al., 2007). Markers of HIV disease progression such as HIV viral load may also be negatively impacted by decreased adherence (Arnsten et al., 2002; Carrico et al., 2007; Rodriguez-Arenas et al., 2006). Stimulant use has also been shown to decrease HAART adherence (Carrico et al., 2007; Hinkin et al., 2007) leading to drug resistance including resistance to non-nucleoside reverse transcriptase inhibitors, a specific class of antiretroviral drugs used to treat HIV infection (Colfax et al., 2007; Gorbach et al., 2008).

HAART therapy has improved outcomes for individuals with HIV; however, these benefits may be significantly decreased in those using intravenous drugs. Studies indicate that IDU increases the rate of progression to AIDS, increases the incidence of AIDS defining illnesses such as *Pneumocystis carinii* or Kaposi's sarcoma, and increases the mortality rate in this population (Baum et al., 2010; Malta et al., 2009; Porter et al., 2003; Rodriguez-Arenas et al., 2006). Three-year survival rates are lower for HIV patients with IDU than nonusers (Grigoryan et al., 2009).

While IDU is concerning, individuals with drug use by routes other than injection are at risk as well. Those individuals with NIDU (including those who use alcohol and nicotine), like those with IDU, progress more quickly to AIDS than non-drug users (Kapadia et al., 2005). In addition, those with NIDU have an increased risk of developing opportunistic infections due to their impaired immune system (Lucas, Griswold, et al., 2006), increased mortality (Cook et al., 2008; Lucas, Cheever, Chaisson, & Moore, 2001), and a negative impact on markers of HIV disease progression such as greater decline in white blood cell (CD4+) count and increased HIV viral load as compared to HIV-positive individuals who do not use drugs (Baum et al., 2010; Carrico et al., 2008; Cook et al., 2008; Lucas et al., 2001).

HIV progression in substance abusers may also be affected by homelessness (Gore-Felton & Koopman, 2008), and poor nutrition (McGowan et al., 2011), as well as comorbid infections including tuberculosis (Gore-Felton & Koopman, 2008), hepatitis C virus infection (Braitstein et al., 2006) and other sexually transmitted diseases (Wong, Chaw, Kent, & Klausner, 2005). In addition, HIV-infected individuals who use nicotine are more likely than nonsmokers to be hospitalized with the HIV-associated pneumonia, *P. carinii* or community acquired pneumonia (Miguez-Burbano et al., 2005). HIV-positive individuals who have substance use disorders are more likely to screen positive for comorbid psychiatric disorders than individuals who do not abuse substances (Bansil et al., 2009; Bing et al., 2001; Gaynes, Pence, Eron, & Miller, 2008; Tegger et al., 2008). Clearly, substance abuse in patients with HIV is concerning and contributes to a variety of concerning issues.

Assessment of substance use should be included in any mental health evaluation and is a critical component of medical history taking when clinicians are assessing individuals presenting with HIV. A thorough clinical assessment includes a detailed history of drug use including age of first use, which substances have been or are being used (keeping in mind that polysubstance use is not uncommon), experience with alcohol or drug rehabilitation programs (including the 12-step program Alcoholics Anonymous (AA)), periods of abstinence or sobriety, history of withdrawal and associated problems such as delirium tremens or seizures, social support and social contact (i.e., other users), legal problems associated with drug use, and current use (Table 2). If a substance use disorder is suspected it is useful to determine the individual's stage of willingness to change through common behavioral treatments including motivational interviewing (Rollnick, Miller, & Butler, 2008).

Improvements in antiretroviral adherence and medical outcomes are improved when substance users stop using (Altice, Kamarulzaman, Soriano, Schechter, & Friedland, 2010; Lucas, Griswold, et al., 2006; Lucas, Mullen, et al., 2006). Appropriate individuals should be referred to substance abuse treatment programs including inpatient hospitalizations, day program, and/or AA/narcotics anonymous (Berg, Michelson, & Safren, 2007). In addition, needle exchange programs can decrease the risk of HIV seroconversion (Wodak & Cooney, 2006) and individuals should be educated regarding using sterile needles or disinfecting injection equipment with bleach. Behavioral interventions and talk therapy may also be beneficial. Suggesting and coordinating case management which can provide a single point of contact for social services, medical and psychiatric care, and substance abuse treatment (Samet, Walley, & Bridden, 2007) may be helpful for some people.

Medication assisted therapy for HIV-infected drug users may improve access and adherence to antiretroviral therapy (ART) and decrease risky behaviors (Spire, Lucas, & Carrieri, 2007). For example, methadone and buprenorphine are opioid replacement medication therapies that reduce cravings for narcotic drugs (opioids), block euphoric effects if individuals use opioids, and treat withdrawal symptoms (Samet et al., 2007). Methadone treatment has been shown to improve HIV medication adherence, HIV virus suppression, and CD4+ count maintenance (Palepu et al., 2006). There can be significant drug interactions between methadone or buprenorphine and HIV drugs and treating clinicians should be aware of these and closely monitor this treatment (Samet et al., 2007). Other medication assisted therapy options include naltrexone for opioid and alcohol dependence and acamprosate and disulfram for alcohol dependence.

The use of directly observed therapy programs may also increase adherence in individuals with HIV infection (Lucas, Mullen, et al., 2006; Mitty et al., 2005; Smith-Rohrberg, Mezger, Walton, Bruce, & Altice, 2006). Evidence suggests that access to appropriate support services can increase adherence to ART and therefore increase the likelihood of a good outcome for HIV-positive individuals who present with substance use problems (Malta, Strathdee, Magnanini, & Bastos, 2008).

Table 2 Elements of the clinical assessment of substance use

History of substance use	Age of first use
	Substances used
	Rehabilitation programs
	Periods of abstinence/sobriety
	History of withdrawal
	History of legal problems associated with substance use
Current substance use	Which substances? How much? How often?
	Social contacts (i.e., associating with other substance users)
	Social supports
	Insight into problem
	Stage of willingness/readiness to change

Issues Specific to Children, Adolescents, and Families

Assessment of children and adolescents with HIV should include developmental, environmental, social, and family factors including collateral information from school and family members. A psychiatric history including recent stressors should be taken (Benton, 2010). Multiple factors including effects of the HIV virus on the central nervous system (CNS), genetic factors, prenatal exposure to substances, and opportunistic infections can affect the presentation of psychiatric symptoms in this population (Benton et al., 2010; Donenberg & Pao, 2005; Lwin & Melvin, 2001).

Although congenitally acquired HIV is rare in the United States where highly active antiretroviral therapy (HAART) is readily available, 59 cases were reported to the Centers for Disease Control and Prevention (CDC) in 2003 (Centers for Disease Control and Prevention, 2007) and it is still a problem worldwide. Transmission of HIV from mother to child may occur during pregnancy, childbirth or breastfeeding. Routine, voluntary HIV screening for pregnant women (Branson et al., 2006) and the use of reverse transcriptase inhibitors (a class of antiretroviral drug used to treat HIV infection) during pregnancy and breast-feeding has decreased mother to child transmission of HIV (Benton, 2011). Infants presenting with HIV may have cognitive, language, motor, and behavioral impairments and, in severe forms, can exhibit a rapidly progressive course characterized by an acute encephalopathy leading to brain injury and loss of previously acquired skills with eventual loss of brain tissue (cortical atrophy) and learning disabilities (Burchett & Pizzo, 2003; Wolters & Brouwers, 2005).

Between 2006 and 2009 there was an estimated 21% increase in HIV incidence for people between the ages of 13 and 29 with the highest increase (48%) in African American young men who have sex with men (Centers for Disease Control and Prevention, 2011). Children living with HIV may have to deal with a myriad of emotional and physical issues including dealing with their medical illness, missing school and activities for appointments or hospitalizations, stigma when HIV status is known or disclosed, and blaming themselves for perinatally acquired HIV (Benton, 2011). Additional stressors may include poverty, an unstable home life, family stress, parental mental illness or substance abuse, and limited social support (Donenberg & Pao, 2005; Gaughan et al., 2004). Fears associated with chronic disease and mortality, body image issues associated with delayed development, dermatologic issues, and lipodystrophy (a condition in which body fat is redistributed and can lead to changes in body shape) can also affect HIV-infected youth (Brown, Lourie, & Pao, 2000; DeLaMora, Aledort, & Stavola, 2006).

Psychiatric problems are often seen in this population (Chernoff et al., 2009; Mellins et al., 2009). Children with HIV/AIDS are at an increased risk of being psychiatrically hospitalized compared with children in the general population (Gaughan et al., 2004), although some studies suggest no difference in psychiatric or behavioral problems between HIV-infected youth and peers living in similar conditions (Gadow et al., 2010; Mellins et al., 2003). HIV-negative adolescents with psychiatric or substance use problems may be at a particularly high risk of seroconversion due to risky sexual behavior (Brown, Danovsky, Lourie, DiClemente, & Ponton, 1997; Lehrer, Shrier, Gortmaker, & Buka, 2006; Tubman, Gil, Wagner, & Artigues, 2003) including the use of drugs or alcohol (Donenberg & Pao, 2005).

Diagnosis of psychiatric disorders should be assessed taking into consideration medical status, antiretroviral drug adherence and/or resistance and recent stressors (Benton, 2010). Adherence to antiretroviral therapies (ART) presents a significant problem for adolescents with up to 24% nonadherence seen in 15–18-year olds (Williams et al., 2006). Decreased or nonadherence presents the risk of increased viral load (a marker of HIV disease progression), acquisition of viral drug resistance (which can limit drug treatment options), and an increased risk for central nervous system (CNS) disease (Benton, 2011; Van Dyke et al., 2002; Williams et al., 2006). A combination of nonadherence, high risk sexual behavior, mental health and substance abuse problems more often seen in patients with behaviorally acquired HIV may increase the risk of HIV transmission to sexual or drug partners as well as lead to poor medical and quality of life outcomes (Koenig et al., 2010; Mellins et al., 2011).

HIV-infected youth with depression or anxiety may have an increased risk of acquiring other sexually transmitted diseases or becoming pregnant due to increased high-risk sexual behaviors (Murphy, Durako, et al., 2001). High rates of depression, up to four times greater than that seen in the general adolescent population, have been noted in youth with HIV (Misdrahi et al., 2004; Pao et al., 2000; Scharko, 2006). Adolescent depression presents similarly to that in adults, and making a formal psychiatric diagnosis requires two weeks of depressive symptoms with impairment in functioning or significant distress (American Psychiatric Association, 2000). However, symptoms of the medical illness and side effects of HIV medications may be difficult to differentiate from biologically based depressive symptoms including loss of appetite or fatigue (Benton, 2011). Untreated depression can cause impairments in social functioning and increase the risk of suicide, and in HIV-infected individuals may contribute to negative effects on markers of HIV progression including CD4 counts and viral loads (DeLaMora et al., 2006). Anxiety disorders including phobias, separation anxiety, agoraphobia, generalized anxiety disorder, panic disorder and obsessive compulsive disorder are not uncommon in HIV-infected children and adolescents (Mellins, Brackis-Cott, Dolezal, & Abrams, 2006). Providers working with HIV infected children and adolescents should routinely screen for depression and anxiety.

Pharmacotherapeutic treatment of depression and anxiety in children and adolescents is typically with specific serotonin reuptake inhibitors (SSRIs). All SSRIs carry an FDA (Food and Drug Administration) black box warning for risk of increased suicidality in children and adolescents; accordingly, adolescents started on SSRIs should be closely monitored. Tricyclic antidepressants drugs (TCAs), while FDA approved for the treatment of depression in adolescents, can be sedating and toxic in overdose and are rarely used in most clinical practice settings. In addition, the HIV drug ritonavir inhibits TCA's metabolism via interactions with liver enzymes, thereby increasing its potential for toxicity (De Maat et al., 2003). Depression has been associated with decreased adherence to ART (Murphy et al., 2005; Murphy, Wilson et al., 2001; Williams et al., 2006) and effectively treating depression may improve adherence and overall outcomes for HIV-infected youth. In treating any psychiatric disorder, the benefits must outweigh the risks from taking psychotropic medications.

Substance abuse is found in up to 59% of HIV-positive adolescents (Pao et al., 2000) and may contribute to high-risk sexual behaviors (Elkington, Bauermeister, Brackis-Cott, Dolezal, & Mellins, 2009). Considering that there is an association between lower levels of alcohol and drug use and improved adherence (Comulada, Swendeman, Rotheram-Borus, Mattes, & Weiss, 2003; Murphy et al., 2005), HIV-infected youth should be assessed for substance use disorders and treated as appropriate.

Other psychiatric disorders including bipolar disorder, attention deficit-hyperactivity disorder (ADHD), posttraumatic stress disorder (PTSD), conduct disorders and psychotic disorders are not as extensively studied in HIV-infected youth as in HIV-negative youth. Bipolar disorder in children has a presentation that is similar to that seen in adults with decreased need for sleep, grandiosity, racing thoughts and hypersexuality, but has not been examined in HIV-positive youth (Benton 2010; Geller et al., 2002). Treatment for bipolar disorder is generally with mood stabilizers. As with all psychiatric drugs, drug interactions, liver toxicity, and side effects should be monitored (Geller et al., 2002; Kowatch & DelBello, 2006).

Rates of ADHD, which is characterized by inattention, hyperactivity, and impulsivity, may be higher in HIV-infected children and adolescents than in their HIV-negative peers (American Psychiatric Association, 2000; Mellins et al., 2009; Scharko, 2006). Stimulant medications including amphetamine and methylphenidate are used in the treatment of ADHD in the same manner as used in non-HIV-infected children and have few drug interactions (Benton, 2010). Rates of conduct disorders, manifested by a persistent pattern of violating the basic rights of others or societal norms (American Psychiatric Association, 2000), have been found to be nearly 30% in HIV-positive adolescents (Pao et al., 2000), although this rate is similar to that found in HIV-negative individuals (Mellins et al., 2009).

Diagnosis of a life-threatening illness is considered a precipitating event for the diagnosis of PTSD in children, and youth with HIV may experience PTSD symptoms including avoidance, reexperiencing, and hyperarousal (American Psychiatric Association, 2000). It has been suggested that individuals with pediatric HIV who also exhibit symptoms of PTSD may have a greater risk of medication nonadherence than those without PTSD (Radcliffe et al., 2007). Appropriate screening and diagnosis should be done to ensure appropriate treatment for PTSD in this population. PTSD treatment includes adequate pain management, psychopharmacology, cognitive behavioral therapy and psychodynamic psychotherapy (Stuber & Shemesh, 2006). In addition, it is important to be aware that parents of children with life-threatening illness may also suffer from PTSD associated with their child's diagnosis and prognosis (Stuber & Shemesh, 2006) and appropriate support and treatment should be offered.

Up to 62% of parents of HIV-infected children have psychiatric disorders or hospitalizations, substance abuse issues or incarceration (thereby exposing the child to heritable factors, in utero risks, and stressful home environments) which increase the risk of children growing up in these homes having their own psychiatric and substance abuse problems (Pao et al., 2000). Simply living with a parent with HIV can lead to increased depressive symptoms, somatic complaints, distress, irritability and anger in adolescents (Rotheram-Borus, Weiss, Alber, & Lester, 2005). Separation from parents due to parental loss from death due to HIV or other causes is not uncommon (DeLaMora et al., 2006; Mellins et al., 2006).

The role of the family in HIV is important, complex and affects all members. Acceptance of a chronic and eventually fatal illness, caring for children while ill, adherence to complicated medical regimens, facing stigma, planning for death and care of children, living with chronically ill parents or children and dealing with comorbid mental health or substance abuse problems are just a few of the issues families must address (Benton, 2011).

Routine mental health screening should be incorporated into health care practices dealing with children and adolescents who are HIV-positive (Mellins et al., 2011) and coordinated care with psychiatric caregivers should be undertaken (Spiegel & Futterman, 2009). In addition, clinicians should be aware that children exposed to HIV in utero have been found to have higher rates of anxiety and depression than their nonexposed peers, but may not have their mental health care needs adequately addressed since they are not necessarily seen in the HIV care system (Esposito et al., 1999; Mellins et al., 2009). Support groups may improve quality of life for children and families (Spiegel & Futterman, 2009) and interventions that are family-focused and coping-skills oriented may benefit adolescents, especially with regard to decreasing substance use (Rotheram-Borus, Stein, & Lester, 2006). In addition, disclosure of information regarding HIV status and treatment should be undertaken at an appropriate level based on the child's age and be a combined effort of the medical caregiver, the parents and the family (Burchett & Pizzo, 2003). Adherence with both psychiatric and HIV treatments may be increased by case management services, education, reminder systems, directly observed therapy, simplifying regimes, parental support and incentives for adherence (Simoni et al., 2007).

Conclusion

Many individuals with HIV/AIDS experience comorbid mental conditions that need to be considered in the context of HIV or other medical status and treatments, individual preferences and needs, as well as the individual's social and cultural context. Mental disorder nearly always complicates illness management. However, there is strong evidence that appropriate and assessment of comorbid mental conditions can optimize overall health outcomes. While there has been some growth in the extant literature on the topic of how best to assess and treat comorbid mental illness in people with HIV/AIDS, more attention and research is clearly needed to better inform future interventions for this most vulnerable group of individuals.

Related Topics: Adherence, antiretroviral therapy, caregiving and caregivers, case management, children, cognitive impairment, coping, cytomegalovirus, harm reduction, HIV-related dementia, protease inhibitors, social support, stigma and stigmatization, suicide and suicidal ideation.

References

Altice, F. L., Kamarulzaman, A., Soriano, W., Schechter, M., & Friedland, G. H. (2010). Treatment of medical, psychiatric, and substance-use comorbidities in people infected with HIV who use drugs. *Lancet, 376*(9738), 367–387.

American Psychiatric Association. (2000). *Diagnostic and statistical manual of mental disorders, fourth edition, text revision (DSM-IV-TR)*. Washington, DC: American Psychiatric Association.

Arendt, G., de Nocker, D., von Giesen, H. J., & Nolting, T. (2007). Neuropsychiatric side effects of efavirenz therapy. *Expert Opinion on Drug Safety, 6*(2), 147–154. doi:10.1517/14740338.6.2.147.

Arnsten, J. H., Demas, P. A., Grant, R. W., Gourevitch, M. N., Farzadegan, H., Howard, A. A., et al. (2002). Impact of active drug use on antiretroviral therapy adherence and viral suppression in HIV-infected drug users. *Journal of General Internal Medicine, 17*(5), 377–381.

Azar, M. M., Springer, S. A., Meyer, J. P., & Altice, F. L. (2010). A systematic review of the impact of alcohol use disorders on HIV treatment outcomes, adherence to antiretroviral therapy and health care utilization. *Drug and Alcohol Dependence, 112*(3), 178–193. doi:10.1016/j.drugalcdep. 2010.06.014.

Baillargeon, J. G., Paar, D. P., Wu, H., Giordano, T. P., Murray, O., & Raimer, B. G. (2008). Psychiatric disorders, HIV infection and HIV/hepatitis co-infection in the correctional setting. *AIDS Care, 20*, 124–129.

Bansil, P., Jamieson, D. J., Posner, S. F., & Kourtis, A. P. (2009). Trends in hospitalizations with psychiatric diagnoses among HIV-infected women in the USA, 1994–2004. *AIDS Care, 21* (11), 1432–1438. doi:10.1080/09540120902814387.

Baum, M. K., Rafie, C., Lai, S., Sales, S., Page, J. B., & Campa, A. (2010). Alcohol use accelerates HIV disease progression. *AIDS Research and Human Retroviruses, 26*(5), 511–518. doi:10.1089/aid.2009.0211.

Benton, T. D. (2010). Treatment of psychiatric disorders in children and adolescents with HIV/AIDS. *Current Psychiatry Reports, 12*(2), 104–110. doi:10.1007/s11920-010-0092-z.

Benton, T. D. (2011). Psychiatric considerations in children and adolescents with HIV/AIDS. *Pediatric Clinics of North America, 58*(4), 989–1002. doi:10.1016/j.pcl.2011.06.013. xii.

Benton, T., Lynch, K., Dube, B., Gettes, D. R., Tustin, N. B., Ping Lai, J., Metzger, D. S., Blume, J., Douglas, S. D., & Evans, D. L. (2010). Selective serotonin reuptake inhibitor suppression of HIV infectivity and replication. *Psychosomatic Medicine, 72*(9), 925–932. doi:10.1097/PSY.0b013e3181f883ce.

Berg, C. J., Michelson, S. E., & Safren, S. A. (2007). Behavioral aspects of HIV care: Adherence, depression, substance use, and HIV-transmission behaviors. *Infectious Disease Clinics of North America, 21*(1), 181–200. doi:10.1016/j.idc.2007.01.005. x.

Bing, E. G., Burnam, M. A., Longshore, D., Fleishman, J. A., Sherbourne, C. D., London, A. S., et al. (2001). Psychiatric disorders and drug use among human immunodeficiency virus-infected adults in the United States. *Archives of General Psychiatry, 58*(8), 721–728.

Blumberg, S. J., & Dickey, W. C. (2003). Prevalence of HIV risk behaviors, risk perceptions, and testing among U.S. adults with mental disorders. *Journal of Acquired Immune Deficiency Syndromes (1999), 32*(1), 77–79.

Braitstein, P., Justice, A., Bangsberg, D. R., Yip, B., Alfonso, V., Schechter, M. T., et al. (2006). Hepatitis C coinfection is independently associated with decreased adherence to antiretroviral therapy in a population-based HIV cohort. *AIDS (London, England), 20*(3), 323–331. doi:10.1097/01.aids.0000198091.70325.f4.

Branson, B. M., Handsfield, H. H., Lampe, M. A., Janssen, R. S., Taylor, A. W., Lyss, S. B., et al. (2006). Revised recommendations for HIV testing of adults, adolescents, and pregnant women in health-care settings. *Morbidity and Mortality Weekly Report: Recommendations and Reports/Centers for Disease Control*, 55(RR-14), 1–17 (quiz CE1-4).

Brogan, K., & Lux, J. (2009). Management of common psychiatric conditions in the HIV-positive population. *Current HIV/AIDS Reports, 6*(2), 108–115.

Brown, L. K., Danovsky, M. B., Lourie, K. J., DiClemente, R. J., & Ponton, L. E. (1997). Adolescents with psychiatric disorders and the risk of HIV. *Journal of the American Academy of Child & Adolescent Psychiatry, 36*(11), 1609–1617. doi:10.1016/S0890-8567(09)66573-4.

Brown, L. K., Lourie, K. J., & Pao, M. (2000). Children and adolescents living with HIV and AIDS: A review. *Journal of Child Psychology and Psychiatry, and Allied Disciplines, 41*(1), 81–96.

Burchett, S. K., & Pizzo, P. A. (2003). HIV infection in infants, children, and adolescents. *Pediatrics in Review/American Academy of Pediatrics, 24*(6), 186–194.

Carrico, A. W., Johnson, M. O., Morin, S. F., Remien, R. H., Riley, E. D., Hecht, F. M., et al. (2008). Stimulant use is associated with immune activation and depleted tryptophan among HIV-positive persons on anti retroviral therapy. *Brain, Behavior, and Immunity, 22*(8), 1257–1262. doi:10.1016/j.bbi.2008.07.010.

Carrico, A. W., Johnson, M. O., Moskowitz, J. T., Neilands, T. B., Morin, S. F., Charlebois, E. D., et al. (2007). Affect regulation, stimulant use, and viral load among HIV-positive persons on anti-retroviral therapy. *Psychosomatic Medicine, 69*(8), 785–792. doi:10.1097/PSY.0b013e318157b142.

Centers for Disease Control and Prevention (CDC). (2007, June). *HIV/AIDS surveillance report, 2005. Vol. 17. rev ed.* Atlanta, GA: U.S. Department of Health and Human Services.

Centers for Disease Control and Prevention (CDC). (2011). *HIV surveillance in injection drug users (through 2009).* Retrieved November 29, 2011 from http://www.cdc.gov/hiv/idu/resources/slides/index.htm

Chernoff, M., Nachman, S., Williams, P., Brouwers, P., Heston, J., Hodge, J., et al. (2009). Mental health treatment patterns in perinatally HIV-infected youth and controls. *Pediatrics, 124*(2), 627–636. doi:10.1542/peds.2008-2441.

Ciesla, J. A., & Roberts, J. E. (2001). Meta-analysis of the relationship between HIV infection and risk for depressive disorders. *The American Journal of Psychiatry, 158*(5), 725–730.

Coleman, S. M., Blashill, A. J., Gandhi, R. T., Safren, S. A., & Freudenreich, O. (2012). Impact of integrated and measurement-based depression care: Clinical experience in an HIV clinic. *Psychosomatics, 53*(1), 51–57. doi:10.1016/j.psym.2011.07.004.

Colfax, G. N., Vittinghoff, E., Grant, R., Lum, P., Spotts, G., & Hecht, F. M. (2007). Frequent methamphetamine use is associated with primary non-nucleoside reverse transcriptase inhibitor resistance. *AIDS (London, England), 21*(2), 239–241. doi:10.1097/QAD.0b013e3280114a29.

Comulada, W. S., Swendeman, D. T., Rotheram-Borus, M. J., Mattes, K. M., & Weiss, R. E. (2003). Use of HAART among young people living with HIV. *American Journal of Health Behavior, 27*(4), 389–400.

Cook, J. A., Burke-Miller, J. K., Cohen, M. H., Cook, R. L., Vlahov, D., Wilson, T. E., et al. (2008). Crack cocaine, disease progression, and mortality in a multicenter cohort of HIV-1 positive women. *AIDS (London, England), 22*(11), 1355–1363. doi:10.1097/QAD.0b013e32830507f2.

Cournos, F., Guido, J. R., Coomaraswamy, S., Meyer-Bahlburg, H., Sugden, R., & Horwath, E. (1994). Sexual activity and risk of HIV infection among patients with schizophrenia. *The American Journal of Psychiatry, 151*(2), 228–232.

Cournos, F., Horwath, E., Guido, J. R., McKinnon, K., & Hopkins, N. (1994). HIV-1 infection at two public psychiatric hospitals in New York City. *AIDS Care, 6*(4), 443–452. doi:10.1080/09540129408258659.

Cournos, F., McKinnon, K., & Sullivan, G. (2005). Schizophrenia and comorbid human immunodeficiency virus or hepatitis C virus. *The Journal of Clinical Psychiatry, 66*(Suppl. 6), 27–33.

Cruess, D. G., Douglas, S. D., Petitto, J. M., Have, T. T., Gettes, D., Dube, B., et al. (2005). Association of resolution of major depression with increased natural killer cell activity among HIV-seropositive women. *The American Journal of Psychiatry, 162*(11), 2125–2130. doi:10.1176/appi.ajp. 162.11.2125.

Dalessandro, M., Conti, C. M., Gambi, F., Falasca, K., Doyle, R., Conti, P., et al. (2007). Antidepressant therapy can improve adherence to antiretroviral regimens among HIV-infected and depressed patients. *Journal of Clinical Psychopharmacology, 27*(1), 58–61. doi:10.1097/JCP.0b013e31802f0dd1.

de la Garza, C. L., Paoletti-Duarte, S., Garcia-Martin, C., & Gutierrez-Casares, J. R. (2001). Efavirenz-induced psychosis. *AIDS (London, England), 15*(14), 1911–1912.

De Maat, M. M. R., Ekhart, G. C., Huitema, A. D. R., Koks, C. H. W., Mulder, J. W., & Beijnen, J. H. (2003). Drug interactions between antiretroviral drugs and comedicated agents. *Clinical Pharmakokinetics, 42*(3), 223–282.

De Ronchi, D., Bellini, F., Cremante, G., Ujkaj, M., Tarricone, I., Selleri, R., et al. (2006). Psychopathology of first-episode psychosis in HIV-positive persons in comparison to first-episode schizophrenia: A neglected issue. *AIDS Care, 18*(8), 872–878. doi:10.1080/09540120500307842.

De Ronchi, D., Faranca, I., Forti, P., Ravaglia, G., Borderi, M., Manfredi, R., et al. (2000). Development of acute psychotic disorders and HIV-1 infection. *International Journal of Psychiatry in Medicine, 30*(2), 173–183.

DeLaMora, P., Aledort, N., & Stavola, J. (2006). Caring for adolescents with HIV. *Current HIV/AIDS Reports, 3*(2), 74–78.

Dew, M. A., Becker, J. T., Sanchez, J., Caldararo, R., Lopez, O. L., Wess, J., et al. (1997). Prevalence and predictors of depressive, anxiety, and substance use disorders in HIV-infected and uninfected men: A longitudinal evaluation. *Psychological Medicine, 27*, 395–409.

Dodig, M., & Tavill, A. S. (2001). Hepatitis C and human immunodeficiency virus coinfections. *Journal of Clinical Gastroenterology, 33*(5), 367–374.

Donenberg, G. R., & Pao, M. (2005). Youths and HIV/AIDS: Psychiatry's role in a changing epidemic. *Journal of the American Academy of Child and Adolescent Psychiatry, 44*(8), 728–747. doi:10.1097/01.chi.0000166381.68392.02.

Dyer, T. P., Stein, J. A., Rice, E., & Rotheram-Borus, M. J. (2012). Predicting depression in mothers with and without HIV: The role of social support and family dynamics. *AIDS and Behavior*. doi:10.1007/s10461-012-0149-6.

Elkington, K. S., Bauermeister, J. A., Brackis-Cott, E., Dolezal, C., & Mellins, C. A. (2009). Substance use and sexual risk behaviors in perinatally human immunodeficiency virus-exposed youth: Roles of caregivers, peers and HIV status. *The Journal of Adolescent Health: Official Publication of the Society for Adolescent Medicine, 45*(2), 133–141. doi:10.1016/j.jadohealth.2009.01.004.

Ellen, S. R., Judd, F. K., Mijch, A. M., & Cockram, A. (1999). Secondary mania in patients with HIV infection. *The Australian and New Zealand Journal of Psychiatry, 33*(3), 353–360.

Esposito, S., Musetti, L., Musetti, M. C., Tornaghi, R., Corbella, S., Massironi, E., et al. (1999). Behavioral and psychological disorders in uninfected children aged 6 to 11 years born to human immunodeficiency virus-seropositive mothers. *Journal of Developmental and Behavioral Pediatrics, 20*(6), 411–417.

Evans, D. L., Leserman, J., Perkins, D. O., Stern, R. A., Murphy, C., Zheng, B., et al. (1997). Severe life stress as a predictor of early disease progression in HIV infection. *The American Journal of Psychiatry, 154*(5), 630–634.

Fauci, A. S., Mavilio, D., & Kottilil, S. (2005). NK cells in HIV infection: Paradigm for protection or targets for ambush. *Nature Reviews. Immunology, 5*(11), 835–843. doi:10.1038/nri1711.

Ferguson, M. C. (2011). Current therapies for chronic hepatitis C. *Pharmacotherapy, 31*(1), 92–111. doi:10.1592/phco.31.1.92.

Ferrando, S. J. (2005). Managing depression in HIV disease, viral hepatitis, and substance abuse. *The PRN Notebook, 10*(4). Retrieved April 23, 2012 from http://www.prn.org/images/pdfs/70_663_ferrando_stephen_v10_n4.pdf

Foster, R., Olajide, D., & Everall, I. P. (2003). Antiretroviral therapy-induced psychosis: Case report and brief review of the literature. *HIV Medicine, 4*(2), 139–144.

Freudenreich, O., Goforth, H. W., Cozza, K. L., Mimiaga, M. J., Safren, S. A., Bachmann, G., et al. (2010). Psychiatric treatment of persons with HIV/AIDS: An HIV-psychiatry consensus survey of current practices. *Psychosomatics, 51*(6), 480–488. doi:10.1176/appi.psy.51.6.480.

Gadow, K. D., Chernoff, M., Williams, P. L., Brouwers, P., Morse, E., Heston, J., et al. (2010). Co-occuring psychiatric symptoms in children perinatally infected with HIV and peer comparison sample. *Journal of Developmental and Behavioral Pediatrics, 31*(2), 116–128. doi:10.1097/DBP.0b013e3181cdaa20.

Gaughan, D. M., Hughes, M. D., Oleske, J. M., Malee, K., Gore, C. A., Nachman, S., et al. (2004). Psychiatric hospitalizations among children and youths with human immunodeficiency virus infection. *Pediatrics, 113*(6), e544–e551.

Gaynes, B. N., Pence, B. W., Eron, J. J., Jr., & Miller, W. C. (2008). Prevalence and comorbidity of psychiatric diagnoses based on reference standard in an HIV+ patient population. *Psychosomatic Medicine, 70*(4), 505–511. doi:10.1097/PSY.0b013e31816aa0cc.

Geller, B., Zimerman, B., Williams, M., Delbello, M. P., Frazier, J., & Beringer, L. (2002). Phenomenology of prepubertal and early adolescent bipolar disorder: Examples of elated mood, grandiose behaviors, decreased need for sleep, racing thoughts and hypersexuality. *Journal of Child and Adolescent Psychopharmacology, 12*(1), 3–9. doi:10.1089/10445460252943524.

Gewirtz, G., Horwath, E., Cournos, F., & Empfield, M. (1988). Patients at risk for HIV. *Hospital & Community Psychiatry, 39*(12), 1311–1312.

Gorbach, P. M., Drumright, L. N., Javanbakht, M., Pond, S. L., Woelk, C. H., Daar, E. S., et al. (2008). Antiretroviral drug resistance and risk behavior among recently HIV-infected men who have sex with men. *Journal of Acquired Immune Deficiency Syndromes (1999), 47*(5), 639–643. doi:10.1097/QAI.0b013e3181684c3d.

Gore-Felton, C., & Koopman, C. (2008). Behavioral mediation of the relationship between psychosocial factors and HIV disease progression. *Psychosomatic Medicine, 70*(5), 569–574. doi:10.1097/PSY.0b013e318177353e.

Gottesman, I. I., & Groome, C. S. (1997). HIV/AIDS risks as a consequence of schizophrenia. *Schizophrenia Bulletin, 23*(4), 675–684.

Grigoryan, A., Hall, H. I., Durant, T., & Wei, X. (2009). Late HIV diagnosis and determinants of progression to AIDS or death after HIV diagnosis among injection drug users, 33 US states, 1996–2004. *PLoS One, 4*(2), e4445. doi:10.1371/journal.pone.0004445.

Hansen, B. A., Greenberg, K. S., & Richter, J. A. (1996). Ganciclovir-induced psychosis. *The New England Journal of Medicine, 335*(18), 1397. doi:10.1056/NEJM199610313351814.

Harris, M. J., Jeste, D. V., Gleghorn, A., & Sewell, D. D. (1991). New-onset psychosis in HIV-infected patients. *The Journal of Clinical Psychiatry, 52*(9), 369–376.

Heinssen, R. K., Liberman, R. P., & Kopelowicz, A. (2000). Psychosocial skills training for schizophrenia: Lessons from the laboratory. *Schizophrenia Bulletin, 26*(1), 21–46.

Hendershot, C. S., Stoner, S. A., Pantalone, D. W., & Simoni, J. M. (2009). Alcohol use and antiretroviral adherence: Review and meta-analysis. *Journal of Acquired Immune Deficiency Syndromes (1999), 52*(2), 180–202. doi:10.1097/QAI.0b013e3181b18b6e.

Hinkin, C. H., Barclay, T. R., Castellon, S. A., Levine, A. J., Durvasula, R. S., Marion, S. D., et al. (2007). Drug use and medication adherence among HIV-1 infected individuals. *AIDS and Behavior, 11*(2), 185–194. doi:10.1007/s10461-006-9152-0.

Hoffman, R. G., Cohen, M. A., Alfonso, C. A., Weiss, J. J., Jones, S., Keller, M., et al. (2003). Treatment of interferon-induced psychosis in patients with comorbid hepatitis C and HIV. *Psychosomatics, 44*(5), 417–420. doi:10.1176/appi.psy.44.5.417.

Houston, E., Sandfort, T., Dolezal, C., & Carballo-Dieguez, A. (2012). Depressive symptoms among MSM who engage in bareback sex: Does mood matter? *AIDS and Behavior*. doi:10.1007/s10461-012-0156-7.

Hriso, E., Kuhn, T., Masdeu, J. C., & Grundman, M. (1991). Extrapyramidal symptoms due to dopamine-blocking agents in patients with AIDS encephalopathy. *The American Journal of Psychiatry, 148*(11), 1558–1561.

Johannessen, D. J., & Wilson, L. G. (1988). Mania with cryptococcal meningitis in two AIDS patients. *Journal of Clinical Psychiatry, 49*(5), 200–201.

Kalichman, S. C., Kelly, J. A., Johnson, J. R., & Bulto, M. (1994). Factors associated with risk for HIV infection among chronic mentally ill adults. *The American Journal of Psychiatry, 151*(2), 221–227.

Kapadia, F., Cook, J. A., Cohen, M. H., Sohler, N., Kovacs, A., Greenblatt, R. M., et al. (2005). The relationship between non-injection drug use behaviors on progression to AIDS and death in a cohort of HIV seropositive women in the era of highly active antiretroviral therapy use. *Addiction (Abingdon, England), 100*(7), 990–1002. doi:10.1111/j.1360-0443.2005.01098.x.

Kelly, J. A., Murphy, D. A., Bahr, G. R., Brasfield, T. L., Davis, D. R., Hauth, A. C., et al. (1992). AIDS/HIV risk behavior among the chronic mentally ill. *The American Journal of Psychiatry, 149*(7), 886–889.

Kelly, J. A., Murphy, D. A., Bahr, G. R., Koob, J. J., Morgan, M. G., Kalichman, S. C., et al. (1993). Factors associated with severity of depression and high-risk sexual behavior among persons diagnosed with human immunodeficiency virus (HIV) infection. *Health Psychology: Official Journal of the Division of Health Psychology, American Psychological Association, 12* (3), 215–219.

Kieburtz, K., Zettelmaier, A. E., Ketonen, L., Tuite, M., & Caine, E. D. (1991). Manic syndrome in AIDS. *The American Journal of Psychiatry, 148*(8), 1068–1070.

Koblin, B. A., Husnik, M. J., Colfax, G., Huang, Y., Madison, M., Mayer, K., et al. (2006). Risk factors for HIV infection among men who have sex with men. *AIDS (London, England), 20*(5), 731–739. doi:10.1097/01.aids.0000216374.61442.55.

Koenig, L. J., Pals, S. L., Chandwani, S., Hodge, K., Abramowitz, S., Barnes, W., et al. (2010). Sexual transmission risk behavior of adolescents with HIV acquired perinatally or through risky behaviors. *Journal of Acquired Immune Deficiency Syndromes (1999), 55*(3), 380–390. doi:10.1097/QAI.0b013e3181f0ccb6.

Kowatch, R. A., & DelBello, M. P. (2006). Pediatric bipolar disorder: Emerging diagnostic and treatment approaches. *Child and Adolescent Psychiatric Clinics of North America, 15*(1), 73–108. doi:10.1016/j.chc.2005.08.013.

Lampinen, T. M., Mattheis, K., Chan, K., & Hogg, R. S. (2007). Nitrite inhalant use among young gay and bisexual men in vancouver during a period of increasing HIV incidence. *BMC Public Health, 7*, 35. doi:10.1186/1471-2458-7-35.

Lehrer, J. A., Shrier, L. A., Gortmaker, S., & Buka, S. (2006). Depressive symptoms as a longitudinal predictor of sexual risk behaviors among US middle and high school students. *Pediatrics, 118*(1), 189–200. doi:10.1542/peds.2005-1320.

Leserman, J. (2008). Role of depression, stress, and trauma in HIV disease progression. *Psychosomatic Medicine, 70*(5), 539–545.

Levine, A. B., Aaron, E. Z., & Criniti, S. M. (2008). Screening for depression in pregnant women with HIV infection. *The Journal of Reproductive Medicine, 53*(5), 352–356.

Lombardi, D., Mizuno, L. T., & Thornberry, A. (2010). The use of the zung self-rating depression scale to assist in the case management of patients living with HIV/AIDS. *Care Management Journals: Journal of Case Management; The Journal of Long Term Home Health Care, 11*(4), 210–216.

Lopes, M., Olfson, M., Rabkin, J., Hasin, D. S., Alegria, A. A., Lin, K. H., et al. (2012). Gender, HIV status, and psychiatric disorders: Results from the national epidemiologic survey on alcohol and related conditions. *The Journal of Clinical Psychiatry, 73*(3), 384–391. doi:10.4088/JCP.10m06304.

Lowenhaupt, E. A., Matson, K., Qureishi, B., Saitoh, A., & Pugatch, D. (2007). Psychosis in a 12-year-old HIV-positive girl with an increased serum concentration of efavirenz. *Clinical Infectious Diseases: An Official Publication of the Infectious Diseases Society of America, 45*(10), e128–e130. doi:10.1086/522764.

Lucas, G. M., Cheever, L. W., Chaisson, R. E., & Moore, R. D. (2001). Detrimental effects of continued illicit drug use on the treatment of HIV-1 infection. *Journal of Acquired Immune Deficiency Syndromes (1999), 27*(3), 251–259.

Lucas, G. M., Griswold, M., Gebo, K. A., Keruly, J., Chaisson, R. E., & Moore, R. D. (2006). Illicit drug use and HIV-1 disease progression: A longitudinal study in the era of highly active antiretroviral therapy. *American Journal of Epidemiology, 163*(5), 412–420. doi:10.1093/aje/kwj059.

Lucas, G. M., Mullen, B. A., Weidle, P. J., Hader, S., McCaul, M. E., & Moore, R. D. (2006). Directly administered antiretroviral therapy in methadone clinics is associated with improved HIV treatment outcomes, compared with outcomes among concurrent comparison groups. *Clinical Infectious Diseases: An Official Publication of the Infectious Diseases Society of America, 42*(11), 1628–1635. doi:10.1086/503905.

Lwin, R., & Melvin, D. (2001). Paediatric HIV infection. *Journal of Child Psychology and Psychiatry, and Allied Disciplines, 42*(4), 427–438.

Lyketsos, C. G., Hanson, A. L., Fishman, M., Rosenblatt, A., McHugh, P. R., & Treisman, G. J. (1993). Manic syndrome early and late in the course of HIV. *The American Journal of Psychiatry, 150*(2), 326–327.

Lyketsos, C. G., Schwartz, J., Fishman, M., & Treisman, G. (1997). AIDS mania. *The Journal of Neuropsychiatry and Clinical Neurosciences, 9*(2), 277–279.

Mainie, I., McGurk, C., McClintock, G., & Robinson, J. (2001). Seizures after buproprion overdose. *Lancet, 357*(9268), 1624. doi:10.1016/S0140-6736(00)04770-X.

Malta, M., Bastos, F. I., da Silva, C. M., Pereira, G. F., Lucena, F. F., Fonseca, M. G., et al. (2009). Differential survival benefit of universal HAART access in Brazil: A nation-wide comparison of injecting drug users versus men who have sex with men. *Journal of Acquired Immune Deficiency Syndromes (1999), 52*(5), 629–635. doi:10.1097/QAI.0b013e3181b31b8a.

Malta, M., Strathdee, S. A., Magnanini, M. M., & Bastos, F. I. (2008). Adherence to antiretroviral therapy for human immunodeficiency virus/acquired immune deficiency syndrome among drug users: A systematic review. *Addiction (Abingdon, England), 103*(8), 1242–1257. doi:10.1111/j.1360-0443.2008.02269.x.

Martin, S. J., & Bowden, F. J. (2007). Ethambutol toxicity manifesting as acute onset psychosis. *International Journal of STD & AIDS, 18*(4), 287–288. doi:10.1258/095646207780658863.

McGowan, C. C., Weinstein, D. D., Samenow, C. P., Stinnette, S. E., Barkanic, G., Rebeiro, P. F., et al. (2011). Drug use and receipt of highly active antiretroviral therapy among HIV-infected persons in two U.S. clinic cohorts. *PLoS One, 6*(4), e18462. doi:10.1371/journal.pone.0018462.

McKinnon, K., Cournos, F., Sugden, R., Guido, J. R., & Herman, R. (1996). The relative contributions of psychiatric symptoms and AIDS knowledge to HIV risk behaviors among people with severe mental illness. *The Journal of Clinical Psychiatry, 57*(11), 506–513.

Meade, C. S. (2006). Sexual risk behavior among persons dually diagnosed with severe mental illness and substance use disorder. *Journal of Substance Abuse Treatment, 30*(2), 147–157. doi:10.1016/j.jsat.2005.11.005.

Meade, C. S., & Sikkema, K. J. (2005). Voluntary HIV testing among adults with severe mental illness: Frequency and associated factors. *AIDS and Behavior, 9*(4), 465–473. doi:10.1007/s10461-005-9033-y.

Mellins, C. A., Brackis-Cott, E., Dolezal, C., & Abrams, E. J. (2006). Psychiatric disorders in youth with perinatally acquired human immunodeficiency virus infection. *The Pediatric Infectious Disease Journal, 25*(5), 432–437. doi:10.1097/01.inf.0000217372.10385.2a.

Mellins, C. A., Brackis-Cott, E., Leu, C. S., Elkington, K. S., Dolezal, C., Wiznia, A., et al. (2009). Rates and types of psychiatric disorders in perinatally human immunodeficiency virus-infected youth and seroreverters. *Journal of Child Psychology and Psychiatry, and Allied Disciplines, 50*(9), 1131–1138. doi:10.1111/j.1469-7610.2009.02069.x.

Mellins, C. A., Smith, R., O'Driscoll, P., Magder, L. S., Brouwers, P., Chase, C., et al. (2003). High rates of behavioral problems in perinatally HIV-infected children are not linked to HIV disease. *Pediatrics, 111*(2), 384–393.

Mellins, C. A., Tassiopoulos, K., Malee, K., Moscicki, A. B., Patton, D., Smith, R., et al. (2011). Behavioral health risks in perinatally HIV-exposed youth: Co-occurrence of sexual and drug use behavior, mental health problems, and nonadherence to antiretroviral treatment. *AIDS Patient Care and STDs, 25*(7), 413–422. doi:10.1089/apc.2011.0025.

Miguez-Burbano, M. J., Ashkin, D., Rodriguez, A., Duncan, R., Pitchenik, A., Quintero, N., et al. (2005). Increased risk of pneumocystis carinii and community-acquired pneumonia with tobacco use in HIV disease. *International Journal of Infectious Diseases: Official Publication of the International Society for Infectious Diseases, 9*(4), 208–217. doi:10.1016/j.ijid.2004.07.010.

Mijch, A. M., Judd, F. K., Lyketsos, C. G., Ellen, S., & Cockram, A. (1999). Secondary mania in patients with HIV infection: Are antiretrovirals protective? *The Journal of Neuropsychiatry and Clinical Neurosciences, 11*(4), 475–480.

Misdrahi, D., Vila, G., Funk-Brentano, I., Tardieu, M., Blanche, S., & Mouren-Simeoni, M. C. (2004). DSM-IV mental disorders and neurological complications in children and adolescents with human immunodeficiency virus type 1 infection (HIV-1). *European Psychiatry: The Journal of the Association of European Psychiatrists, 19*(3), 182–184. doi:10.1016/j.eurpsy.2003.06.009.

Mitty, J. A., Macalino, G. E., Bazerman, L. B., Loewenthal, H. G., Hogan, J. W., MacLeod, C. J., et al. (2005). The use of community-based modified directly observed therapy for the treatment of HIV-infected persons. *Journal of Acquired Immune Deficiency Syndromes (1999), 39*(5), 545–550.

Monahan, P. O., Shacham, E., Reece, M., Kroenke, K., Ong'or, W. O., Omollo, O., et al. (2009). Validity/reliability of PHQ-9 and PHQ-2 depression scales among adults living with HIV/AIDS in western Kenya. *Journal of General Internal Medicine, 24*(2), 189–197. doi:10.1007/s11606-008-0846-z.

Morin, S. F., Myers, J. J., Shade, S. B., Koester, K., Maiorana, A., & Rose, C. D. (2007). Predicting HIV transmission risk among HIV-infected patients seen in clinical settings. *AIDS and Behavior, 11*(5 Suppl), S6–S16. doi:10.1007/s10461-007-9253-4.

Murphy, D. A., Belzer, M., Durako, S. J., Sarr, M., Wilson, C. M., Muenz, L. R., et al. (2005). Longitudinal antiretroviral adherence among adolescents infected with human immunodeficiency virus. *Archives of Pediatrics & Adolescent Medicine, 159*(8), 764–770. doi:10.1001/archpedi.159.8.764.

Murphy, D. A., Durako, S. J., Moscicki, A. B., Vermund, S. H., Ma, Y., Schwarz, D. F., & Adolescent Medicine HIV/AIDS Research Network. (2001). No change in health risk behaviors over time among HIV infected adolescents in care: Role of psychological distress. *The Journal of Adolescent Health: Official Publication of the Society for Adolescent Medicine, 29*(3 Suppl), 57–63.

Murphy, D. A., Wilson, C. M., Durako, S. J., Muenz, L. R., Belzer, M., & Adolescent Medicine HIV/AIDS Research Network. (2001). Antiretroviral medication adherence among the REACH HIV-infected adolescent cohort in the USA. *AIDS Care, 13*(1), 27–40. doi:10.1080/09540120020018161.

Nakimuli-Mpungu, E., Musisi, S., Mpungu, S. K., & Katabira, E. (2006). Primary mania versus HIV-related secondary mania in Uganda. *The American Journal of Psychiatry, 163*(8), 1349–1354. doi:10.1176/appi.ajp. 163.8.1349 (quiz 1480).

Nurutdinova, D., Chrusciel, T., Zerinque, A., Scherrer, J. F., Al-Aly, Z., McDonald, J. R., et al. (2012). Mental health disorders and the risk of AIDS-defining illness and death in HIV-infected veterans. *AIDS, 26*(2), 229–234.

O'Dowd, M. A., & McKegney, F. P. (1988). Manic syndrome associated with zidovudine. *The Journal of the American Medical Association, 260*(24), 3587–3588.

Olatunji, B. O., Mimiaga, M. J., O'Cleirigh, C., & Safren, S. A. (2006). Review of treatment studies of depression in HIV. *Topics in HIV Medicine: A Publication of the International AIDS Society, USA, 14*(3), 112–124.

Ostrow, D. G., Plankey, M. W., Cox, C., Li, X., Shoptaw, S., Jacobson, L. P., et al. (2009). Specific sex drug combinations contribute to the majority of recent HIV seroconversions among MSM in the MACS. *Journal of Acquired Immune Deficiency Syndromes (1999), 51*(3), 349–355. doi:10.1097/QAI.0b013e3181a24b20.

Otto-Salaj, L. L., Heckman, T. G., Stevenson, L. Y., & Kelly, J. A. (1998). Patterns, predictors and gender differences in HIV risk among severely mentally ill men and women. *Community Mental Health Journal, 34*(2), 175–190.

Palepu, A., Tyndall, M. W., Joy, R., Kerr, T., Wood, E., Press, N., et al. (2006). Antiretroviral adherence and HIV treatment outcomes among HIV/HCV co-infected injection drug users: The role of methadone maintenance therapy. *Drug and Alcohol Dependence, 84*(2), 188–194. doi:10.1016/j.drugalcdep. 2006.02.003.

Pao, M., Lyon, M., D'Angelo, L. J., Schuman, W. B., Tipnis, T., & Mrazek, D. A. (2000). Psychiatric diagnoses in adolescents seropositive for the human immunodeficiency virus. *Archives of Pediatrics & Adolescent Medicine, 154*(3), 240–244.

Plankey, M. W., Ostrow, D. G., Stall, R., Cox, C., Li, X., Peck, J. A., et al. (2007). The relationship between methamphetamine and popper use and risk of HIV seroconversion in the multicenter AIDS cohort study. *Journal of Acquired Immune Deficiency Syndromes (1999), 45*(1), 85–92. doi:10.1097/QAI.0b013e3180417c99.

Porter, K., Babiker, A., Bhaskaran, K., Darbyshire, J., Pezzotti, P., Porter, K., et al. (2003). Determinants of survival following HIV-1 seroconversion after the introduction of HAART. *Lancet, 362*(9392), 1267–1274.

Psaros, C., Israel, J., O'Cleirigh, C., Bedoya, C. A., & Safren, S. A. (2011). Psychological co-morbidities of HIV/AIDS. In S. Pagoto (Ed.), *Psychological co-morbidities of physical illness: A behavioral medicine perspective* (pp. 233–273). New York, NY: Springer Science + Business Media LLC.

Purohit, V., Rapaka, R. S., & Shurtleff, D. (2010). Mother-to-child transmission (MTCT) of HIV and drugs of abuse in post-highly active antiretroviral therapy (HAART) era. *Journal of Neuroimmune Pharmacology: The Official Journal of the Society on NeuroImmune Pharmacology, 5*(4), 507–515. doi:10.1007/s11481-010-9242-7.

Radcliffe, J., Fleisher, C. L., Hawkins, L. A., Tanney, M., Kassam-Adams, N., Ambrose, C., et al. (2007). Posttraumatic stress and trauma history in adolescents and young adults with HIV. *AIDS Patient Care and STDs, 21*(7), 501–508. doi:10.1089/apc.2006.0144.

Repetto, M. J., & Petitto, J. M. (2008). Psychopharmacology in HIV-infected patients. *Psychosomatic Medicine, 70*(5), 585–592. doi:10.1097/PSY.0b013e3181777190.

Rodriguez-Arenas, M. A., Jarrin, I., del Amo, J., Iribarren, J. A., Moreno, S., Viciana, P., et al. (2006). Delay in the initiation of HAART, poorer virological response, and higher mortality among HIV-infected injecting drug users in Spain. *AIDS Research and Human Retroviruses, 22*(8), 715–723. doi:10.1089/aid.2006.22.715.

Rollnick, S., Miller, W. R., & Butler, C. E. (2008). *Motivational interviewing in health care*. New York, NY: Guilford.

Romanelli, F., Jennings, H. R., Nath, A., Ryan, M., & Berger, J. (2000). Therapeutic dilemma: The use of anticonvulsants in HIV-positive individuals. *Neurology, 54*(7), 1404–1407.

Rosenberg, S. D., Goodman, L. A., Osher, F. C., Swartz, M. S., Essock, S. M., Butterfield, M. I., et al. (2001). Prevalence of HIV, hepatitis B, and hepatitis C in people with severe mental illness. *American Journal of Public Health, 91*(1), 31–37.

Rothbard, A. B., Miller, K., Lee, S., & Blank, M. (2009). Revised cost of estimates of Medicaid recipients with serious mental illness and HIV/AIDS. *Psychiatric Services (Washington, DC), 60*(7), 974–977.

Rotheram-Borus, M. J., Stein, J. A., & Lester, P. (2006). Adolescent adjustment over six years in HIV-affected families. *The Journal of Adolescent Health: Official Publication of the Society for Adolescent Medicine, 39*(2), 174–182. doi:10.1016/j.jadohealth.2006.02.014.

Rotheram-Borus, M. J., Weiss, R., Alber, S., & Lester, P. (2005). Adolescent adjustment before and after HIV-related parental death. *Journal of Consulting and Clinical Psychology, 73*(2), 221–228. doi:10.1037/0022-006X.73.2.221.

Sacks, M., Dermatis, H., Looser-Ott, S., & Perry, S. (1992). Seroprevalence of HIV and risk factors for AIDS in psychiatric inpatients. *Hospital & Community Psychiatry, 43*(7), 736–737.

Samet, J. H., Walley, A. Y., & Bridden, C. (2007). Illicit drugs, alcohol, and addiction in human immunodeficiency virus. *Panminerva Medica, 49*(2), 67–77.

Sandelowski, M., Voils, C. I., Chang, Y., & Lee, E. J. (2009). A systematic review comparing antiretroviral adherence descriptive and intervention studies conducted in the USA. *AIDS Care, 21*(8), 953–966. doi:10.1080/09540120802626212.

Scharko, A. M. (2006). DSM psychiatric disorders in the context of pediatric HIV/AIDS. *AIDS Care, 18*(5), 441–445. doi:10.1080/09540120500213487.

Schlebusch, L., & Vawda, N. (2010). HIV-infection as a self-reported risk factor for attempted suicide in South Africa. *African Journal of Psychiatry, 13*, 280–283.

Schuster, R., Bornovalova, M., & Hunt, E. (2012). The influence of depression on the progression of HIV: Direct and indirect effects. *Behavior Modification, 36*(2), 123–145. doi:10.1177/0145445511425231; 10.1177/0145445511425231.

Sewell, D. D. (1996). Schizophrenia and HIV. *Schizophrenia Bulletin, 22*(3), 465–473.

Sewell, D. D., Jeste, D. V., Atkinson, J. H., Heaton, R. K., Hesselink, J. R., Wiley, C., et al. (1994). HIV-associated psychosis: A study of 20 cases. San Diego HIV Neurobehavioral Research Center Group. *The American Journal of Psychiatry, 151*(2), 237–242.

Simoni, J. M., Montgomery, A., Martin, E., New, M., Demas, P. A., & Rana, S. (2007). Adherence to antiretroviral therapy for pediatric HIV infection: A qualitative systematic review with recommendations for research and clinical management. *Pediatrics, 119*(6), e1371–e1383. doi:10.1542/peds.2006-1232.

Singh, A. N., Golledge, H., & Catalan, J. (1997). Treatment of HIV-related psychotic disorders with risperidone: A series of 21 cases. *Journal of Psychosomatic Research, 42*(5), 489–493.

Smith-Rohrberg, D., Mezger, J., Walton, M., Bruce, R. D., & Altice, F. L. (2006). Impact of enhanced services on virologic outcomes in a directly administered antiretroviral therapy trial for HIV-infected drug users. *Journal of Acquired Immune Deficiency Syndromes (1999), 43* (Suppl. 1), S48–S53. doi:10.1097/01.qai.0000248338.74943.85.

Spiegel, H. M., & Futterman, D. C. (2009). Adolescents and HIV: Prevention and clinical care. *Current HIV/AIDS Reports, 6*(2), 100–107.

Spire, B., Lucas, G. M., & Carrieri, M. P. (2007). Adherence to HIV treatment among IDUs and the role of opioid substitution treatment (OST). *The International Journal on Drug Policy, 18* (4), 262–270. doi:10.1016/j.drugpo.2006.12.014.

Stahl, S. M., Mignon, L., & Meyer, J. M. (2009). Which comes first: Atypical antipsychotic treatment or cardiometabolic risk? *Acta Psychiatrica Scandinavica, 119*(3), 171–179. doi:10.1111/j.1600-0447.2008.01334.x.

Stuber, M. L., & Shemesh, E. (2006). Post-traumatic stress response to life-threatening illnesses in children and their parents. *Child and Adolescent Psychiatric Clinics of North America, 15*(3), 597–609. doi:10.1016/j.chc.2006.02.006.

Tegger, M. K., Crane, H. M., Tapia, K. A., Uldall, K. K., Holte, S. E., & Kitahata, M. M. (2008). The effect of mental illness, substance use, and treatment for depression on the initiation of highly active antiretroviral therapy among HIV-infected individuals. *AIDS Patient Care and STDs, 22*(3), 233–243. doi:10.1089/apc.2007.0092.

Treisman, G., & Angelino, A. (2007). Interrelation between psychiatric disorders and the prevention and treatment of HIV infection. *Clinical Infectious Diseases: An Official Publication of the Infectious Diseases Society of America, 45*(Suppl. 4), S313–S317. doi:10.1086/522556.

Tubman, J. G., Gil, A. G., Wagner, E. F., & Artigues, H. (2003). Patterns of sexual risk behaviors and psychiatric disorders in a community sample of young adults. *Journal of Behavioral Medicine, 26*(5), 473–500.

UNAIDS. (2011). *UNAIDS world AIDS day report 2011 (No. JC2216E). Joint United Nations Programme on HIV/AIDS*. Retrieved from http://www.unaids.org/en/media/unaids/contentassets/documents/unaidspublication/2011/JC2216_WorldAIDSday_report_2011_en.pdf

Van Dyke, R. B., Lee, S., Johnson, G. M., Wiznia, A., Mohan, K., Stanley, K., et al. (2002). Reported adherence as a determinant of response to highly active antiretroviral therapy in children who have human immunodeficiency virus infection. *Pediatrics, 109*(4), e61.

Vanable, P. A., Carey, M. P., Carey, K. B., & Maisto, S. A. (2007). Differences in HIV-related knowledge, attitudes, and behavior among psychiatric outpatients with and without a history of a sexually transmitted infection. *Journal of Prevention and Intervention in the Community, 33* (1–2), 79–94.

Walkup, J., Crystal, S., & Sambamoorthi, U. (1999). Schizophrenia and major affective disorder among Medicaid recipients with HIV/AIDS in New Jersey. *American Journal of Public Health, 89*(7), 1101–1103.

Walkup, J., McAlpine, D. D., Olfson, M., Boyer, C., & Hansell, S. (2000). Recent HIV testing among general hospital inpatients with schizophrenia: Findings from four New York City sites. *The Psychiatric Quarterly, 71*(2), 177–193.

Walkup, J., Sambamoorthi, U., & Crystal, S. (2001). Incidence and consistency of antiretroviral use among HIV-infected Medicaid beneficiaries with schizophrenia. *The Journal of Clinical Psychiatry, 62*(3), 174–178.

Williams, P. L., Storm, D., Montepiedra, G., Nichols, S., Kammerer, B., Sirois, P. A., et al. (2006). Predictors of adherence to antiretroviral medications in children and adolescents with HIV infection. *Pediatrics, 118*(6), e1745–e1757. doi:10.1542/peds.2006-0493.

Wise, M. E., Mistry, K., & Reid, S. (2002). Drug points: Neuropsychiatric complications of nevirapine treatment. *BMJ (Clinical Research Ed.), 324*(7342), 879.

Wodak, A., & Cooney, A. (2006). Do needle syringe programs reduce HIV infection among injecting drug users: A comprehensive review of the international evidence. *Substance Use & Misuse, 41*(6–7), 777–813. doi:10.1080/10826080600669579.

Wolters, P. L., & Brouwers, P. (2005). Neurobehavioral function and assessment of children and adolescents with HIV-1 infection. In S. L. Zeichner & J. S. Read (Eds.), *Textbook for pediatric care* (pp. 269–284). Cambridge: Cambridge University Press.
Wong, W., Chaw, J. K., Kent, C. K., & Klausner, J. D. (2005). Risk factors for early syphilis among gay and bisexual men seen in an STD clinic: San Francisco, 2002–2003. *Sexually Transmitted Diseases, 32*(7), 458–463.
Yanofski, J., & Croarkin, P. (2008). Choosing antidepressants for HIV and AIDS patients: Insights on safety and side effects. *Psychiatry (Edgmont (PA: Township)), 5*(5), 61–66.

Legal Issues for the HIV-Infected Client

Brandy L. Johnson and Lisa M. Henderson-Newlin

Introduction

The World Health Organization has estimated that there were 33.4 million people living with HIV/AIDS in 2008. In the United States alone, it was estimated that there were 1.1 million people living with a diagnosis of HIV/AIDS in 2011 (Kaiser, 2011). With the recognition of the disease in the early 1980s came the need to protect those with the disease and, at the same time, the need to decrease its rate of transmission to others. To that end, governments and courts have, over time, developed bodies of laws that codify rights and obligations related to those who carry the disease.

Individuals who have HIV/AIDS often find themselves confronted with prejudice, ostracism, and discrimination (Herek, 1999). This is due, at least in part, to its initial association with homosexual men and intravenous drug users (Terrence Higgins Trust, 2001). Fear and a lack of understanding of the disease also have contributed to the stigma, prejudice, and discrimination that many individuals with HIV/AIDS encounter (Aggleton, Wood, Malcolm, Parker, & UNAIDS, 2005). Many governments have attempted to address the prejudice and discrimination by passing laws that provide specific protections to individuals with HIV/AIDS. In 2010, 71% of countries had some form of legislation in place to protect individuals with HIV/AIDS from discrimination (UNAIDS, 2010). Governmental bodies have also put laws into place that attempt to protect the public against the transmission of HIV/AIDS.

This chapter provides an overview of some of the legal rights and protections that are available to individuals living with HIV/AIDS. It also discusses some of the

B.L. Johnson (✉)
Rynearson, Suess, Schnurbusch & Champion, L.L.C., St. Louis, MO, USA
e-mail: bjohnson@rssclaw.com

L.M. Henderson-Newlin
McAnany, Van Cleave & Phillips, P.A., St. Louis, MO, USA

S. Loue (ed.), *Mental Health Practitioner's Guide to HIV/AIDS*,
DOI 10.1007/978-1-4614-5283-6_3, © Springer Science+Business Media New York 2013

ways the law has been used to provide a measure of protection to the public against the transmission of the disease. It is beyond the scope of this chapter to address these issues in great depth, and the reader is referred to additional sources for a more detailed discussion. Additionally, as it is not possible address the laws of every country, this chapter focuses on the laws of the United States.

Instruments Available to Protect Legal Rights

The legal institution of marriage confers on couples various legal rights. These rights include medical decision-making, family visitation, next-of-kin status for emergency medical decisions, funeral decision making, joint parenting, and inheritance (Cross, Palmer, & Smith, 2009). It has been estimated that in 2009, there were 6.7 million unmarried opposite-sex couples and 594,000 same-sex couples cohabitating (Kreider, 2010; Lofquist, 2011). Many of these couples were raising children. Unmarried individuals with HIV/AIDS must give serious thought to whom they would like to confer decision making authority on their behalf if they were to become incapacitated and unable to make the decisions themselves. Additionally, although a number of states now recognize same-sex marriages or civil unions, couples should be aware of the rights being conferred, which vary from state to state and often do not include all of the rights given to married heterosexual couples, and take steps to compensate for the rights that are not extended (Stolarsky, 2009).

Individuals with HIV/AIDS can utilize various legal documents to help ensure that their wishes are followed and to identify the person or persons to whom they wish to grant the power to make decisions. For unmarried couples, and especially same-sex couples, these legal documents can also be utilized to provide visitation rights, the ability to obtain confidential information from medical professionals, and to plan funerals. These documents include powers of attorney, living wills, HIPAA releases, wills and trusts. An additional benefit of utilizing these instruments, besides legal protection, is the fact that the documents permit individuals with HIV/AIDS, who often feel they have little control over the effect the disease has on their bodies, to exert some control over the conduct of doctors, hospitals, family members, and loved ones (Goldfein & Schalman-Bergen, 2010c). The following is a brief discussion of each of these instruments. The reader should be cautioned, however, that most states have statutes addressing the documents' content, the requirements for their proper execution, and what rights can be conferred. Consequently, the reader is encouraged to research the law in his or her geographic area and/or to seek professional advice before executing any of these legal documents.

Power of Attorney

All states recognize two types of powers of attorney (POA): the power of attorney for property and the power of attorney for health care. A POA allows an individual (the "principal") to designate a person who will act as an agent in his or her place. The designee, sometimes called an "attorney-in-fact," need only be a competent adult. The attorney-in-fact does not have to be an actual attorney. An attorney-in-fact is generally expected to act in a manner consistent with what the principal would have wanted (Hickey, 2009).

POAs can be general or limited. A general POA is effective immediately and is most useful for short term matters. A limited, or special, POA specifies what powers the attorney-in-fact can utilize and/or the amount of time for which the authority to act is conferred. Due to the fact that a general POA typically allows the attorney-in-fact to make almost any decision the principal could ordinarily make for him- or herself, the individual executing the POA must decide, after careful consideration, how broad or narrow the powers granted by the document should be (Hickey, 2009).

A POA, except under certain circumstances, terminates when the principal becomes incompetent or dies. However, if the principal executed a "durable power of attorney," the attorney-in-fact can continue to exercise the powers granted despite the principal's incompetence/incapacitation. To make a POA durable, language must be used that clearly conveys that concept (Hickey, 2009). Additionally, durable POAs are usually either immediate or springing. An immediate POA conveys the authority to the attorney-in-fact to act as soon as the POA is executed. Consequently, the attorney-in-fact has the power to start acting on behalf of the principal, competency notwithstanding. A springing durable POA, on the other hand, makes the attorney-in-fact's authority to act contingent upon the principal being found incompetent by a physician or some other triggering event. When a POA is springing in nature, the document should be clear and specific concerning the circumstances triggering the transfer of power to the attorney in fact (Hickey, 2009).

Unless made irrevocable, POAs can be terminated at any time by a competent principal. The POA, itself, may also contain a clause stating when the conveyance of authority to the attorney in fact terminates. Most states have statutory forms for both the POA for Property and the POA for Healthcare.

Power of Attorney for Property. Also known as a power of attorney for finances, this document gives the attorney-in-fact the ability to handle financial affairs on behalf of the individual. The power of attorney usually either permits the attorney-in-fact to do any act the principal could have performed or it is tailored to limited, defined tasks. With a POA for property, the attorney-in-fact can be allowed to perform tasks, including depositing/withdrawing money from a bank account, paying bills, managing real estate, asset/stock/portfolio management, dealing with insurance, filing taxes, selling or buying property, and signing legal documents. Unlimited, the POA for property could also convey to the attorney-in-fact the power to make gifts, change beneficiaries, donate money or assets, and make decisions for any business owned by the principal.

By using a POA for property, an unmarried principal with HIV/AIDS can ensure that a trusted individual has the authority to pay bills, file tax returns, manage investments, and handle insurance matters if the principal becomes too ill to act, is hospitalized, or is too heavily medicated to control financial matters. For married couples, a POA for property can also be useful when a couple has joint property and the principal spouse becomes incapacitated or incompetent. Under such circumstances, the POA permits the attorney-in-fact to act quickly and without court intervention in matters in which the consent of both spouses is required.

Power of Attorney for Healthcare. Similar to a POA for property, a POA for healthcare allows the attorney-in-fact to make decisions for the principal. The powers that can be conferred with this type of POA include, but are not limited to, the ability to consent to procedures and/or treatment, admission to a hospital, placement in a long-term care facility, and selection or change of physicians, healthcare providers, and/or treatment facilitates. The attorney-in-fact can also be granted the power to withhold treatment/procedures, food and fluids, cardiopulmonary resuscitation, life-saving measures, life-prolonging treatment, life-support, and the ability to make decisions concerning the termination of existing treatment or life-sustaining measures. POAs for healthcare can be used in place of, or in conjunction with, a living will. However, POAs for healthcare are more powerful and encompassing than living wills, as the POA is broader and not limited to situations involving terminal conditions (it should be noted that, in some states, the ability of the attorney-in-fact to consent on behalf of the principal to specified forms of treatment for mental illness and/or the withdrawal of a feeding tube may be limited by statute).

The use of a POA for healthcare allows the principal to designate an attorney-in-fact who is willing to follow the principal's wishes concerning treatment and life-sustaining treatment. This is especially important to principals with HIV/AIDS who do not believe their spouses or, when unmarried, next-of-kin will respect their wishes. Moreover, when the principal and attorney-in-fact are an unmarried, heterosexual couple or a same-sex couple, the POA can confer rights to the significant other that are otherwise denied by law (Hickey, 2009).

Besides the rights discussed above, the POA for healthcare can convey the right to sign medical documents, be notified of any change in condition, acquire medical records, visit the principal in the hospital, and obtain information and/or be consulted about the principal's condition, prognosis, and treatment. In some states, a principal can permit the attorney-in-fact the right to make decisions concerning the disposition of the principal's body after death. Depending on the state, this can include authorizing an autopsy, organ donation, or the decision to bury or cremate the body.

Family members may challenge the authority of the attorney-in-fact to make healthcare decisions. This is not uncommon when the family does not approve of the significant other or when emotionally charged decisions, such as the removal of life support, are involved. At times, healthcare professionals may refuse to recognize and honor the POA. An attorney-in-fact should be prepared to turn to the courts to enforce their rights under the POA.

Living Wills

A living will is a legal document that declares the individual's wishes with regard to the types of treatment, if any, that he or she is willing to accept. A living will usually involves incurable, irreversible and/or terminal conditions and takes effect when the individual becomes incompetent or incapable of making his or her decisions known. The document conveys the individual's wishes concerning life-saving or life-prolonging treatment.

A living will addresses what type of treatment should be withheld, provided, and when treatment should be withdrawn. A living will might advise, for example, whether the individual does not want to receive blood transfusions, cardiopulmonary resuscitation, dialysis, medication, antibiotics, food, fluids, palliative care, or placement on a respirator/ventilator. The reader should be aware that the statutory provisions for living wills and what they can contain vary from state to state. In Illinois, living wills are very narrow and can only be used to withhold or withdraw life-prolonging procedures when death is imminent (Illinois Living Will Act, 1988). A living will in Kentucky, in comparison, permits the individual to refuse or request life prolonging treatment, refuse or request artificial feeding/hydration, and express his or her wishes regarding organ donation (Kentucky Living Will Directive Act, 2010). In 2010, a survey showed that only 29% of those interviewed had a living will (Ebeling, 2010).

The information contained in a living will can, and often is, included in a POA for healthcare. An individual can also have both a living will and a POA for healthcare. If an individual does have both documents, however, care should be taken to ensure that the instructions in the two documents do not conflict or cause ambiguity. If an individual with HIV/AIDS who has a POA that provides for artificial feeding if he or she were to be in a vegetative state, were to also execute a living will that forbade food to be given, the individual risks having his or her true wishes disregarded. In states like New Hampshire and Illinois, the POA controls if there is a conflict between the terms of the POA and the living will. Thus, in the above example, if the terms of the living will reflect the individual's true intent concerning artificial feeding, he or she, per the terms of the POA, would receive food intravenously despite his or her opposition to it.

Living wills can be placed in the individual's medical chart. Many healthcare facilities inquire about living wills prior to the admission of the individual for treatment or a procedure. In states like California, advanced directive/living will "registries" have been established and allow people to file their living wills with the state. There are also private organizations that offer living will registries. A living will can be revoked at any time so long as the individual is still competent.

HIPAA Release

Under the Health Insurance Portability and Accountability Act ("HIPAA"), healthcare professionals are prohibited by law from disclosing medical information about a patient to certain individuals. For example, if the patient or client is unmarried, a medical provider will likely refuse to discuss the patient's medical condition with his or her significant other without a power of attorney (Hickey, 2009). However, if the patient has executed a HIPAA release, the healthcare professional/entity will be able to discuss with the designated individual, information about the patient's condition and/or provide medical records. If the patient does not want certain types of information released, such as records relating to mental illness, drug/alcohol abuse, or HIV/AIDS status, the document can be tailored to limit what can be disclosed. Unlike a power of attorney, a HIPAA release does not convey the power to make medical decisions. Rather, it is limited to the receipt of medical information.

Wills

A will is a legal declaration of how an individual's real and/or personal property will be managed after death. When a person dies without a will, also known as dying intestate, the deceased person's property will be disbursed according to the state of residence's statutory scheme. Usually, this will involve the division of property between the deceased's spouse and/or children. If the deceased is unmarried and does not have children, the estate is usually divided between his or her parents or, if they are also deceased, any siblings.

If an individual does not want his or her property divided according to the state's statutory scheme, a will is generally required. By utilizing a will, the individual can specify how property should be distributed and, if he or she so desires, can include gifts to a significant other, friend, charity, or even a beloved pet. Wills further allow an individual to name someone he or she trusts to serve as executor of the estate and ensure that the will's terms are carried out properly.

It should be noted that a will may not address the disposition of all of the decedent's assets. In most states, where a spouse survives, assets can pass free of probate and, despite directives in a will, state statute may protect a surviving spouse or children. In addition, some assets, such as life insurance, retirement accounts, and property held in joint tenancy, will pass to the named beneficiary regardless of whether a will exists. Similarly, certain types of accounts, vehicles, or other asset ownership can be designated as "payable on death" or "transfer on death," so that a change in ownership occurs when the individual dies. These types of assets are not considered to be a part of the decedent's estate and their management, therefore, would not be governed by the terms of a will.

A will can be executed by anyone over the age of majority who is mentally competent. The requirements for wills vary from state to state. Although an attorney is not required to draft or execute a legally binding will, consultation with an attorney is usually recommended. Unfortunately, family members who are not pleased with the terms of a will often bring a legal challenge in an attempt to have the will set aside (Goffe, 2009; Knauer, 2010). By having an attorney prepare or review the will, the individual can maximize the likelihood that all of a state's requirements have been met and can decrease the likelihood of a successful will contest.

One of the most difficult, but important, tasks a parent will confront is planning for the future care and custody of a minor child (Goldfein & Schalman-Bergen, 2010a) (it is also important to provide for an adult child who is relatively incapacitated or limited due to severe mental illness. This is discussed in the context of trusts, further below). In executing a will, the decedent can provide for the care of any minor children or dependents by naming a legal guardian who would be charged with said care. Without a will designating a guardian, the courts would have the responsibility of appointing one. Thus, a single parent who does not want the courts deciding who will care for his or her child should utilize a will to name a guardian. This is especially important when the parent has an incurable disease, like HIV/AIDS, that can be fatal. Appointing a guardian allows the parent to choose the person he or she feels is responsible, trustworthy, and best equipped raise the minor. It ensures that an objectionable family member is not appointed guardian and provides some peace of mind.

In 2010, a survey showed that 65% of the participants did not have a will (Ebeling, 2010). However, when an individual has a disease like HIV/AIDS, provisions should be made for the ultimate distribution of assets and the care of any minor children in the event of death. The execution of a will permits the individual to guarantee that the estate's assets are managed in an acceptable manner, specify how the assets should be divided, and address the guardianship of a minor. In doing so, the execution of a will can provide both a sense of comfort and security.

Trusts

A trust is a legal arrangement that determines, depending on the type of trust, how a person's property will be managed and distributed during his or her lifetime and/or upon death. A trust involves one party, often called the settler or trustor, transferring property to a trustee, who then manages it on behalf of the named beneficiary or beneficiaries. There are two main categories of trusts: testamentary trusts and living trusts.

Testamentary Trust. A testamentary trust is established and funded upon the death of the settlor. A testamentary trust and its terms, including the assets being transferred to fund it, is created through the settlor's will. Such trusts are often utilized to provide for the care of minors and dependents. The trustee is directed to use the assets placed in the trust for the care and needs of the trust's beneficiaries.

Due to the fact the trust is created as part of the settlor's will, a probate court has an oversight role. Probate courts monitor how testamentary trusts are managed and trustees are required to submit reports. This supervision has proven to be a deterrent to dishonesty, abuse, neglect, or misappropriation by trustees. Additionally, the involvement of the probate court provides beneficiaries with an avenue to seek redress for problems that may arise with a trust or the trustee.

A testamentary trust can be revoked or modified anytime before the settlor dies. After death, however, the trust is irrevocable. The trust will also become a matter of public record when, after the settlor's death, the will is submitted to the court for probate.

Living Trusts/Inter Vivos Trusts. Unlike testamentary trusts, living trusts are created during the lifetime of the settlor. Living trusts, also known as *inter vivos* trusts, can be used to manage property, provide for the settlor in event of mental or physical incapacity, and/or dispose of property upon death. The trustee of such a trust is responsible for managing the assets, as directed by the settlor, for the benefit of the beneficiaries. After the settlor's death, the trust, depending on its terms, either (1) is terminated and its assets are distributed to the beneficiaries, (2) survives and a trustee continues to manage all the assets, or (3) survives with some assets being distributed and remaining assets continuing under a trustee's management.

The settlor, while physically and mentally capable, can act as the trustee. Often, when this occurs, settlors find there is very little difference in managing their property and managing a trust's property. A settlor who also serves as the trustee can still buy, sell, or give away assets. He or she can still use and enjoy the trust's property. The assets are merely in the name of the trust rather than the settlor. Despite this, for tax purposes, the property is considered to still belong to the settlor. Therefore, income taxes on the trust's assets, during the settlor's lifetime, can be reported on the settlor's income tax return if he or she is also the trustee.

When the settlor also serves as the trustee, the trust documents should provide for a successor trustee who would assume control of the trust if the settlor/trustee becomes incapacitated or dies. By naming a successor trustee, a settlor/trustee who becomes incapacitated may be able to avoid a conservatorship or guardianship of the estate. The reader should be aware that, to avoid a conservatorship or guardianship of the estate, the naming of a successor trustee may need to be coupled with a Power of Attorney for Property to ensure that the trust remains adequately funded. A successor trustee can be an individual or a professional trustee (e.g., a bank).

Living trusts are created through the execution of a legal document. The document is usually called a "trust agreement," "declaration of trust," or "indenture of trust." The trust documents and their execution by the settlor must conform to state law. The trust documents should show a clear intention to create the trust, identify the property funding it, and have the beneficiaries either clearly identified or ascertainable.

The trust can be funded during the lifetime of the settlor, after the settlor's death, or a combination of both. If a settlor chooses to add assets to the living trust after his or her death, he or she would utilize a legal device known as a "pour over" will. Essentially, in the settlor's will, he or she designates the trust as a beneficiary. The property to be distributed to the trust will then "pour over" from the settlor's probate estate into the preexisting living trust.

A living trust can also be funded throughout the lifetime of the settlor. When funding the trust, the settlor is required to take the appropriate steps to transfer ownership of the assets to the trust. Consequently, deeds, titles, stocks, securities, bonds, bank accounts, investment accounts, money market accounts, treasury bills, safety deposit boxes, etc. need to be transferred and/or retitled to the trust's name. Non-titled property can be listed on a trust schedule. Additionally, the beneficiary designation should be changed on any of those assets the settlor wants to go into the trust after his or her death. For example, if the settlor desires the funds from a life insurance policy to become trust property upon the settlor's death, the trust should be listed as the designated beneficiary on the policy.

Living trusts can be revocable or irrevocable. An irrevocable trust cannot be modified or terminated by the settlor after it has been established. Thus, the settlor loses control over the assets that have been used to fund the trust. Irrevocable trusts are usually utilized to help shield the trust's assets from creditors and to avoid or pay lower taxes.

Conversely, revocable trusts can be revoked, amended, or modified by the settlor at any time during his or her lifetime. The settlor of a revocable trust retains the right to change the terms of the trust, the trustee, and/or the trust's assets regardless of whether he or she is also the trustee. This allows the settlor to amend or revoke the trust in the case of divorce or death of a beneficiary. Unlike with wills, an ex-spouse is not automatically disqualified as a beneficiary.

Living trusts can be used as another legal precaution for an individual who faces possible physical incapacity or mentally capacity due to HIV/AIDS or a diagnosed mental illness Utilizing a living trust can help ensure that the financial affairs of the individual with HIV/AIDS or the parent of a child with HIV/AIDS or mental illness are managed by a trustee he or she trusts if the parent's illness causes incapacity. The terms can also ensure that any dependents will have the funds needed for their care after the death of the settlor. As such, a living trust should be considered by individuals with HIV/AIDS and by parents of a child with HIV/AIDS and/or severe mental illness who are planning for illness, incapacity, and death.

In general, trusts are more private and, upon death, can help save in probate expenses. They offer settlors a measure of control over how assets are managed, who is managing them, and how they are distributed. However, trusts are not a substitute for other legal documents, such as wills and powers of attorney. For example, a trust may be established to care for minors after the settlor's death, but a will is still needed to name the minors' guardian. Consequently, trusts should be viewed as one weapon in the arsenal of legal mechanisms that can be used to protect their assets and rights.

Guardianship and Conservatorship

Guardianship is a legal relationship between a competent adult and a person who has been judged unable to manage his or her own affairs (i.e., the ward). Through a guardianship, the guardian is charged with the responsibility of managing the personal affairs of ward. Thus, a guardian is charged with the care and protection of the ward. This can include the ward's personal care, clothing, transportation, and access to nutrition. To this end, the guardian can make decisions concerning the ward's residence, health care, counseling, and therapeutic care. The guardian can consent to, or deny, medical treatment, release confidential information, and make end-of-life decisions.

Similar to a guardianship, a conservatorship is a legal relationship between a competent adult and a person who has been judged unable to manage his or her own affairs. However, unlike a guardianship, in many states a conservatorship only permits the management of ward's financial affairs. In those states, conservators have no authority over the ward's health or personal affairs. Instead, conservators have the right to manage and protect the ward's assets and estate. This would include real and personal property. The conservator may be able, among other things, to obtain property appraisals, receive estate income, give gifts, lend money, borrow money, make a will, handle legal actions, pay bills, and make other disbursements.

The reader should be aware the terms "guardianship" and "conservatorship" are sometimes used interchangeably. While some states use the term "guardianship" for personal affairs and "conservatorship" for financial affairs, other states will utilize only one of the terms for both financial and personal affairs. For instance, in California, courts appoint "conservators of the person" and "conservators of the estate" (Guardianship-Conservatorship Law, 2008). Conversely, Illinois recognizes "guardians of the person" and "guardians of the estate" (Illinois Probate Act of 1975, 1979). Some states, such as Wisconsin, allow for "conservators of the estate," "guardians of the estate," and "guardians of the person" (Guardianships and Conservatorships, 2005).

Guardianship and conservatorship are most frequently utilized for the care of minors, but can be used for adults who do not have the capacity to make, or communicate, decisions concerning their person or property. Often, guardianship/conservatorship is ordered due to conditions such as mental illness, mental deterioration, chronic intoxication, physical incapacity, or developmental disability.

The laws of each state vary with regard as to what is required for the necessary finding of incapacity. For example, in Washington state, a person is considered incapacitated if there is a significant risk of personal harm based on an inability to adequately manage nutrition, health, housing, physical safety, property, or financial affairs (Washington Trust Act of 1984, 2008). Illinois considers individuals to be disabled for the purposes of guardianship if they (a) because of mental deterioration or physical incapacity, are not fully able to manage either personal or financial affairs; (b) have a mental illness or developmental disability that prevents the full management of either personal or financial affairs; (c) because of gambling, idleness, debauchery or excessive use of intoxicants/drugs, spend or waste their estates to such an extent that it exposes them or their families to want or suffering; or (d) have a diagnosis of fetal alcohol syndrome or fetal alcohol effects (Illinois Probate Act of 1975, 1979).

Although the process will vary from state to state, guardianships and conservatorships are typically established by petitioning a court and alleging that the potential ward is incompetent. A hearing may follow, wherein the court will decide (1) whether the potential ward is incapacitated under the laws of the state, (2) who or what entity will be appointed the guardian/conservator, and (3) what authority will be granted to the guardian/conservator. During this legal process, a report or testimony may be required, usually from a medical professional, that certifies that the potential ward has some disability and, as a result, needs a guardian/conservator. A *guardian ad litem*, an unbiased individual who represents the interests of the potential ward in the legal proceedings, may be appointed to investigate, obtain medical opinions, and make recommendations to the court. A guardianship/conservatorship proceeding can be costly, complex, and cumbersome (Goldfein & Schalman-Bergen, 2010b). If a guardianship or conservatorship is granted, the guardian/conservator is required to submit reports to the court.

Again, the requirements to become a guardian/conservator will depend on the state's statute, but the guardian/conservator will have to be a legal adult of sound mind. Some states' statutes, such as Washington, will not appoint someone who has been convicted of a serious crime (Washington Trust Act of 1984, 2008). Although family may be given priority, the best interest of the ward is often, if not always, considered by the court (Legal Information Institute, 2010). A private or public institution can be made a guardian/conservator, and, when involving only the estate, so can a financial institution. Most courts will respect a ward's nomination of a guardian/conservator if it was made while the ward was competent (Goldfein & Schalman-Bergen, 2010b). The nomination should be in writing and comply with state statutory requirements (Goldfein & Schalman-Bergen, 2010b).

Guardianships and conservatorships can be temporary or permanent in nature. They may also be limited. Under a limited guardianship or conservatorship, the court specifies what authority is being conferred. The ward retains all other rights. The authority being conferred under a guardianship or conservatorship should be given serious consideration, as the legal arrangement will remove some, or all, of the ward's civil rights and impose personal limitations. Among other things, the ward can lose the ability to vote, marry, hold a driver's license, or object to commitment in an institutional setting. Consequently, the ward should be afforded the least restrictive guardianship or conservatorship appropriate to his or her condition.

Due to the fact guardianships and conservatorships can strip an individual of numerous rights, it should be viewed as a last resort and alternatives should be considered when possible (Goldfein & Schalman-Bergen, 2010b). Guardianship/conservatorship may be avoided if the ward has executed a power of attorney for health care and/or a power for attorney of property (Goldfein & Schalman-Bergen,

2010b). A living will, a health care surrogacy, joint bank accounts, and trusts are also alternatives that may help prevent a guardianship/conservatorship. Case management, community agencies/services, veteran administration benefits, and community advocacy programs are other resources that can be explored. Through them, it may be possible to arrange respite care, adult day care, home health care, home-delivered meals, mental health services, tenant support, or appointment of a financial fiduciary/designated payee. Another possible alternative is the use of a representative payee to manage any Social Security benefits.

Guardianships and conservatorships can be reviewed, modified, or removed by the court. A petition to review the guardianship or conservatorship can be filed with the court by the ward or someone on the ward's behalf. After a hearing on the issue, the court could order the guardian/conservator to take certain acts or measures, remove the guardian/conservator, or replace the guardian/conservator. If the ward is able to show regained capacity, the court can modify or terminate the guardianship or conservatorship.

Unfortunately, individuals with HIV/AIDS can become ill, and possibly incapacitated, quickly (Goldfein & Schalman-Bergen, 2010c). If an individual with HIV/AIDS becomes too ill from any medical condition to care for him- or herself, it is possible that a guardianship and/or conservatorship could be pursued and granted. Thus, the individual risks a court deciding who should make personal and financial decisions on his or her behalf. Although the guardian and/or conservator should act in the ward's best interest, the decisions made may be inconsistent with what the ward would have preferred. Therefore, as a part of preparing for any serious illness or incapacity, a person with HIV/AIDS should consider this possibility and, if he or she objects to guardianship and/or conservatorship, be proactive. A person with HIV/AIDS can exert a measure of control over what will happen if he or she becomes incapacitated by utilizing the available legal alternatives. If the person with HIV/AIDS chooses to nominate a guardian and/or conservator, strict attention should be paid to the state's statutory requirements and the proper execution of the required steps.

Funeral Arrangements

Providing for funeral and burial arrangements in advance is most important for unmarried individuals (Goffe, 2009). All of the states have laws addressing the disposition of remains. Upon death, funeral arrangements are typically made by the deceased's spouse or, if unmarried, the next-of-kin (Knauer, 2010). In most states, an individual's significant other, if unmarried, would have no right to make, or participate in, the funeral arrangements (Knauer, 2010). Individuals can take steps, however, to plan for the disposal of their remains or appoint an agent to make the arrangements. This is especially important when an unmarried individual has no family or does not want the funeral/burial arrangements to be made by the next-of-kin. Such steps would also be beneficial when an individual does not believe that his or her spouse will act in manner consistent with the individual's wishes. For example, although a man may want his body donated to science, his wife may indicate that she will only consider burial.

One way to dictate the manner of disposition of one's body and/or the funeral arrangements is to include the instructions in a will. The reader should be cautioned, however, that utilizing a will in this manner is not always advisable (Goffe, 2009). Wills are often read after the funeral (Goffe, 2009). Some states will recognize and uphold written documents, like Funeral Planning Declarations, that specify the deceased's wishes (Knauer, 2010). Depending on the state, a power of attorney may permit an attorney-in-fact limited rights concerning the disposition of bodily remains. These documents can be used alone or in conjunction with a will. If multiple documents are used, steps should be taken to ensure the instructions in the documents do not conflict.

Major Laws Applicable to Protect Individuals with HIV/AIDS

Although many states have laws that protect the rights of individuals with HIV/AIDS, this chapter will discuss two of the federal laws that have been passed to help protect the rights of such individuals. These laws have been chosen due to their breadth and the purpose. This writer encourages the reader to research his or her state's laws on the subject, but also cautions that the protections afforded to individuals with HIV/AIDS will vary from state to state. The laws discussed below, due to their federal nature, apply regardless of state lines.

Americans with Disabilities Act

The Americans with Disabilities Act (ADA) is a federal law that was enacted in 1990 to protect the rights of individuals with disabilities. The ADA prohibits discrimination based on disability in employment, public accommodations, commercial facilities, transportation, telecommunications, and by state and local governments (Americans with Disabilities Act, 1990). It was most recently amended on September 25, 2008, by the ADA Amendments Act of 2008 (ADAA). While the ADA has five separate titles, this chapter examines the two most well-known titles.

To be protected by the ADA, an individual has to (1) have a physical or mental impairment that substantially limits one or more major life activities ("actual disability" prong), (2) have a record of such an impairment ("record of" prong), or (3) be regarded as having such an impairment ("regarded as" prong). After the ADAA (2008), the "regarded as" prong requires that an individual be subjected to an action prohibited by the ADA due to an actual or perceived impairment that is not both "transitory and minor" (Regulations to Implement the Equal Employment Provisions of the Americans with Disabilities Act, 2010).

The Equal Employment Opportunity Commission (EEOC) has defined a physical impairment to include any physiological disorder or condition, cosmetic disfigurement, or anatomical loss affecting one or more body systems (Regulations to Implement the Equal Employment Provisions of the Americans with Disabilities Act, 2010). Likewise, it defined mental impairment to include any mental or psychological disorder (Regulations to Implement the Equal Employment Provisions of the Americans with Disabilities Act, 2010). An impairment that is episodic or in remission, such as HIV/AIDS or a severe mental illness, can still be considered a disability if it would substantially limit a major life activity when active (ADA Amendments Act, 2008).

For an impaired individual to be protected under the ADA, it must be shown there is a major life activity that is, or has a record of being, substantially limited by the impairment. Major life activities have been found to include the following: (1) caring for oneself, performing manual tasks, seeing, hearing, eating, sleeping, walking, standing, sitting, reaching, lifting, bending, speaking, breathing, learning, reading, concentrating, thinking, communicating, interacting with others, and working; and (2) the operation of major bodily functions such as the immune system, special sense organs, skin, cell growth, bladder, bowel, brain, respiration, circulation, cardiovascular system, endocrine system, hemic system, lymphatic system, digestive system, neurological system, musculoskeletal system, reproduction, and the operation of an individual organ within a body system (ADA Amendments Act, 2008; Regulations to Implement the Equal Employment Provisions of the Americans with Disabilities Act, 2010). It should be noted the above is not an inclusive list of every a major life activity for the purposes of the ADA (Regulations to Implement the Equal Employment Provisions of the Americans with Disabilities Act, 2010).

Although the ADA does not specify all of the impairments that would be given coverage, the EEOC has provided a list of conditions it regards as virtually always imposing a substantial limitation on a major life activity (Regulations to Implement the Equal Employment Provisions of the Americans with Disabilities Act, 2010). The EEOC has found that it should be easily concluded that (1) deafness substantially limits hearing; (2) blindness substantially limits seeing; (3) an intellectual disability, cerebral palsy, and autism substantially limit brain function; (4) partially or completely missing limbs or mobility impairments requiring the use of a wheelchair substantially limit musculoskeletal function; (5) cancer substantially limits normal cell growth; (6) diabetes substantially limits endocrine function; (7) epilepsy, multiple sclerosis, and muscular dystrophy substantially limit neurological function; (8) HIV infection substantially limits immune function; and (9) major depressive disorder, bipolar disorder, posttraumatic stress disorder, obsessive compulsive disorder, and schizophrenia substantially limit brain function (Regulations to Implement the Equal Employment Provisions of the Americans with Disabilities Act, 2010).

The U.S. Department of Justice, Congress, and the EEOC recognize HIV/AIDS, both symptomatic and asymptomatic, as being covered by the ADA (Equal Employment Opportunities Commission, 2008; House Report, 1990; Nondiscrimination on the Basis of Disability by Public Accommodations, 2010; Senate Report,

1989; United States Department of Justice, 2002). The United States Supreme Court first examined the issue in *Bragdon v. Abbott* (1998). In *Bragdon*, the Court held Sidney Abbott's asymptomatic HIV infection was a physical impairment that substantially limited the major life activity of reproduction (*Bragdon v. Abbott*, 1998). In deciding *Bragdon*, the Court did not find HIV/AIDS is a disability *per se* for the purposes of the ADA (*Bragdon v. Abbott*, 1998). Since the *Bragdon* decision, courts have tended to treat HIV/AIDS as an "impairment," but require a showing that a major life activity is substantially limited (Corporate Counsel's Guide, 2011). In *Horgan v. Simmons* (2010), the Seventh Circuit held that, under the ADAA, an HIV positive status is a condition that substantially limits a major life activity (*Horgan v. Simmons*, 2010). In this case the impaired major life activity was the functioning of the immune system.

Under the ADA, a "mental impairment" includes any mental or psychological disorder. (Equal Employment Opportunity Commission's Americans With Disability Act Employment Regulations, 1996). This includes emotional or mental illness like major depression, bipolar disorder, schizophrenia, and personality disorders (Equal Employment Opportunity Commission, 1997). Anxiety disorders, such as panic disorders, obsessive compulsive disorder, and posttraumatic stress disorder, are also recognized (Equal Employment Opportunity Commission, 1997). The American Psychiatric Association's 2000 *Diagnostic and Statistical Manual of Mental Disorders* is relevant in identifying these disorders (Equal Employment Opportunity Commission, 1997). It must be remembered showing the existence of one of these conditions is not enough to trigger the protections afforded by the ADA. Instead, the impairment of a major life activity must also be demonstrated.

Title I. Under Title I of the ADA, employers are prohibited from discriminating against qualified individuals with disabilities. Title I applies to private employers with 15 or more employees (ADA Amendments Act, 2008). All public entities, regardless of the number of employees, are also subject to the ADA through Title II of the Act (Nondiscrimination on the Basis of Disability in State and Local, 2010).

Employers cannot discriminate in their job application procedures, hiring decisions, job training, job assignments, promotions, or firing decisions (ADA Amendments Act, 2008; Equal Employment Opportunity Commission, 2008). For individuals with disabilities like HIV/AIDS, this prevents employers from asking certain disability-related questions during the application process, establishing policies where they refuse to hire or promote employees with HIV/AIDS, or firing employees solely due to their HIV/AIDS status or the possibility they will become too ill to work in the future (United States Department of Justice, 2002). Other employment-related activity, such as wages, leave, and insurance benefits, are also protected by the ADA (ADA Amendments Act, 2008; Equal Employment Opportunity Commission, 2008). Consequently, an employer cannot contract with an insurance carrier that places a cap on the benefit amount available for HIV/AIDS treatment but not on any other type of treatment.

The above protections also extend to individuals with mental illness or psychiatric disabilities. Employers are prohibited from making blanket inquiries into an applicant's mental health or psychiatric history. Therefore, a prospective employer cannot ask whether applicant has received psychiatric treatment, the type of treatment, or if the treatment is ongoing. The employer can, however, make objective inquiries to help it determine whether the applicant can perform the essential duties of the job. Thus, an employer can ask about the applicant's ability to come to work regularly, appear at work on-time, interact with others, and stay on task.

It should be noted Title I only makes it unlawful to discriminate against "qualified" individuals with disabilities (ADA Amendments Act, 2008). A "qualified individual with a disability" is a person who meets the legitimate skill, experience, education, and/or other requirements of a job position and can perform the "essential functions" of the position with, or without, reasonable accommodation (ADA Amendments Act, 2008; *School Board of Nassau County v. Arline*, 1987). The "essential functions" of a job are the core duties that are the reason the job position exists (United States Department of Justice, 2002). The essential function of a taxi driving position, for example, is the ability to drive. By requiring that the person be able to complete the essential functions of a job, the ADA prevents employers from adding tasks to a position that are designed to disqualify disabled individuals (United States Department of Justice, 2002). Whether an individual meets the definition of a "qualified individual with a disability" must be decided on a case-by-case basis (*School Board of Nassau County v. Arline*, 1987).

A "reasonable accommodation" is a modification or adjustment that enables a qualified individual with a disability to perform the essential functions of the job, participate in the application process, and/or enjoy the benefits/privileges of the employment (United States Department of Justice, 2002). An accommodation is "reasonable" if it is feasible or plausible (Office of Legal Counsel, 2002). An illustration of a reasonable accommodation is the provision of a stool for a grocery store clerk who, because of AIDS, had difficulty standing for long periods of time. It should be noted that employers are generally only required to accommodate actual, known disabilities (Equal Employment Opportunity Commission, 2008; United States Department of Justice, 2002). As such, the responsibility falls to the disabled individual to request the accommodation (United States Department of Justice, 2002). If an appropriate accommodation is not readily apparent, the employer must make a reasonable effort determine accommodations that could be provided (Equal Employment Opportunity Commission, 2008). This might include talking to the disabled individual, the EEOC, and/or vocational professionals (Equal Employment Opportunity Commission, 2008). Additionally, the employer does not have to provide the specific accommodations requested by the disabled individual but, instead, is only required to provide an effective accommodation that meets the individual's needs (Equal Employment Opportunity Commission, 2008; United States Department of Justice, 2002). If the disabled individual refuses a reasonable, necessary accommodation, he or she could be considered not qualified (Equal Employment Opportunity Commission, 2008; *Hankins v. The Gap, Inc.*, 1996).

An employer's responsibility to not discriminate against a qualified disabled individual, however, is not without limitation. Employers are not required to hire or retain a qualified individual with a disability if that person poses a direct threat to the health or safety of others. A "direct threat" is defined as "a significant risk to the health or safety of others that cannot be eliminated by reasonable accommodation" (ADA Amendments Act, 2008). Before an employer can rely on this provision of the ADA, it must establish through objective, medically supportable methods that there is a significant risk that substantial harm could occur in the workplace (United States Department of Justice, 2002). As an example, an individual with a diagnosis of paranoid schizophrenia who is nonadherent to medications that control his hallucinations and paranoia and has a record of harming others might be considered to pose a significant risk to the safety of others.

An individual's HIV/AIDS status will not pose a direct threat in a majority of employment settings (United States Department of Justice, 2002). HIV/AIDS is most commonly transmitted through sexual contact, sharing needles with an infected person, exposure to infected blood/blood products, organ transplantation, or perinatally during pregnancy, birth, or breast feeding (Centers for Disease Control and Prevention, 2010). A human bite, wherein the skin is broken and there is severe trauma with the presence of blood, presents only a remote risk of transmission (Centers for Disease Control and Prevention, 2010). HIV cannot be transmitted by casual, everyday contact (Centers for Disease Control and Prevention, 2010). Contact with saliva alone has never been shown to result in the transmission of HIV/AIDS and scratches present no risk of transmission (Centers for Disease Control and Prevention, 2010). Given the above, HIV cannot be transmitted through ordinary workplace contacts in most occupations (Analysis and guidelines—AIDS, 2011; Centers for Disease Control and Prevention, 2010).

Despite the fact the individual's HIV/AIDS status, by itself, does not usually pose a direct threat, employment action may be justified if having HIV/AIDS impairs the individual's ability to safely perform functions of the job and, as a result, creates a direct threat to the health or safety of others. For example, if a bus driver's HIV/AIDS condition causes dizziness, he or she may pose a direct threat to the health and safety of others.

Further, an individual's HIV/AIDS status may be a direct threat in certain health care professions. Although the risk of transmission in most health care professions is low, courts have found that some health care professionals pose a direct threat to the health and safety of others. In *Estate of Mauro v. Borgess Medical Center* (1998), Mr. Mauro was fired from his job as a surgical technician due to his HIV status (*Estate of Mauro v. Borgess Medical Center*, 1998). The Court found that Mr. Mauro's job would require him to, at times, have his hands in or near an operative site, where visibility is poor, in the presence of sharp instruments (*Estate of Mauro v. Borgess Medical Center*, 1998). As the job might require Mr. Mauro to engage in invasive, exposure-prone activities, the Court believed that Mr. Mauro's position as a surgical technician posed a direct threat to the health and safety of others (*Estate of Mauro v. Borgess Medical Center*, 1998).

Under Title I, an employer's responsibility to accommodate a qualified disabled individual is not without limitation. An employer is not required to make an accommodation that would impose an undue hardship on the operation of the business (ADA Amendments Act, 2008). An "undue hardship" is an action that requires significant difficulty or expense in relation to the size of the employer, the resources available, and the nature of the operation (ADA Amendments Act, 2008). Undue hardships exist when the provision of an accommodation would be unduly costly, extensive, substantial, disruptive, or would fundamentally alter the nature or operation of the business (Equal Employment Opportunity Commission, 2008). The installation of an elevator into a small book store owned by a sole proprietor would likely qualify as an undue hardship. Conversely, the provision of a dedicated parking spot close to the book store would probably not qualify as an undue hardship. Whether the provision of an accommodation would constitute an undue hardship is determined on a case-by-case basis (Office of Legal Counsel, 2002; United States Department of Justice, 2002). However, the fears and/or prejudices of customers or co-workers and the possible negative effect on morale are not valid considerations (Equal Employment Opportunity Commission, 2002; Regulations to Implement the Equal Employment Provisions of the Americans with Disabilities Act, 2010; United States Department of Justice, 2002). Thus, according to the U.S. Department of Justice, the loss of customers and/or co-workers due to the employment of someone with HIV/AIDS would not constitute an undue hardship (United States Department of Justice, 2002).

When making employment decisions, Title I prevents employers from making pre-offer inquiries about a disability (ADA Amendments Act, 2008). Instead, inquiries can only be made into the individual's ability to perform specific job functions (ADA Amendments Act, 2008). Employers are also prohibited from requiring the applicant to undergo a medical evaluation before making a job offer (ADA Amendments Act, 2008). After an offer of employment has been made, however, the employer can require a medical evaluation if it is also required of all employees entering the job (ADA Amendments Act, 2008). While an employer can condition the job offer on a satisfactory post-offer medical exam, an individuals' HIV status alone will rarely be a legitimate basis for an adverse hiring decision (ADA Amendments Act, 2008; United States Department of Justice, 2012). During the course of the employment, medical examinations or inquiries of an employee can be conducted if they are job-related and consistent with business necessity (ADA Amendments Act, 2008). Medical examinations can be conducted, for example, when there is evidence of a job performance or safety problem, when required by other federal laws, when necessary to determine the employee's current "fitness" to perform a particular job, and/or when voluntary examinations are part of employee health programs (United States Department of Justice, 2002).

Title III. Title III of the ADA prevents discrimination on the basis of disability with regard to the full and equal enjoyment of the goods, services, facilities, privileges, advantages, or accommodations of any place of public accommodation (ADA Amendments Act, 2008). The Title applies to any person who owns, leases, or operates a place of public accommodation (ADA Amendments Act, 2008). The Act defines a public accommodation:

If the operations of such entities affect commerce—

(a) An inn, hotel, motel, or other place of lodging, except for an establishment located within a building that contains not more than five rooms for rent or hire and that is actually occupied by the proprietor of such establishment as the residence of such proprietor.
(b) A restaurant, bar, or other establishment serving food or drink.
(c) A motion picture house, theater, concert hall, stadium, or other place of exhibition or entertainment.
(d) An auditorium, convention center, lecture hall, or other place of public gathering.
(e) A bakery, grocery store, clothing store, hardware store, shopping center, or other sales or rental establishment.
(f) A laundromat, dry-cleaner, bank, barber shop, beauty shop, travel service, shoe repair service, funeral parlor, gas station, office of an accountant or lawyer, pharmacy, insurance office, professional office of a health care provider, hospital, or other service establishment.
(g) A terminal, depot, or other station used for specified public transportation.
(h) A museum, library, gallery, or other place of public display or collection.
(i) A park, zoo, amusement park, or other place of recreation.
(j) A nursery, elementary, secondary, undergraduate, or postgraduate private school, or other place of education.
(k) A day care center, senior citizen center, homeless shelter, food bank, adoption agency, or other social service center establishment.
(l) A gymnasium, health spa, bowling alley, golf course, or other place of exercise or recreation (ADA Amendments Act, 2008).

Thus, under this Title, disabled individuals must be given an equal opportunity to use or enjoy the public accommodation's goods, services, or facilities. A restaurant, then, could not refuse to serve a customer with HIV/AIDS or charge more for the meal. However, disabled individuals can be excluded when they pose a direct threat to the health and safety of others (ADA Amendments Act, 2008). Private clubs and religious organizations are exempted from this Title's requirements (ADA Amendments Act, 2008).

Covered public accommodations have a responsibility to remove any architectural barriers and communication barriers, which are structural in nature, to existing facilities when it is readily achievable (ADA Amendments Act, 2008). Readily achievable is defined as "easily accomplishable and able to be carried out without much difficulty or expense" (ADA Amendments Act, 2008). Any new construction, modifications, or alterations to a facility must comply with the Americans with Disabilities Act Accessibility Guidelines. Under Title III, a public accommodation may be required to install ramps, widen doors, install power doors, and provide disabled parking spaces. Individuals with HIV/AIDS may suffer weakness, fatigue, loss of eyesight, or require the use or a wheelchair. Title III helps ensure that such individuals do not lose access to public facilities and services.

The Ryan White CARE Act

The Ryan White CARE Act (CARE Act) was passed in 1990 to provide medical assistance and funding to those living with HIV/AIDS that otherwise could not afford the care. It also provides funding to medical facilities who provide care to those affected by the virus. It is named after Ryan White, a young man who died from AIDS in 1990 (Health Resources and Services Administration HIV/AIDS Programs, n.d.b). Ryan White was a thirteen year old hemophiliac who acquired HIV through a blood transfusion and died at the age of 18 (Health Resources and Services Administration HIV/AIDS Programs, n.d.b).

The purpose of the CARE Act was to increase the availability of care for victims of HIV/AIDS who have a low-income, are uninsured, or are underinsured and their families (Health Resources and Services Administration HIV/AIDS Programs, n.d. c). Administered by the Health Resource and Services Administration, the CARE Act's programs fund treatment when no other resources are available and provide services for more than half a million people a year (Kaiser, 2006). It is the third largest source, after Medicare and Medicaid, of public funding of HIV/AIDS care in the United States (Kaiser, 2006).

In 2004, approximately three-quarters, or 72%, of recipients had annual household incomes at, or below, the poverty level (Kaiser, 2006). Thirty-one percent of recipients had no medical insurance and 55% were covered by public insurance programs (Kaiser, 2006). Recipients of the CARE Act's funding are primarily males between the ages of 25 and 44 (Kaiser, 2006). The majority of recipients are also people of color (Kaiser, 2006).

The CARE Act is divided into five main parts. The types of entities eligible for funds through the Act include states, cities, directly funded public and private providers, and other organizations (Kaiser, 2006). Of the funds distributed under the CARE Act, approximately 55% is given to states, 30% to cities, and the remainder to organizations directly (Kaiser, 2006).

Part A. Part A of the CARE Act allows for funding to assist eligible metropolitan areas (EMA) that are affected by HIV/AIDS. In order for an area to qualify as an EMA, it must (1) have a cumulative total of more than 2,000 reported AIDS cases over the most recent 5-year period; (2) be a "transitional grant area," which is an area with a reported 1,000–1,999 AIDS cases over the most recent 5-year period; and (3) have a population of at least 50,000 (Health Resources and Services Administration HIV/AIDS Programs, n.d.d). The numbers are based upon the reported AIDS cases reported to the Centers for Disease Control (Ryan White Comprehensive AIDS Resources Emergency Act of 1990, 1990).

In 2006, 30% of the funding under the CARE Act was allocated for Part A (Kaiser, 2006). Funds distributed under Part A are given out under either a formula grant or a supplemental grant (Health Resources and Services Administration HIV/AIDS Programs, n.d.d). Formula grants are based on an EMA's share of those estimated to be living AIDS cases and make up half of the funding distributed under Part A (Kaiser, 2006). The remainder of the funding is distributed through supplemental grants that are awarded competitively based on severe need (Kaiser, 2006).

Those who are awarded the assistance must use at least 75% of the funds on core services for the virus. Core services include AIDS drug assistance, AIDS pharmaceutical assistance, oral health services, early intervention services, health insurance premiums and cost sharing assistance for low-income individuals, medical nutrition therapy, hospice, home and community-based health services, mental health services, substance abuse outpatient care, home health care, medical case management, and outpatient and ambulatory medical care (Health Resources and Services Administration HIV/AIDS Programs, n.d.d).

The remainder of the funds, but no more than 25%, can be used on support services for those infected with the virus if those services are linked to medical outcomes (Health Resources and Services Administration HIV/AIDS Programs, n.d.d). Support services include medical transportation, case management, and referrals to health care providers (Health Resources and Services Administration HIV/AIDS Programs, n.d.d).

In each EMA city, a planning council must be established to formulate a strategy for identifying those affected and how to assist them (Health Resources and Services Administration HIV/AIDS Programs, n.d.d). The planning council must be comprised of people who have expertise in areas affected by HIV/AIDS such as healthcare, housing for the homeless, and substance abuse and mental health treatment (Health Resources and Services Administration HIV/AIDS Programs, n.d.d).

Part B. Part B of the CARE Act provides funding for services such as prescription drugs, health insurance purchasing and continuation, home health care, early intervention activities, and direct health and support services (Kaiser, 2006). In 2006, 55% of the funding under the CARE Act was allocated for Part B (Kaiser, 2006). Funds are distributed to all 50 states, the District of Columbia, Puerto Rico, Guam, and the U.S. Virgin Islands (Kaiser, 2006).

Funding distribution under Part B includes base funding, the AIDS Drug Assistance Program (ADAP), and Emerging Communities Grants (Kaiser, 2006). The base funding is determined according to a formula that considers a state's share of the estimated living with AIDS cases (Kaiser, 2006). ADAP funds are earmarked by Congress to provide medication or health insurance that provides for medication (Kaiser, 2006). Additionally, 5% of the earmark is reserved for supplemental grants to states and territories found to have a severe need that prevents the provision of medication (Health Resources and Services Administration HIV/AIDS Programs, n.d.e). States provide services to clients directly or through an association of organizations set up to plan for and deliver HIV care (Health Resources and Services Administration HIV/AIDS Programs, n.d.e). Finally, a portion of funds under Part B is allocated for grants to metropolitan areas that have reached a minimum level of reported AIDS cases but do not yet qualify as EMAs (Kaiser, 2006).

Part C. Part C of the CARE Act provides funds directly to service providers in order to support outpatient HIV early intervention services and ambulatory care (Health Resources and Services Administration HIV/AIDS Programs, n.d.f). Early intervention services include HIV testing, case management, and risk reduction counseling (Kaiser, 2006). Funds under this title are also used to fund planning grants and capacity development grants (Health Resources and Services Administration HIV/AIDS Programs, n.d.f). These grants provide support to organizations for both the planning for service delivery and building the capacity to provide services (Kaiser, 2006). In 2006, 10% of the funding under the CARE Act was allocated for Part C (Kaiser, 2006).

Part D. Part D of the CARE Act provides direct funding for family-centered and community-based medical care for those living with HIV/AIDS (Health Resources and Services Administration HIV/AIDS Programs, n.d.g). Funds under this title are typically used for women, infants, children and youth living with the virus (Health Resources and Services Administration HIV/AIDS Programs, n.d.g). The services provided by the organizations receiving funding include outreach, prevention, primary and specialty medical care, and psychosocial services (Kaiser, 2006). In 2006, four percent of the funding under the CARE Act was allocated for Part D (Kaiser, 2006).

Funding under Part D often goes to organizations that are trying to enhance their response to the virus in their community (Health Resources and Services Administration HIV/AIDS Programs, n.d.g). Organizations must, as a condition of the funding, provide education to the clients of their facilities about available research opportunities and how to enroll in them (Health Resources and Services Administration HIV/AIDS Programs, n.d.g).

Part F. In this title of the CARE Act, funding is provided for AIDS Education and Training Center (AETCs), the Special Projects of National Significance (SPNS) program, and the Dental Reimbursement Program (Health Resources and Services Administration HIV/AIDS Programs: Living History, n.d.a). In 2006, 2% of the CARE Act's funds was allocated for AETCs and 1% for the dental portion under Part F (Kaiser, 2006).

SPNSs advance health and support services to areas with underserved populations dealing with HIV (Health Resources and Services Administration HIV/AIDS Programs: Living History, n.d.a). Some of those special projects include one project for Hepatitis C treatment and another for promoting the development of electronic client data (Health Resources and Services Administration HIV/AIDS Programs: Living History, n.d.a). AETCs are national and regional centers dedicated to educating and training health care providers who provide treatment to individuals with HIV/AIDS (Kaiser, 2006).

The Dental Reimbursement Program provides funding to help alleviate the costs of uncompensated care provided to individuals with HIV/AIDS by academic dental institutions (Health Resources and Services Administration HIV/AIDS Programs: Living History, n.d.a). In 2000, the Community-Based Dental Partnership Program was also added. This program supports collaborations between dental education programs, community-based dentists, and dental clinics to further increase the reach of services into communities that lack academic dental institutions (Health Resources and Services Administration HIV/AIDS Programs: Living History, n.d.a).

Due to advances in the treatment of HIV, a slower progression from HIV infection to AIDS is more common (Buchanan & Hatcher, 2007). The slower progression can make it difficult for an individual with HIV to meet the criteria necessary to receive Medicaid (Buchanan & Hatcher, 2007). Despite having a low income, most individuals will not qualify for Medicaid until they become disabled by AIDS. As a result, the need for programs like those provided under the CARE Act has grown (Buchanan & Hatcher, 2007). Without funding from programs under the CARE Act, many individuals with HIV/AIDS would find themselves locked out of the services they may desperately need (Buchanan & Hatcher, 2007).

Laws to Protect the Public Against HIV/AIDS

At the end of 2008, there were an estimated 1,178,350 Americans aged 13 and older living with HIV (Centers for Disease Control and Prevention, 2011a, 2011b, 2011c). To fight the epidemic, governments and legislators have sought ways to limit exposure to others and reduce the number of transmissions of the virus every year. As a result, states and civilians have turned to the courts to impute criminal and civil liability upon those who, without disclosure, knowingly expose others to the virus. The following is a brief discussion of the criminal and civil causes of action being utilized.

Criminalization of the Failure to Disclose

In many states, if an individual knows that he or she has HIV and exposes others to the disease without full disclosure, the individual can be charged with a criminal offense. Although the cases usually involve a sexual partner, the donation of infected blood or organs has also been criminalized. As of 2008, there were 36 states in the United States that had prosecuted individuals for criminal transmission or exposure to HIV (AVERT, n.d.).

Only some of these states have statutes that specifically address HIV (AVERT, n.d.). The statutes may either create separate crimes for intentional HIV exposure or enhance existing criminal penalties when the crime is committed by someone with HIV (Wolf & Venzia, 2004). In California, for instance, the law makes it a crime to engage in unprotected, uninformed sex with the specific intent to infect another person with HIV (Communicable Disease Prevention and Control Act, 2004).

However, not all states have passed laws that specifically make infecting others with HIV a crime. Instead, many states utilize existing, general laws, such as assault and attempted murder, to prosecute offenders (Wolf & Venzia, 2004). In 2010, for example, the State of Texas tried a man for aggravated assault with a deadly weapon, i.e., his penis, and aggravated assault after he raped one woman and transmitted the virus to another woman through uninformed, consensual sex (Emily, 2010).

Additionally, the states' laws vary with regard to the severity of charges. The charges can range from misdemeanors to serious felonies that carry significant prison sentences. Often, the severity of the charge may depend on the type of exposure. In Georgia, a person can be charged with a misdemeanor if he or she causes bodily harm to, or endangers the bodily safety of, another person "by consciously disregarding a substantial and unjustifiable risk that his act or omission will cause harm or endanger the safety" of another and the disregard "constitutes a gross deviation from the standard of care which a reasonable person would exercise in the situation" (Criminal Code of Georgia, 2003). However, if the individual knowingly engages in sexual acts, shares hypodermic needles/syringes, or donates blood, blood products, bodily fluids, or body parts, he or she can be charged with a felony and sentenced to up to 10 years in prison (Criminal Code of Georgia, 2003).

The criminalization of HIV exposure and/or transmission typically focuses on intentional and reckless actions. The intentional transmission of HIV involves the deliberate or willful transmission of the virus. Examples include a medical technician in Missouri who, in 1998, deliberately injected his son with HIV infected blood and received a sentence of life in prison (Usborne, 1989). Similarly, in 2009, Dennis Rios was charged in California for intentionally infecting women with HIV through uninformed, sexual activity (McMillan, 2009).

Reckless exposure, on the other hand, occurs when there is exposure or the virus is transmitted through carelessness rather than an intent to do so (AVERT, n.d.). By way of illustration, in 2011, a Missouri man was convicted of four counts of reckless exposure to HIV and sentenced to 30 years in prison after failing to disclose his HIV status to his sexual partner and infecting her with the virus (O'Connell, 2009).

In addition to criminalizing the above mentioned activities, the biting of an individual by an HIV-infected person is another act that has been made a crime. In May 2011, a Florida male was charged with criminal transmission of HIV for trying to bite a police officer (Alvarez, 2011). Likewise, an HIV positive Oklahoma man and Missouri woman were criminally charged after biting a police officer in 2011 (Anon, 2011; Grummer, 2011).

Preventive measures and disclosure are the only real defenses to these types of crimes. However, only a small minority of states take preventive measures into account in their statutes (Wolf & Venzia, 2004). California, for example, has limited the scope of its statute to sexual acts without a condom (Communicable Disease Prevention and Control Act, 2004). The Missouri statute, on the other hand, states that the use of a condom is not a defense (Health & Welfare, AIDS, 2002).

Disclosure appears to be the best defense. Ten of the states that criminalize intentional HIV exposure through sexual activity list the failure to disclose as an element of the crime and, therefore, a requirement for a successful prosecution (Wolf & Venzia, 2004). Other states permit consent to be put forth as an affirmative defense if the victim knew the accused had HIV and the activity could result in the transmission of HIV (Wolf & Venzia, 2004). Finally, some states fail to mention consent at all, leaving the possibility of prosecution either way (Wolf & Venzia, 2004).

Civil Ramifications of Contact with Others Without Disclosing HIV Positive Status

In addition to the criminal ramifications possible for failing to disclose one's HIV status when engaging with others in contact that could expose them to virus, there can also be civil liability. Regardless of whether a criminal prosecution of the offender is successful, the party exposed to HIV can file civil claims against the offender and seek monetary compensation. As the estimated lifetime cost of treating HIV is approximately $355,000, a person infected with the virus suffers a large monetary loss. Thus, the civil court system can be used to attempt to recover some of the cost of the medical care that may be needed in the future (Schackman et al., 2006). It should be noted that the realization of a civil recovery is restricted by the defendant's finances and the limits of any available insurance policy.

There is no one specific type of civil claim that must be filed against the offender. Rather, the affected party has the typical claims available under tort law and, over the years, there have been a wide variety of claims in different jurisdictions for different tortuous offenses. The examples outlined below are in no way exhaustive of the types of civil claims that can be filed against an individual who exposes another to the HIV virus.

Infliction of Emotional Distress. Emotional distress occurs when someone experiences mental, emotional, or psychological pain. When the emotional distress is the result of the act of another, the victim may have a civil cause of action against the perpetrator. Two tortious actions potentially available are the intentional infliction of emotional distress (IIED) and the negligent infliction of emotional distress (NIED).

IIED allows for recovery of damages from the development of emotional distress when the wrongful act was intentional and a physical injury occurred (*Restatement (Second) of Tort*, 1977). It must be shown that the act was intentional, and the acting party intended to inflict harm or distress (*Restatement (Second) of Tort*, 1977). It is not enough to claim only mental distress; an actual physical injury must have resulted from the wrongful act (*Restatement (Second) of Tort*, 1977). The physical injury need not be significant, but there must be some physical manifestation of injury. This can be a difficult burden to prove, as some individuals can suffer from mental distress but never manifest physical injury. In fact, many IIED claims fail because of this requirement.

NIED is similar to IIED, but lacks the element of intent. Instead of showing intent, the claimant may only need to show, for example, that he or she suffered emotional distress through the other party's carelessness. In some jurisdictions, a plaintiff may have a cause of action for negligent infliction of emotional distress despite the absence of physical injury (Maroulis, 1993). In such cases the claimant must prove that the defendant breached some duty of care owed to the claimant and, as a result, the claimant suffered severe emotional distress (Maroulis, 1993).

IIED claims often involve claimants who have sued after engaging in sexual intercourse with HIV positive partners and the courts have addressed them in varying ways. Consider the case of *In re Louie* (1997). In that case, the plaintiff and the defendant were in a long-term relationship and agreed to live together as a married couple (*In re Louie*, 1997). The defendant was HIV-positive and failed to disclose that to the plaintiff (*In re Louie*, 1997). The plaintiff later discovered the defendant's HIV status and terminated the relationship (*In re Louie*, 1997). The plaintiff then sued for various torts including unwanted sexual touching and IIED (*In re Louie*, 1997). The plaintiff's IIED claim ultimately failed because he tested negative for HIV six months after exposure (*In re Louie*, 1997). The court found that the plaintiff had no damages, but the decision suggested that the plaintiff could have proceeded with the IIED claim if the test for HIV had been positive (*In re Louie*, 1997).

In contrast, the court in *J.B v. Antoinette Bohonovsky* (1993) did not share the *Louie* court's analysis for IIED. In *J.B. v. Bohonovsky* (1993), the plaintiff alleged IIED after he discovered his prior sexual partner, who was deceased at the time of the lawsuit, was HIV positive (*J.B. v. Bohonovsky*, 1993). The plaintiff did not contract HIV (*J.B. v. Bohonovsky*, 1993). In this case, the Court did not appear to focus on the plaintiff's negative HIV status (*J.B. v. Bohonovsky*, 1993). Instead, the Court found the plaintiff had to prove that his distress was so severe that no reasonable person could endure it (*J.B. v. Bohonovsky*, 1993). The Court found that the plaintiff did not do so and dismissed the case (*J.B. v. Bohonovsky*, 1993).

There are very few IIED cases that have been successful. Aetna v. Sheft (1993) is one of the few cases where the claimant (plaintiff) prevailed. In Aetna v. Sheft (1993), Marc Sheft filed an IIED claim against the estate of celebrity Rock Hudson. Mr. Sheft alleged he suffered IIED once he discovered Mr. Hudson was HIV-positive (Aetna v. Sheft, 1993). Although Mr. Sheft never contracted HIV, a jury awarded him damages based upon his distress and fear of contracting HIV over an eight month period (Aetna v. Sheft, 1993).

If one is unaware of his or her HIV status, an argument can be made that there was not an intentional transmission of the virus to another person. This could be a viable defense under the IIED theory. However, a court could still find a viable NIED claim.

This was recognized in John B. v. Superior Court (2006). In that case, a wife, after that discovering her husband was HIV positive, sued him for IIED and NEID (John B. v. Superior Court, 2006). The court permitted discovery that was intended to determine whether the husband knew, or had reason to know, of his HIV status while engaging in sexual relations with his wife (John B. v. Superior Court, 2006). Thus, the wife was allowed to try and determine if her husband should have known of his HIV status and was, therefore, negligent (John B. v. Superior Court, 2006).

Like IIED, the courts' treatment of claims for the NIED vary. In *Heiner v. Moretuzzo* (1995), the Ohio Supreme Court held that a claim for NIED would fail if the distress is caused by a nonexistent physical peril (*Heiner v. Moretuzzo*, 1995). In that case, the plaintiff was misdiagnosed as having HIV (*Heiner v. Moretuzzo*, 1995). As the plaintiff did not, indeed, have HIV, the Court found no physical peril and did not permit any recovery for the NIED (*Heiner v. Moretuzzo*, 1995).

A different result was reached in *Brown v. New York City Health and Hospitals Corp.* (1996). In *Brown v. New York City Health and Hospitals Corp.*, a nurse sued for NIED after being stuck with a hypodermic needle that was left in the crib of an HIV-positive infant. In analyzing the cause of action, the Court held that the plaintiff could proceed even in the absence of a physical injury if a duty was owed and breached (*Brown v. New York City Health and Hospitals Corp.*, 1996). However, the Court recognized that the circumstances under which one could recover for purely emotional harm are extremely limited and must generally be premised upon a breach of a duty owed directly to the plaintiff that either endangered his or her physical safety or caused fear for his or her physical safety (*Brown v. New York City Health and Hospitals Corp.*, 1996). In NIED cases involving HIV/AIDS, the Court found that plaintiffs who have not tested positive must offer proof of actual exposure (*Brown v. New York City Health and Hospitals Corp.*, 1996). Actual exposure was defined as proof of both a scientifically accepted method of transmission and that the source of the allegedly transmitted blood/fluid was HIV-positive (*Brown v. New York City Health and Hospitals Corp.*, 1996). Finally, the Court imposed a limitation on the plaintiff's ability to recover if, after 6 months, he or she tested HIV-negative (*Brown v. New York City Health and Hospitals Corp.*, 1996). Under such circumstances, the Court appeared to limit damages to the first six months, finding that a plaintiff's initial, reasonable fear of contracting HIV/AIDS becomes unreasonable after he or she continues to test negative for HIV antibodies six months after the exposure (*Brown v. New York City Health and Hospitals Corp.*, 1996).

The courts' treatment of claims for HIV exposure brought under either theory of emotional distress is far from settled. The requirements and treatment of such cases will vary from state to state and, at times, from jurisdiction to jurisdiction within a state. For example, the treatment of such cases may differ between state courts in New York and state courts in Ohio, and may even differ between state courts in northern Ohio and the southern part of the same state. The analysis employed by the courts is extremely fact specific and, as a result, the outcome will differ from case to case. Undoubtedly, plaintiffs who test HIV positive appear to have more success with emotional distress claims.

In general mental health professionals may want to advise their clients that disclosure of their HIV-positive status to a prospective sexual partner before-the-fact can be both a preventive measure and the best defense to claims of IIED and

NIED. Ultimately, regardless of whether an IIED or NIED claim would be viable, individuals with HIV/AIDS should be aware of the causes of action that are available and that have been litigated. And, even if the plaintiff's claim against the HIV-infected person fails, the defendant is forced to expend time, money, and energy to defend against the claim.

Battery. The tort of battery describes an intentional, unwanted or offensive touching of another person without permission that results in physical or emotional harm (American Jurisprudence, n.d.). The exact definition of battery and what must be proven will vary from state to state. However, as no physical harm is required, battery claims can be successful where IIED claims fail.

The transmission of HIV may constitute an intentional tort and lead to the recovery of damages (Maroulis, 1993). In cases where there was only a fear of transmission, a claim for battery may be pursued when there was a deliberate attempt to infect another with the virus or an individual engages in sexual relations without disclosing his or her HIV status (Maroulis, 1993).

The key element in battery cases involving exposure to HIV is the element of intent. Courts seem to focus on whether the offender knew about the HIV status when the contact occurred. For example, in *In re Louie*, the plaintiff's civil claim for unwanted sexual touching/sexual battery was viable (*In re Louie*, 1997). The Court held that, although the sexual conduct was consensual at the time, the subsequent revelation that the defendant had HIV and the plaintiff may have been infected by HIV was enough to reasonably cause emotional distress (*In re Louie*, 1997).

Significantly, this case suggests that someone could pursue a sexual battery tort claim, at least in California, against an individual with HIV even if the virus was not transmitted. It is surprising, then, there have not been a larger number of tortuous battery claims filed against HIV positive sexual partners. However, given the possibility of recovery regardless of transmission, claimants may utilize this cause of action more in the future. Again, it is important that mental health care providers advise their clients of the potential consequences if they fail to inform a sexual partner of their HIV status.

Conclusion

Despite medical advances, the unfortunate reality is that individuals with HIV/AIDS often face medical complications, illness, and premature death. Further, fear of discrimination, stigma, rejection, and social isolation results in a reluctance to be tested for HIV and to disclose an HIV-positive status. The reluctance to be tested leads to a higher early death rate. The reluctance to disclose one's HIV status increases the transmission rate of the virus.

To protect themselves and their dependents, loved ones, and estates, individuals with HIV should explore and utilize the legal mechanisms available to them. Such individuals should also be aware of the legal protections afforded to them through state and federal legislation. Likewise, individuals with HIV/AIDS should be aware of the criminal and civil ramifications of exposing others to the virus, especially without disclosure beforehand. An awareness of legal rights and obligations will help ensure that individuals with HIV/AIDS are able to pursue their livelihoods and the best quality of life possible without legal ramifications.

Related Topics: Confidentiality laws, contact tracing, disability laws, disclosure, disclosure laws, discrimination, partner notification, Ryan White Health Care Act.

References

6 American Jurisprudence, 2d. (1963, Suppl. 1983). *Assault and battery, Section 3.*

ADA Amendments Act of 2008 (2008, September 25). Pub. L. No. 110–32.

Aetna v. Sheft, 989 F.2d 1105. (9th Dist. 1993).

Aggleton, P., Wood, K., Malcolm, A., Parker, R., & UNAIDS. (2005). *HIV-related stigma, discrimination and human rights violations: Case studies of successful programmes*. Geneva, Switzerland: Joint United Nations Programme on HIV/AIDS (UNAIDS). Retrieved October 30, 2011 from http://data.unaids.org/publications/irc-pub06/jc999-humrightsviol_en.pdf

Alvarez, D. (2011). BSO accused man with HIV of trying to bite deputy. *Sun Sentinel*. Retrieved October 30, 2011 from http://articles.sun-sentinel.com/2011-05-31/health/fl-home-depot-hiv-20110531_1_hiv-bso-deputy

Americans with Disabilities Act of 1990, 42 U.S.C. §§ 12101–12300 (1990).

American Psychiatric Association. (2000). *Diagnostic and statistical manual, fourth edition, text revision*. Washington, DC: Author.

Analysis and guidelines—AIDS. (2011). *Workers' compensation guide* § 4:77.

Anon. (2011). *Man with HIV charged with biting O'Fallon police officer*. Retrieved October 30, 2011 from http://www.kmov.com/news/local/Man-with-HIV-charged-with-biting-OFallon-Missouri-police-officer-117739179.html

AVERT. (n.d.). *Criminal transmission of HIV*. Retrieved October 30, 2011 from http://www.avert.org/criminal-transmission.htm

Bragdon v. Abbott (1998). 524 U.S. 624.

Brown v. New York City Health and Hospitals Corp., 225 A.D.2d 36. (N.Y. 1996).

Buchanan, R., & Hatcher, W. (2007). Compassionate conservatism: Federal funding for the Ryan White CARE Act during the Bush administration. *American Journal of Public Health, 97*(11), 2013–2016.

Centers for Disease Control and Prevention. (2011). *Diagnoses of HIV infection and AIDS in the United States and dependent areas, 2009*. Retrieved October 30, 2011 from http://www.cdc.gov/hiv/surveillance/resources/reports/2009report/index.htm

Centers for Disease Control and Prevention. (2010). *HIV transmission*. Retrieved October 30, 2011 from http://www.cdc.gov/hiv/resources/qa/transmission.htm

Centers for Disease Control and Prevention. (2011). *Morbidity and Mortality Weekly Report, HIV Surveillance—United States, 1981–2008*, 60(21) 689–693. Retrieved October 30, 2011 from http://www.cdc.gov/mmwr/preview/mmwrhtml/mm6021a2.htm

Centers for Disease Control and Prevention. (2011). *Occupational HIV transmission and prevention among health care workers*. Retrieved October 30, 2011 from http://www.cdc.gov/hiv/resources/factsheets/hcwprev.htm

Communicable Disease Prevention and Control Act, California Health & Safety Code Annotated § 120291 (2004).

Criminal Code of Georgia, Georgia Code § 16-5-60 (2003).

Cross, J., Palmer, N., & Smith, C. (2009). Families redefined: Kinship groups that deserve benefits. *Mississippi Law Journal, 79*, 791–831.

Ebeling, A. (2010). Americans lack basic estate plans. *Forbes*. Retrieved October 30, 2011 from http://www.forbes.com/2010/03/01/estate-tax-living-will-schiavo-personal-finance-no-estate-plans.html?boxes=Homepagechannels

Emily, J. (2010). HIV carrier who endangered women pleads guilty in the midst of trial. *Dallas Morning News*. Retrieved October 30, 2011 from http://www.dallasnews.com/news/community-news/dallas/headlines/20100716-hiv-carrier-who-endangered-women-pleads-guilty-in-midst-of-trial.ece

Equal Employment Opportunity Commission. (2008). *The ADA: Your responsibilities as an employer*. Retrieved October 30, 2011 from http://www.eeoc.gov/facts/ada17.html

Equal Employment Opportunity Commission. (1997). *EEOC Enforcement Guidance on the Americans with Disabilities Act and Psychiatric Disabilities*. Retrieved December 13, 2011 from http://www.eeoc.gov/policy/docs/psych.html

Equal Employment Opportunity Commission's Americans With Disability Act Employment Regulations, 29 Code of Federal Regulations § 1630.2(h)(2) (1996).

Estate of Mauro v. Borgess Medical Center (1998). 137 F.3d, 398.

Goffe, W. (2009). *Estate planning for the unmarried adult*. Retrieved October 30, 2011 from http://www.cepcweb.org/Chicago-IL/Library/Speaker%20Outline%20-%20Goffe%20April%2023.pdf

Goldfein, R., & Schalman-Bergen, S. (2010a). Preparation for illness, incapacity, and death—Health, funeral, and estate planning. Additional considerations for parents. *Sexual Orientation & the Law*, *2*, § 15:19.

Goldfein, R., & Schalman-Bergen, S. (2010b). Preparation for illness, incapacity, and death—Health, funeral, and estate planning. Critical documents-Nomination of a guardian or conservator. *Sexual Orientation & the Law, 2*, § 15:12.

Goldfein, R., & Schalman-Bergen, S. (2010c). Preparation for illness, incapacity, and death—Health, funeral, and estate planning. Health, financial, and estate planning. *Sexual Orientation & the Law*, *2*, § 15:9.

Grummer, J. (2011). HIV-positive inmate accused of biting jailer. *The Times Record*. Retrieved October 30, 2011 from http://www.swtimes.com/news/article_976c2328-7266-11e0-9ec0-001cc4c03286.html

Guardianship-Conservatorship Law, California Probate Code §§ 2350–2410 (2008).

Guardianships and Conservatorships, Wisconsin Statures Ch. 54 (2005).

Hankins v. The Gap Inc. (1996). 84 F.3d, 797.

Herek, G. (1999). AIDS & stigma. *American Behavioral Scientist, 42*(7), 1106–1116.

Health & Welfare, AIDS, Revised Statutes of Missouri. §191.677 (2002).

Health Resources and Services Administration HIV/AIDS Programs. (n.d.a). *A living history—Part F: A diverse portfolio for an evolving epidemic*. Retrieved October 30, 2011 from http://hab.hrsa.gov/livinghistory/programs/Part-F.htm

Health Resources and Services Administration HIV/AIDS Programs. (n.d.b). *About Ryan White*. Retrieved October 30, 2011 from http://hab.hrsa.gov/abouthab/ryanwhite.html

Health Resources and Services Administration HIV/AIDS Programs. (n.d.c). *Legislation*. Retrieved October 30, 2011 from http://hab.hrsa.gov/abouthab/legislation.html

Health Resources and Services Administration HIV/AIDS Programs. (n.d.d). *Part A—Grants to emerging metropolitan & transitional areas*. Retrieved October 30, 2011 from http://hab.hrsa.gov/abouthab/parta.html

Health Resources and Services Administration HIV/AIDS Programs. (n.d.e). *Part B—AIDS Drug Assistance Program*. Retrieved October 30, 2011 from http://hab.hrsa.gov/abouthab/partbdrug.html

Health Resources and Services Administration HIV/AIDS Programs. (n.d.f). *Part C*. Retrieved October 30, 2011 from http://hab.hrsa.gov/abouthab/partc.html

Health Resources and Services Administration HIV/AIDS Programs. (n.d.g). *Part D—Services for women, infants, children, youth & their families*. Retrieved October 30, 2011 from http://hab.hrsa.gov/abouthab/partd.html

Heiner v. Moretuzzo, 652 N.E.2d 664 (Ohio 1995).

The Henry J. Kaiser Family Foundation. (2011). *HIV/AIDS policy, fact sheet: The HIVAIDS epidemic in the United States*. Retrieved October 30, 2011 from http://www.kff.org/hivaids/upload/3029-12.pdf

The Henry J. Kaiser Family Foundation. (2006). *HIV/AIDS policy, fact sheet: Ryan White Comprehensive AIDS Resources Emergency Act*. Retrieved October 30, 2011 from http://www.kff.org/hivaids/upload/7582s.pdf

Hickey, M. (2009). Estate planning for cohabitants. *Journal of the American Academy of Matrimonial Law, 22*, 1–28.

House Report No. 101–485, pt. 2, 101st Cong., 2nd Sess. 52 (1990).

Horgan v. Simmons (N.D. Ill. 2010). 704 F. Supp. 2d, 814.

Illinois Living Will Act, 755 Illinois Complied Statutes 35/2(h) (1988).

Illinois Probate Act of 1975, 755 Illinois Complied Statutes 5/11-5/30-3 (1979).

In re Louie, 213 B.R. 754 (N.D. Cal. 1997).

J.B v. Antoinette Bohonovsky, 835 F.Supp.796 (D. N.J. 1993) *John B. v. Superior Court*, 137 P.3d 153 (Cal. 2006).

Kentucky Living Will Directive Act of 1994, Kentucky Revised Statutes 311.623 (2010).

Knauer, N. (2010). Gay and lesbian elders: Estate planning and end-of-life decision making. *Florida Costal Law Review, 12*, 163–213.

Kreider, R.M. (2010). Housing and Household Economics Statistics Division working paper: Increase in opposite-sex cohabiting couple from 2009 to 2010 in the Annual Social and Economic Supplement (ASRC) to the Current Population Survey (CPS). Washington, DC: United States Bureau of the Census. http://www.census.gov/population/www/socdemo/Inc-Opp-swx-2009-to-2010.pdf. Accessed 12 Oct 2012.

Legal Information Institute. (2010). *Guardian*. Retrieved October 30, 2011 from http://www.law.cornell.edu/wex/guardian

Lofquist, D. (2011). American Community Survey Briefs: Same-sex couple households [ACSBR/10-03]. Washington, DC: United States Bureau of the Census. http://www.census.gov/prod/2011pubs/acsbr10-03.pdf. Accessed 11 Oct 2012.

Maroulis, J. (1993). Can HIV-negative plaintiffs recover emotional distress damages or their fear of AIDS? *Fordham Law Review, 62*(1), 225–263.

McMillan, R. (2009). Man intentionally infects women with HIV. *Inland Empire News*. Retrieved October 30, 2011 from http://abclocal.go.com/kabc/story?section=news/local/inland_empire&id=7006846

Nondiscrimination on the Basis of Disability by Public Accommodations, 28 Code of Federal Regulations § 36.104(1)(iii) (2010).

Nondiscrimination on the Basis of Disability in State and Local, 28 Code of Federal Regulations § 35.140(b)(1) (2010).

O'Connell, P. (2009). Northwoods man charged in HIV case. *Stltoday.com*. Retrieved October 30, 2011 from http://www.stltoday.com/news/local/crime-and-courts/article_939b9889-f8fb-5cfd-9004-430cca57ebfd.html

Office of Legal Counsel, Equal Employment Opportunity Commission, ADA Division. (2002). *EEOC enforcement guidance* (No. 915.002). Retrieved October 30, 2011 from http://www.eeoc.gov/policy/docs/accommodation.html#index

Publisher's Editorial Staff. (2011). AIDS under the ADA-AIDS as a disability. *Corporate Counsel's Guide to Americans with Disabilities Act*, 1 §4.

Regulations to Implement the Equal Employment Provisions of the Americans with Disabilities Act, 29 Code of Federal Regulations §1630.2 (2010).

Restatement of Torts (Second): Intentional Infliction of Emotional Distress (Outrage), § 46(1) (1977).

Ryan White Comprehensive AIDS Resources Emergency Act of 1990, 42 U.S.C. §§ 300Ff-300Ff-140. (1990).

Schackman, B. R., Gebo, K. A., Walensky, R. P., et al. (2006). The lifetime cost of current human immunodeficiency virus care in the United States. *Medical Care, 44*(11), 990–997.

School Board of Nassau County v. Arline (1987). 480 U.S. 273.

Senate Report No. 116, 101st Cong., 1st Sess. 22 (1989).

Stolarsky, M. (2009). Advanced directives in same-sex relationships. *Ohio Probate Law Journal, 19*, 132–141.

Terrence Higgins Trust, Policy Campaigns & Research Division. (2001). *Prejudice, discrimination, & HIV: A report.* Retrieved October 30, 2011 from http://www.tht.org.uk/information-resources/publications/policyreports/prejudicereport581.pdf

UNAIDS. (2010). *Global report, UNAIDS report on the global AIDS epidemic 2010.* Geneva, Switzerland: Joint United Nations Programme on HIV/AIDS (UNAIDS). Retrieved October 30, 2011 from http://www.unaids.org/globalreport/documents/20101123_GlobalReport_full_en.pdf

United States Department of Justice, Civil Rights Division, Disability Rights Section. (2002). *Questions and answers: The Americans with Disabilities Act and persons with HIV/AIDS.* Retrieved October 30, 2011 from http://www.ada.gov/pubs/hivqanda.txt

United States Department of Justice. (2012). Questions and answers: The Americans with Disabilities Act and persons with HIV/AIDS. Washington, DC: Author. http://www.ada.gov/aids/ada_q&a_aids.pdf. Accessed 11 Oct 2012.

Usborne, D. (1998). Man injected son with AIDS blood. The Independent, Dec. 7. http://www.independent.co.uk/news/man-injected-son-with-aids-blood-1189843.html. Accessed 11 Oct 2012.

Washington Trust Act of 1984, Revised Code of Washington Ann., Chapter *11.88 et seq.* (2008).

Wolf, L., & Venzia, R. (2004). Crime and punishment: Is there a role for criminal law in HIV prevention policy? *Whittier Law Review, 25*, 826–827. Retrieved October 30, 2011 from http://ari.ucsf.edu/programs/policy/crime_and_punishment.pdf.

World Health Organization. (2009). *AIDS epidemic update.* Retrieved October 30, 2011 from http://www.unaids.org/en/media/unaids/contentassets/dataimport/pub/report/2009/jc1700_epi_uupdat_2009_en.pdf

Access to Care

Daniel J. O'Shea

An International Perspective

At the beginning of the fourth decade of the epidemic, HIV continues to remain a complex global public health challenge, with universal access to HIV prevention, treatment, care and support an elusive target. In 2009, the Joint United Nations Programme on HIV/AIDS (UNAIDS) reported 33.3 million people living with HIV (PLWH) worldwide, including 2.6 million newly infected with HIV; in the same year 1.8 million people died of AIDS. Before the development of effective antiretroviral therapies (ART) beginning in the mid-to-late 1990s, PLWH could progress to AIDS and even death in just a few years. Currently, people can live much longer—even decades—with HIV before they develop AIDS if they have access to appropriate medications and care. ART has continued to evolve at a breathtaking speed, as new medications are developed and additional data from clinical trials are presented. Even so, efforts to address the epidemic through access to care have historically been challenged by the availability and cost of treatment, clinical challenges of the disease itself and its toll on the health and well-being of those infected, and the many social/psychosocial issues linked with the communities that it has heavily impacted, all affecting access to and retention in care. While ART can dramatically improve the health of PLWH and slow progression from HIV infection to AIDS, existing treatments may need to be taken daily for the rest of a person's life, need to be carefully monitored, and come with potential side effects.

Since the mid-to-late 1990s, ART has been readily accessible in the developed, high-income countries (USA, Canada, Western and Central Europe, and Australia), resulting in dramatic declines in AIDS diagnoses (end stage of HIV disease) and deaths. On the other hand, for the majority of PLWH in the developing world (two-thirds of PLWH are in sub-Saharan Africa, followed by 14% in East, South and

D.J. O'Shea (✉)
Public Health Service, County of San Diego, San Diego, CA, USA
e-mail: Dan.OShea@sdcounty.ca.gov

S. Loue (ed.), *Mental Health Practitioner's Guide to HIV/AIDS*,
DOI 10.1007/978-1-4614-5283-6_4, © Springer Science+Business Media New York 2013

Southeast Asia), ART was historically unavailable, primarily due to very high drug prices sustained by international patents. In 2001, the tide began to turn as special terms in international trade law allowed drug manufacturers in developing countries to produce generic drugs at vastly reduced prices, and several countries passed bills to legally purchase generic drugs from abroad. These efforts paved the way for expansion of HIV treatment on a global scale. The Medicines Patent Pool, set up in July 2008 by the global health financing mechanism UNITAID, increased access to newer antiretroviral medicines by creating a pool of patents and intelligence on ART production and by promoting price reductions of existing antiretroviral drugs, stimulating the production of newer first- and second-line drugs and increasing the number of generic producers of these medicines. In September 2010, the US National Institutes of Health became the first patent holder to share intellectual property on ART with the pool.

Through these international efforts, by 2010 UNAIDS reported some success in halting and even reversing the spread of HIV with significantly improved access to ART. In 2009, of the estimated 15 million PLWH in low- and middle-income countries *in need of treatment* (with CD4 cell count <350 cells/mm^3), 36% (approximately 5.2 million) received ART. This represented a 30% overall increase over 2008 and a 13-fold increase since 2004. By geographic region, this encompassed 37% of PLWH *in need of treatment* in sub-Saharan Africa receiving ART, 42% in Central and South America, 51% in Oceania (Australia, New Zealand, Micronesia, Melanesia and Polynesia), 48% in the Caribbean, and 19% in Eastern Europe and Central Asia. Eight countries—Botswana, Cambodia, Croatia, Cuba, Guyana, Namibia, Romania, and Rwanda—achieved ART coverage of 80% or more. Expanded access to treatment contributed to a 19% decline in deaths among PLWH between 2004 and 2009, with an estimated 14.4 million life-years gained by providing ART since 1996. The number of health facilities delivering ART increased by 36% in 2009, averaging 274 individuals receiving ART per facility in 2009, up from 260 in 2008, according to data submitted by 99 countries.

While significant, progress remains fragile and dependent on continuing joint international support and funding. Although more people are receiving ART in all regions of the world than at any previous time in the epidemic, progress remains mixed, with inequitable coverage and substantially greater gains in some settings and on certain aspects of treatment, care, and support than in others. Progress in scaling up tuberculosis (TB) services for PLWH is very slow and the availability of palliative and home-based care services for PLWH remains uneven. Children and marginalized populations at higher risk are less likely to receive ART than the population at large. Few data are available regarding access to care by sex workers, men who have sex with men, and injection drug users. Most countries do not collect data on these groups, and some report that health care workers' negative attitudes deter people at high risk of HIV infection from seeking treatment. Many countries limit access to ART by incarcerating PLWH or PLWH who inject drugs. Laws in some countries with sizeable immigrant populations may also limit ART access to legal citizens only.

Despite a modest decline in HIV prevalence among adults worldwide and increasing access to ART, there has not been a decline in the number of children (0–17 years of age) orphaned by HIV/AIDS. That number actually increased from 14.6 million in 2005 to 16.6 million in 2009, with almost 90% living in sub-Saharan Africa. In contrast, one of the most remarkable contributions to the global response to HIV is the formal and informal systems and networks established to support children orphaned by the epidemic. As a result, orphaned children are nearly as likely to attend school as other children.

In 2010, the World Health Organization (WHO) issued revised HIV treatment guidelines, which included the following elements: (1) *start antiretroviral therapy earlier* at CD4 cell counts <350 cells/mm^3; (2) *use less toxic and more patient-friendly options*, thereby reducing the risk of adverse events and improving adherence by using less toxic drugs and fixed-dose ART combinations; (3) *improve management of coinfections between HIV and TB or hepatitis B*, initiating ART in all PLWH with active TB and chronic active hepatitis B disease regardless of CD4 cell count; and (4) *promote strategic use of laboratory monitoring* such as CD4 and viral load counts to improve the efficiency and quality of HIV treatment and care.

While recognizing a major worldwide public health achievement with 5.2 million PLWH in low- to middle-income countries receiving treatment in 2009, reaching the remaining two thirds of people who need but are not accessing care, and financing the cost of this expanded HIV therapy, will require a sustained global commitment. In response, in 2010 UNAIDS outlined "Treatment 2.0," a comprehensive approach to simplify and improve access to HIV treatment, reduce treatment costs and the burden on health systems, and improve the quality of life for PLWH and their families. The ultimate goals are to decrease deaths from AIDS by ten million by 2025 and reduce new infections by up to one million annually if countries provide ART to everyone who needs it according to the 2010 WHO treatment guidelines. Treatment 2.0 necessitates advances in five areas: 1. *Optimize drug regimens*: develop less toxic, longer-acting and easier to use pharmaceuticals, combined with dose optimization and improved sequencing of first and second line regimens to simplify treatment protocols and improve effectiveness. 2. *Provide access to point of care diagnostics*: simplify diagnostic tools to provide viral load and CD4 cell counts at the point of care to reduce the burden and cost on health systems and increase PLWH access to treatment. 3. *Reduce costs*: drugs, inclusive of first and second line regimen, must continue to become more affordable, along with reducing the non-drug-related treatment costs (such as hospitalization, monitoring treatment, and out-of-pocket expenses), currently twice the cost of the drugs themselves. 4. *Adapt delivery systems*: further decentralize and integrate service delivery systems, reducing repetition and complexity, and facilitating a more effective continuum of care which includes taskshifting and strengthening procurement and supply systems. 5. *Mobilize communities*: involve the community in managing treatment programs to strengthen the demand and uptake for testing; improve treatment access, adherence and coverage; and reduce the burden on health systems and costs for extensive outreach.

Poverty, inequities in gender, health and socio-economic status, discrimination against marginalized groups, and unequal resource pathways all impact access to care. In addition to thereby addressing underlying societal structures, beliefs and value systems, ensuring global access to HIV care will also require widespread awareness of the value of testing and subsequent treatment; life-long commitment to ART and supporting PLWH to adhere to a daily regimen; adequate health infrastructure and staff; and supply chains of effective drugs.

Having faced an evolving and seemingly unstoppable epidemic over the course of three decades, the subsequent experience, scientific and social knowledge and resources available today demonstrate that investments in the HIV response can deliver the treatment, care, and support required to extend and improve the lives of PLWH worldwide. Sustaining and expanding upon these efforts and best practices could ultimately make real the vision of eliminating the toll that HIV imposes on human life. As a radically simplified treatment platform, Treatment 2.0 supports the promise to achieve that goal.

Access to Care in the USA

According to 2010 US Census Bureau data, 16.3% (49.9 million) of Americans are uninsured; 15.9% (48.6 million) of Americans are covered by Medicaid, the federal-state program that provides health care benefits to people with low income or disabilities, and 14.5% (44.3 million) by Medicare, the federal program for seniors and people with disabilities. Overall rates for uninsured vary significantly in the USA by race/ethnicity: 20.8% of African Americans/Blacks and 30.7% of Latinos/Hispanics are uninsured compared with 11.7% of non-Hispanic Whites/Caucasians. Without adequate healthcare coverage, many will not access care until absolutely necessary, when very sick, at clinics or emergency departments. Within this context, access to care for US PLWH is even more limited. According to the US Department of Health and Human Services, fewer than one in five (13%) PLWH have private insurance and nearly 24% have no coverage. Medicaid, Medicare and the Ryan White Program, a federal assistance program for PLWH without any other or enough coverage or financial means, are major resources for healthcare for PLWH. Under the Ryan White model of care, PLWH receive a variety of medical and nonmedical support services; this integrated delivery system has been recommended by the Institute of Medicine as a model for future care. Ryan White also finances the AIDS Drug Assistance Program for PLWH who cannot afford ART and other medications to treat AIDS-related diseases and conditions. Increased opportunities for health care coverage are expected as implementation of the Affordable Care Act moves forward.

Substantial numbers of US PLWH have never received HIV medical care despite availability, benefits and substantial outreach efforts. While improved over time, disparities in access continue among PLWH. Not surprisingly, individuals of lower socioeconomic status and/or who belong to groups historically disenfranchised from care (such as people of color and women) access care in lower proportions. Although there is no population-based system to estimate the number of people who have never received HIV care or to monitor the reasons that care is delayed, a CDC pilot study in five states and local health department jurisdictions from September 2005 through September 2010 indicates that 20–25% of people reported as HIV-infected three to 15 months previously never received HIV medical care; those not in care were more likely to be younger, African American, and Latino/Hispanic than those diagnosed in the same period who were documented as having received care. These demographics clearly mirror the census data for uninsured. Data from San Diego County needs assessments of both providers and PLWH who were not using HIV primary care or who have ever been out of care indicate the following barriers to accessing HIV care: self-assessment of good health status ("feel/felt healthy"), *substance use/abuse*, *mental health issues*, unwillingness to deal with HIV status, socioeconomic instability, side effects of medications, stigma, homelessness and not knowing where to find services. Change in health status (onset of illness or symptoms), case management, access to mental health services, substance abuse detoxification and treatment, housing, transportation services, and one-stop coordinated services centers were identified as strong motivators to get and keep PLWH/A in HIV primary care.

Through efforts and federal funding in alignment with a new National HIV/AIDS Strategy, more PLWH continue to be identified and provided the care they need. Although improved access increases costs in the short run, savings are achieved in the long run by avoiding hospitalizations and emergency department visits, by preventing complications, and by reducing lost productivity due to HIV-related disabilities. The challenge remains to reduce or eliminate existing barriers, address any new barriers, and create a system capable of meeting the needs of all PLWH.

Mental health care providers should assess the ability of their HIV positive clients to access medically appropriate HIV care and medications and be aware of available treatment options and resources, including Ryan White, if the client has no or limited insurance coverage. Providers should be particularly aware of challenges for HIV-positive people of color, women and/or those of lower socioeconomic status. Ideally, linkages or collaborative relationships should be established with HIV primary care and HIV case management (assists clients to access HIV care and other needed services) providers for mutual client referral to ensure integration of services and better client care. Mental health providers should also be aware of potential interaction between psychiatric and HIV medications, and, as needed, consult with an HIV specialist.

Related Topics: AIDS service organizations, antiretroviral therapy, case management, Medicaid, Medicare, prevention strategies, protease inhibitors, Ryan White Care Act, stigma and stigmatization.

Suggested Reading

Fagan, J., Bertolli, J., & McNaghten, A. D. (2010). Understanding people who have never received HIV medical care: A population-based approach. *Public Health Reports, 125*(4), 520–527.

Suggested Resources

AVERT—Averting HIV and AIDS—AIDS & HIV Information from AVERT.org. (2011a). *AIDS, drug prices and generic drugs*. Horsham, West Sussex, UK. Retrieved December 30, 2011 from http://www.avert.org/generic.htm

AVERT—Averting HIV and AIDS—AIDS & HIV Information from AVERT.org. (2011b). *Universal access to AIDS treatment: Targets and challenges*. Horsham, West Sussex, UK. Retrieved December 30, 2011 from http://www.avert.org/universal-access.htm

Centers for Disease Control and Prevention. (2011). *HIV/AIDS*. Atlanta, GA. Retrieved October 22, 2011 from http://www.cdc.gov/hiv/

Healthcare.gov. (2011, November 9). *How the affordable care act helps people living with HIV/AIDS: 2011 and beyond*. Washington, DC: U.S. Department of Health and Human Services. Retrieved February 6, 2012 from http://www.healthcare.gov/news/factsheets/2011/11/hiv-aids11092011a.html

Joint United Nations Programme on HIV/AIDS (UNAIDS) & World Health Organization (WHO). (2009). *AIDS epidemic update 2009*. Geneva (November 2010). Retrieved October 22, 2011 from http://www.unaids.org/en/KnowledgeCentre/HIVData/EpiUpdate/EpiUpdArchive/2009/default.asp

Joint United Nations Programme on HIV/AIDS (UNAIDS) & World Health Organization (WHO). (2010). *UNAIDS report on the global AIDS epidemic 2010*. Geneva. Retrieved October 22, 2011 from http://www.unaids.org/globalreport/Global_report.htm

Shapiro, M. F., Morton, S. C., McCaffrey, D. F., Senterfitt, J. W., Fleishman, J., Perlman, J. F., et al. (2000). *Access to HIV care: Initial results from the HIV cost and services utilization study*. Rand Corporation. Retrieved February 6, 2012 from: http://www.rand.org/pubs/research_briefs/RB4530/index1.html

Adherence

Stefani Parrisbalogun

Adherence in HIV patients is a key predictor of morbidity and mortality in this patient population. Adherence is also the most important factor affecting treatment outcomes. Specifically, poor adherence to antiretroviral therapy results in development of viral resistance, viral cross resistance, progression to AIDS and opportunistic infections, in addition to reduced quality of life. Comorbid psychiatric disorders, especially Axis I diagnoses such as active substance abuse, depression, and anxiety, also adversely affect adherence outcomes, further impacting disease progression and quality of life negatively. In fact, the lifetime prevalence of psychiatric illnesses in HIV-infected persons can range from 1 to 2.5 times that of the general population, underscoring the need for consistent and routine psychiatric screening as well as treatment in this patient population. Moreover, poor adherence also hinders risk reduction and other prevention strategies.

Adherence to HIV therapy and management varies among age groups, socioeconomic classes, social support systems, and according to access to care. Medication adherence in HIV patients can be suboptimal in as much as 70%. Patients who are younger and who have less access to care and limited support are at a greater risk for nonadherence. Other risk factors for nonadherence include the following: decreased health literacy; personal beliefs; maladaptive coping strategies; social stigma; stressful and/or traumatic life events such as abuse; depression; anxiety; hopelessness; housing, financial, occupational, and legal psychosocial stressors; and substance abuse/dependence. Other factors include cognitive disorders such as dementia, delirium, psychosis, and personality disorders. Together, these factors act not only as barriers to adherence in antiretroviral therapy but overall health care in HIV patients.

Furthermore, management of other chronic comorbid illnesses such as hepatitis and renal disease can impact adherence negatively in terms of increased medical-related stress with increased physical dependency, medication/pill burden,

S. Parrisbalogun (✉)
Department of Psychiatry, University Hospitals Case Medical Center, Cleveland, OH, USA
e-mail: Stefani.Parrisbalogun@UHhospitals.org

S. Loue (ed.), *Mental Health Practitioner's Guide to HIV/AIDS*,
DOI 10.1007/978-1-4614-5283-6_5,

drug–drug interactions, medication side effects, neuropsychiatric sequelae and reduced quality of life. Again, delirium, dementia, and other cognitive disorders commonly seen in HIV patients also highlight the need for a biopsychosocial approach to increasing adherence. Psychotropic medication adherence in HIV patients is also fraught with many of the same hindrance factors as antiretroviral therapy. However, the self-discontinuation rate may be higher with psychotropic medications due to the perceived acuity of the and non-life-threatening nature of the psychiatric illness.

Adherence to both psychiatric and medical management in HIV patients is paramount. Multidisciplinary teams of health care professionals including social work/case management, psychiatry, psychology, infectious disease, and primary care specialists are essential in providing patient education, treatment, medication management and psychoeducation to identify adherence barriers, increase community and social support, as well as access to community resources.

Related Topics: Access to care, antiretroviral therapy, case management, mental health comorbidity and HIV/AIDS, protease inhibitors, social support.

Suggested Reading

Berg, C. J., Michelson, S. E., & Safren, S. A. (2007). Behavioral aspects of HIV care: Adherence, depression, substance use, and HIV-transmission behaviors. *Infectious Disease Clinics of North America, 21*, 181–200.

Cohen, M. A., & Gorman, J. M. (2008). *Comprehensive textbook of AIDS psychiatry*. New York, NY: Oxford University Press.

Malta, M., Strathdee, S. A., Magnanini, M., Coutinho, E., & Bastos, F. I. (2008). Adherence to antiretroviral therapy for human immunodeficiency virus/acquired immune deficiency syndrome among drug users: A systematic review. *Addiction, 103*(8), 1242–1247.

Mugavero, M. J., Raper, J. L., Reif, S., Whetten, K., Leserman, J., Thielman, N. M., et al. (2009). Overload: Impact of incident stressful events on antiretroviral medication adherence and virologic failure in a longitudinal, multisite human immunodeficiency virus cohort study. *Psychosomatic Medicine, 71*(9), 920–926.

Suggested Resources

APA treating HIV/AIDS: A quick reference guide.

African Americans

Sana Loue

Incidence and Prevalence of HIV/AIDS

The first cases of HIV among African Americans were diagnosed in the early 1980s. However, portrayals of HIV/AIDS as a disease affecting White gay men led to an initial belief that the infection would not affect African Americans. The public acknowledgement of HIV infection by several high profile African Americans, including the TV anchor Max Robinson, the tennis player Arthur Ashe, and the former basketball player Earvin "Magic" Johnson, led to an increased awareness and underscored the serious impact of HIV on African Americans.

African Americans are disproportionately impacted by HIV/AIDS. Although Blacks represented only 12% of the US population in 2009, they accounted for 44% of all new HIV infections that year and 48% of all individuals diagnosed with AIDS that year. The rate of new infections among Black men is 6.5 times the rate for White men and 2.5 times the rate for Black women. The risk of contracting HIV is frighteningly high: it is estimated that 1 out of every 16 Black men and 1 out of every 32 Black women will contract HIV during their lifetimes.

Black men accounted for 70% of the new infections in 2009. In 2007, HIV was the fourth leading cause of death for Black men ages 24–44. Almost three-quarters (73%) of all new infections among Black men are attributable to unprotected sex with men. Young Black men who have sex with men and who are between the ages of 13 and 29 are particularly impacted. There has been a continuing increase in new infections among this age group of Black men who have sex with men, with an increase of 48% between 2006 and 2009. One study in five major US cities found that 46% of Black gay and bisexual men were HIV-positive, compared to 21% of non-Hispanic White and 17% of Latino gay and bisexual men.

S. Loue (✉)
Department of Epidemiology and Biostatistics, Case Western Reserve University, Cleveland, OH, USA
e-mail: sana.loue@case.edu

S. Loue (ed.), *Mental Health Practitioner's Guide to HIV/AIDS*,
DOI 10.1007/978-1-4614-5283-6_6, © Springer Science+Business Media New York 2013

The majority of new HIV infections among Black women are attributable to unprotected heterosexual relations. The rate of new HIV infections among Black women is 15 times as high as among White women. AIDS is now the leading cause of death for African American women between the ages of 25 and 34; African American women are more than 21 times as likely as non-Hispanic White women to die from HIV/AIDS.

Teenagers ages 13–19 are also at particularly high risk. Black teens account for 17% of all teenagers in the USA. However, in 2009, they accounted for 68% of all new AIDS diagnoses among teens.

In 2008, almost three-quarters (72%) of Blacks living with AIDS resided in 10 states: New York, Florida, Georgia, Maryland, Texas, California, New Jersey, Pennsylvania, Illinois, and Washington, DC. The majority of individuals newly diagnosed with AIDS live in the South.

Risk Factors for HIV/AIDS

Unprotected sex is the leading cause of HIV transmission among African Americans. Infection with another sexually transmitted disease, such as gonorrhea or Chlamydia, may facilitate HIV transmission. Research indicates that Black Americans have eight times the level of Chlamydia infections and 18 times the level of gonorrhea infections compared to Whites. One study by the Centers for Disease Control and Prevention found that 48% of Black women and 39% of Black men were infected with the herpes virus, compared to 21% of all women and 11.5% of all men in the USA.

Injecting drug use represents the second most common mechanism of transmission among African Americans. Non-injecting drug use may be an indirect risk factor for HIV transmission. For example, the use of some drugs, such as crack cocaine and crystal methamphetamine, may lead to lessened inhibitions, which can increase the likelihood that users will engage in unsafe sexual practices. Additionally, the need for drugs may lead individuals to trade sex for drugs.

Poverty has been found to be associated with HIV. In 2010, 15.1% of all Americans lived in poverty, but an estimated 27.4% of African Americans were living in poverty. Poverty affects HIV risk and progression to AIDS in a number of ways. The HIV Cost and Services Utilization Study found that Blacks are more likely to delay seeking medical care because they did not have transportation or were too ill to go to the doctor. A greater proportion of HIV-infected Blacks are uninsured in comparison with HIV-infected Whites. Blacks who have health care insurance are more likely to be insured through publicly financed health insurance programs, such as Medicaid, in comparison with Whites. At the time of HIV diagnosis, Blacks are less likely than Whites to be insured through any health insurance mechanism. Additionally, individuals may engage in survival sex, trading sexual relations to obtain safety, shelter, and/or food that would otherwise not be available or accessible to them.

Various beliefs regarding the origin of HIV may affect individuals' willingness to engage on safe sex practices and to present for HIV testing, counseling, or care. A large proportion of African Americans believes that HIV is a man-made virus and that a cure for AIDS exists but is being withheld from the poor. Many also believe that the virus was manufactured by the government, that it was disseminated into the population by the Central Intelligence Agency (CIA) of the USA, and that it represents a genocidal attack on Blacks. These beliefs stem from a history of slavery and discrimination at the hands of the US government, and the misuse of African Americans in biomedical research, such as the Tuskegee Syphilis Study.

HIV and Mental Illness

Past research provides strong evidence of the association between mental illness and increased HIV risk. Men who have sex with men, and Black men who have sex with men in particular, may experience an enlarged constellation of health problems, including psychosocial problems, that are positively associated with high risk sexual behavior and HIV infection. African-American men at high risk of HIV have been found to have a higher prevalence of mental illness than is often reported in epidemiologic studies, with behaviorally gay and bisexual men evidencing the highest level of risk for psychiatric disorders. Black, behaviorally gay and bisexual men have reported disproportionately high rates of chronic depression, stress, alcohol and substance abuse, and engaging in sex work for subsistence, all experiences and situations that encourage or facilitate unsafe sexual behavior.

Related Topics: Conspiracy theories, denialism, discrimination, stigma and stigmatization, Tuskegee Syphilis Study.

Suggested Reading

Loue, S. (Ed.). (2008). *Health issues confronting minority men who have sex with men*. New York, NY: Springer.

Richardson, M. A., Myers, H. F., & Bing, E. G. (1997). Substance use and psychopathology in African American men at risk for HIV infection. *Journal of Community Psychology, 25*(4), 353–370.

Stillwaggon, E. (2006). *AIDS and the ecology of poverty*. New York, NY: Oxford University Pres.

Washington, H. A. (2006). *Medical apartheid: The dark history of medical experimentation on Black Americans from colonial times to the present*. New York, NY: Doubleday.

Suggested Resources

Centers for Disease Control and Prevention. (2007). *Epidemiology of STDs in African American communities*. Retrieved from http://www.cdc.gov/std/health-disparities/default.htm

Centers for Disease Control and Prevention. (2011, November). *HIV among African Americans*. Retrieved December 28, 2011 from http://www.cdc.gov/hiv/topics/aa/PDF/aa.pdf

The Henry I Kaiser Family Foundation. (2011, August). *HIV/AIDS policy: Fact sheet: Black Americans and HIV/AIDS*. Retrieved December 28, 2011 from http://www.kff.org/hivaids/upload/6089-09.pdf

United States Department of Health and Human Services, Office on Women's Health. (2010, May 18). *Minority women's health: HIV/AIDS*. Retrieved December 28, 2011 from http://www.womenshealth.gov/minority-health/african-americans/hiv-aids.cfm

Aging

Ana-Gabriela Benghiac

Receiving a diagnosis of HIV infection represents a major stressor in one's life, with implications on the personal, professional, and social levels. Additionally, a diagnosis of HIV infection may raise issues of stigma and discrimination.

With the advancements in HIV drug therapy, HIV-positive individuals live longer now than was possible at the beginning of the HIV epidemic in 1981. That being said, mental health disorders seem to have a more premature onset among HIV-infected individuals compared to healthy individuals of the same age. Moreover, HIV-positive adults above the age of 40 or 50 often report a poorer quality of life compared to those who are not HIV-infected. They may acquire diseases in their 40s and 50s that usually affect HIV-negative individuals in their 70s, such as muscle loss, diseases of the kidney, liver, heart, veins, diabetes and bone fragility. Although not all HIV-infected individuals develop cognitive impairments, approximately 50% of them do. Additionally, some may also develop motor skills impairments.

Significant changes seen in older HIV-infected patients include bone fragility and blood flow alteration. Blood flow in HIV-infected individuals is reduced up to levels seen in much older patients. Osteoporosis and osteopenia have a higher prevalence among HIV-positive older individuals compared to the noninfected population of the same age. It is believed that the drug therapy used to treat HIV infection is associated with bone loss in HIV positive individuals, while dementia and other cognitive impairments are more likely to be related to the virus itself. However, there are other factors involved in the emergence of these conditions such as coinfections and smoking.

Individuals diagnosed with HIV at an older age appear to have a lower survival rate in comparison with those who are diagnosed at a younger age. However, this may be due to the fact that older adults are diagnosed with HIV in more advanced stages of the disease, the existence of specific diseases associated with advancing

A.-G. Benghiac (✉)
Department of Bioethics, Case Western Reserve University, Cleveland, OH, USA
e-mail: dr.gabriela_benghiac@yahoo.com

S. Loue (ed.), *Mental Health Practitioner's Guide to HIV/AIDS*,
DOI 10.1007/978-1-4614-5283-6_7,

age, the multidrug therapy and its side effects, and decreased immune system capacity to cope with all of these factors.

Mental health disorders acquired before the infection may be related to risk behaviors leading to HIV infection, while those acquired after the HIV-positive diagnosis can contribute to the spread of the virus to other individuals. Past sexual abuse has been found to be associated with higher HIV risk behaviors such as substance abuse and unprotected sexual relations, as well as with the emergence of mental illnesses.

One of the primary mental health issues associated with HIV patients is the development of depression. This may be due not only to the severity of the diagnosis, but also to stigmatization, lower financial income, lack of social support, and discrimination. Older HIV-positive individuals are usually more isolated and they tend to avoid other people as a mean of coping with the disease. Anxiety, suicidal ideation, and suicide attempts are more frequent among older HIV-patients in comparison with those who are younger.

It is important for healthcare professionals to provide targeted prevention and patient education to older individuals, as they may not have sufficient information regarding prevention and protection in HIV. Because older individuals may feel too ashamed to recognize that they lack basic knowledge about the disease and do not ask questions, they may unwittingly risk not only their own lives but the lives of other people. Healthcare providers may also assume that older individuals already know detailed information about HIV/AIDS and consequently do not engage them in discussions to assess their knowledge. There is a misconception that older individuals are not sexually active and are therefore not at risk for becoming infected. Many older individuals may also assume that they are not at risk to acquire HIV as they associate the disease with young people and youth behavior in general.

Adherence to treatment has been found to be lower in HIV-infected older adults due to the frequent complexities of multidrug therapy and the comorbidities that may impair their thinking and memory. Thus, many of these individuals not only tend to forget to take their medication, but also simply give up their treatment regimen which can lead to the appearance of drug-resistant strains of HIV. Nonadherence to HIV therapy can also be influenced by substance abuse.

The adoption of various strategies may improve individuals' quality of life and disease management. It is recommended that they have a healthy diet and lifestyle, practice appropriate exercises, avoid weight gain, reduce smoking and alcohol intake, avoid mind-altering substances, adhere to the prescribed medication regimen, monitor and treat other illnesses (such as hypertension), and engage in safe sex when they have sexual relations. The American Academy of HIV Medicine (AAHIVM), the American Geriatrics Society (AGS) and the AIDS Community Research Initiative of America (ACRIA) developed *The HIV and Aging Consensus Project: Recommended Treatment Strategies for Clinicians Managing Older Patients with HIV* as a guideline for healthcare professionals who provide treatment to HIV-positive old individuals. Clinicians are advised to encourage HIV-positive older patients to complete a durable power of attorney for healthcare and an advanced directive, to refer patients, if necessary, to counseling programs for abuse or dependence disorders, to perform screening for depressive disorders, cognitive impairments, hepatitis A, B, and C, cancers, diabetes, an cardiovascular disease, to routinely monitor CD4 cell counts and HIV RNA levels, and to perform an annual review of medication and dose adjustments.

Related Topics: Cognitive impairment.

Suggested Reading

Nichols, J. E., Speer, D. C., Watson, B. J., Watson, M. J., Vergon, T. L., Vallee, C. M., et al. (2002). *Aging with HIV: Psychological, social and health issues*. San Diego, CA: Academic.

Suggested Resources

The American Academy of HIV Medicine (AAHIVM), The AIDS Community Research Initiative of America (ACRIA), & The American Geriatrics Society (AGS). (n.d.). *The HIV and aging consensus project: Recommended treatment strategies for clinicians managing older patients with HIV*. Retrieved February 11, 2012 from http://www.aahivm.org/Upload_Module/upload/HIV%20and%20Aging/

Aging %20report%20working%20document%20FINAL%2012.1.pdf

Anon. (n.d.). *Aging and HIV*. Retrieved February 11, 2012 from http://www.aidsmeds.com/articles/2614_20293.shtml

France, D. (2009, November). Another kind of AIDS crisis. *New York Magazine*, 1. Retrieved February 11, 2012 from http://nymag.com/health/features/61740/

Kelly, J. C. (2012). *HIV speeds brain aging*. Retrieved February 11, 2012 from http://www.medscape.com/viewarticle/716221

AIDS Activism

Daniel J. O'Shea

The first decade of AIDS was characterized by death and activism, the second by effective new treatments and optimism, and the third by renewed activism on a global scale to improve access to prevention, care and treatment in the developing world. AIDS activism emerged in the 1980s in epicenters of the epidemic, including New York City, San Francisco, London, and Paris and later in Rio de Janeiro, Sydney, Cape Town, Bangkok, and elsewhere. In the context of accelerating and deadly local epidemics, activists confronted governments and other institutions to demand attention, rights, protection and funding for science research, prevention, and treatment. Often highly educated and sophisticated, activists drew the attention of the public, the political establishment, academics and the media through marches, public demonstrations, lawsuits, legislation and media manipulation. This new science-informed, community-based treatment activism ultimately led to scientists and activists working together to secure the resources for research that led to breakthroughs in diagnosis, prevention, and most dramatically, treatment. Activism in response to the AIDS epidemic changed the relationship both between physicians and patients and between clinical research and patients, including patient involvement in the initiation, design, recruitment, conduct and evaluation of clinical trials, which was virtually nonexistent prior to the late 1980s.

AIDS activism began as a self-empowerment movement for people with AIDS (PWA) who desired to be active participants in their own healthcare. In May 1983, a spontaneous meeting of PWA during the Second National AIDS Forum at the Lesbian and Gay Health Conference in Denver resulted in what became known as the Denver Principles for PWA self-empowerment. These included recommendations for PLA to form caucuses to deal with the media, choose their own agenda and plan their own strategies, and to be involved at every level of AIDS decision-making and included in all AIDS forums with equal credibility. Participants returned to their home cities and created local PWA coalitions and a

D.J. O'Shea (✉)
Public Health Service, County of San Diego, San Diego, CA, USA
e-mail: Dan.OShea@sdcounty.ca.gov

S. Loue (ed.), *Mental Health Practitioner's Guide to HIV/AIDS*,
DOI 10.1007/978-1-4614-5283-6_8, © Springer Science+Business Media New York 2013

national association. Some of the first coordinated AIDS activism was subsequently organized in New York City in 1985 by the media-oriented Gay and Lesbian Alliance Against Defamation (GLAAD) and a gay-rights group called the Lavender Hill Mob in 1986, which demanded stronger legal protections for PWA facing eviction, faster approval of anti-HIV drugs, and no mandatory testing for HIV.

The premier AIDS activist group, ACT UP (AIDS Coalition to Unleash Power), was born on March 10, 1987 when author/activist Larry Kramer seized the attention of 250 people at the Lesbian and Gay Community Services Center in New York by declaring that most of them might be dead in 5 years. In response to his follow-up question whether they wanted to start a new organization devoted solely to political action, the answer was a resounding "yes!" Kramer's speech and its aftermath galvanized the population of sick, dying, frightened, and dispirited people. At a follow-up meeting two days later, 300 people committed to direct action to end the AIDS crisis. The logo became the pink triangle worn by homosexuals in concentration camps of Hitler's Germany, but with the point up and a grim motto: "Silence = Death," underscoring the basic premise of AIDS activism of the late 1980s and early 1990s, that that action equaled life.

ACT UP's first demonstration occurred 2 weeks later, with protestors converging on and stopping traffic on Wall Street to denounce the exorbitant price of AZT and government inaction on AIDS research. Shortly afterward, the US Food and Drug Administration (FDA) announced that it would shorten its drug approval process by 2 years. For the first time, the "victims" of a disease successfully began to organize a political and investigative revolution, challenging and bucking the governmental and medical establishments.

By early 1988, ACT UP chapters appeared throughout the USA, with ultimately more than 100 in US cities, including Boston, Los Angeles, Portland, Seattle, Houston, and New Orleans, and international cities such as Sydney, London, Berlin, Amsterdam, Montreal, and Paris. Other groups drew inspiration from the ACT UP without formally assuming the name.

ACT UP demonstrations at the FDA in October 1988 and at the US National Institutes of Health (NIH) in March 1990 led to significant changes in the way that research was conducted, including expanded access to experimental drugs; involvement of activists and people living with HIV/AIDS (PLWH/A) in all aspects and levels of developing and monitoring clinical trials; the formation of local, national, and drug company community advisory boards, including PLWH/A; and expedited approval of new drugs. Faster approval drew more drug companies into the field which spurred development of more drugs that could be studied as combinations, ultimately resulting in clinically effective triple-therapy combinations. With viral load measurement technology developed to monitor the efficacy of combination therapy, highly active antiretroviral therapy (ART) emerged in 1996. Within 2 years, rates of AIDS-related death decreased by 67% in the USA and other developed resource-rich nations. Activists also focused on promoting research on drugs to prevent and treat major HIV-related opportunistic infections and by the end of the 1990s, most were controllable. ACT UP was instrumental in reducing health insurance costs, and in making needle exchange a viable policy.

ACT UP's activity occurred on many levels, including raucous general meetings; media sound bites; spectacularly choreographed direct actions and street theater; and intensive study to become "lay experts" in their own right. It had a significant influence on public policy, making considerable inroads into the health and medical science establishment bureaucracy. Members graduated from being unwelcome guests "crashing" major scientific meetings and public hearings to become respected invited presenters with a voice and seat at the table. Although ACT UP began to decline as an organization in the mid-1990s, its influence lives on in many areas with former members and others influenced by their activism holding lead positions in AIDS service organizations, political groups, professional organizations, and many other venues today.

As the second decade of the epidemic came to an end, AIDS treatment activism found a new focus in the challenge of providing access to ART in the developing world. At the International AIDS Conference in Durban in 2000, US-based activists began to work with the Treatment Action Campaign (TAC) in South Africa and with the other international treatment access activists. Strong activism and massive scientific investment boosted the global response to AIDS, leading to the Global Fund to Fight AIDS, Tuberculosis, and Malaria (2002), the US President's Emergency Program for AIDS Relief (PEPFAR; 2003), the World Health Organization-led movement to treat three million persons with ART by the end of 2005 ("3 × 5"), and the later United Nations-endorsed goal of universal access by 2010. These efforts led to the unprecedented fact that by 2009, of the estimated 15 million PLWH in low- and middle-income countries in need of treatment (with CD4 cell count less than 350 cells/mm^3), 36 % (approximately 5.2 million) received ART. This represented a 13-fold increase since 2004.

It is critical that these successes be sustained and reach the remaining two thirds of people who need but are not accessing care, finance the cost of this expanded HIV therapy and ultimately achieve universal access to HIV prevention, treatment, care and support. Accordingly, activists and scientists will need to build upon the alliances forged and lessons learned over the past 30 years to convince the leaders of today and tomorrow to work together to mobilize the necessary resources. Opportunities continue to exist that call for the participation and activism of HIV-infected individuals. As an example, the centers for AIDS Research that are funded by the National Institutes of Health require that community advisory boards be established and include representatives from the community who are HIV-infected. Many cities have nonprofit organizations dedicated to the delivery of services to the HIV-infected community, that welcome the participation of HIV-infected individuals as staff members, volunteers, and board members.

Related Topics: AIDS service organizations, coping, human rights.

Suggested Reading

Achmat, Z. (2006). Science and social justice: The lessons of HIV/AIDS activism in the struggle to eradicate tuberculosis. *International Journal of Tuberculosis and Lung Disease, 10*(12), 1312–1317.

Arno, P. S., & Feiden, K. L. (1992). *Against the odds: The story of AIDS, drug development, politics and profits*. New York, NY: HarperCollins Publishers, Inc.

Harrington, M. (2010). From HIV to tuberculosis and back again: A tale of activism in 2 pandemics. *Clinical Infectious Diseases, 50*(S3), S260–S266.

Smith, R., & Ciplon, P. (2006). *Drugs into bodies: A history of AIDS treatment activism*. Westport, CT: Praeger.

Suggested Resources

ACT UP (AIDS Coalition to Unleash Power). (2011). New York, NY. Retrieved December 18, 2011 from http://www.actupny.org

Halsall, P. (Ed.). (1997). *People with a history: An online guide to lesbian, gay, bisexual and trans history*. Last updated April 10, 2007. Retrieved January 22, 2012 from http://www.fordham.edu/halsall/pwh/index-am.asp#c23

AIDS Service Organizations

Oscar Grusky

Organizations are goal-oriented social systems that have the capacity to acquire resources and use them for a variety of purposes and are the chief way of getting things done that are beyond the reach of individuals. AIDS service organizations are designed to provide their clients or patients with needed medical and other services throughout the course of this illness. Not surprisingly, the availability of services is much greater in developed than in the less-developed countries. The range of services that these organizations provide the more than 33 million persons currently living with HIV worldwide is numerous in many *highly developed nations* (particularly in large urban high prevalence communities) and include medical resources such as clinics, substance use/drug assistance and treatment, home health, skilled nursing, mental health, peer support, case management, dental services, educational, food and nutrition, HIV/AIDS testing, hotlines/crisis lines, housing, language services, legal services, prevention, public benefits, infants' and children's services, spiritual services, support groups, thrift stores, transportation, treatment adherence, utility discounts, women's services, work-related including disability services, youth assistance, advocacy, and planning groups. Some organizations provide only a single service while others provide many services. The mix of services provided by a variety of organizations such as hospital-based clinics, local health departments, and many community-based service agencies, can confuse patients and providers and produce fragmentation and service duplication.

Co-occurrence of HIV with other health conditions is frequent and should be detected and treated but too often it is neither detected nor treated and collaboration in the coordinated care of patients does not happen. Although organizations often develop mutual exchanges with other organizations in order to strengthen their resource base by finding other units that may provide resources for them or provide markets for their outputs, there is a worldwide need for improved coordination and integration of services so that there are effective and efficient systems of care. Much

O. Grusky (✉)
Department of Sociology, University of California Los Angeles, Los Angeles, CA, USA
e-mail: grusky@ucla.edu

S. Loue (ed.), *Mental Health Practitioner's Guide to HIV/AIDS*,
DOI 10.1007/978-1-4614-5283-6_9, © Springer Science+Business Media New York 2013

of the research on AIDS service organizations has been conducted in English-speaking developed nations. These studies have found service needs such as lack of rapid HIV testing availability, barriers to coinfection medical services and practices, lack of knowledge of legal rights, and lack of housing availability. Overall the range of services and service organizations available to persons living with HIV in *less-developed nations* for the estimated 68% of people worldwide living with HIV who are from Sub-Saharan Africa (even though only 13% of the global population are in this region) are sparse for both adults and children. These nations need major buildup of their medical and other services' infrastructure. For example, South Africa has more persons living with HIV than any other nation (5.6 million). More than nine out of ten (92%) of children with HIV reside in Sub-Saharan Africa. Consequently, service organization needs are markedly different for those who reside in the less developed areas. For these persons the primary immediate needs are HIV antiretroviral treatment, medical care for co-occurring conditions such as nutritional deficiencies, tuberculosis, malaria and other diseases, and follow-up. For example, as of 2009 almost half (44%) of those with HIV in Sub-Saharan Africa who needed antiretroviral treatment did not have access to it.

Related Topics: Access to care, AIDS activism, case management, HIV testing, HIV counseling, social support.

Suggested Reading

Institute of Medicine. (2006). *Improving the quality of health care for mental and substance-use conditions*. Washington, DC: The National Academies Press.

Kwait, J., Valente, T., & Celentano, D. D. (2001). Interorganizational relationships among HIV/AIDS service organizations in Baltimore: A network analysis. *Journal of Urban Health, 78*(3), 468–487.

Perry, D. F., Kaufman, R. K., & Knitzer, J. (Eds.). (2007). *Social and emotional health in early childhood: Building Bridges between services and systems*. Baltimore, MD: Paul H. Brookes.

Suggested Resources

Journal of HIV/AIDS and Social Services 9: 2010, Special Issue on Improving Service Delivery and Care to HIV-Infected Populations. Taylor & Francis Group, LLC.

Kaiser Family Foundation. (2011). *Fact sheets and U.S. global health policy on HIV/AIDS*. Retrieved June 30, 2011 from http://www.kff.org/hivaids

Alternative and Traditional Healing

Mihaela-Catalina Vicol

Background

Traditional medicine refers to a wide range of practices, from herbal treatments to spiritualism. The use of traditional medicine is a subject of controversy around the world, due to few promising results of the research in the area compared with the outcomes associated with the use of evidence-based medicine. This brings even more controversy in the context of diseases for which allopathic medicine has no cure, such as HIV/AIDS.

According to the UNAIDS Global Report 2010, new HIV infections are declining (2.6 million people in 2009, comparing to 3.1 million people in 1999), due to antiretroviral therapy and to HIV prevention education. However, in low developed and poor countries like South Africa, the availability of antiretroviral therapy is low. In addition, the use of antiretroviral therapy is expensive and it requires an expensive medical infrastructure that not many countries can afford to implement. Antiretroviral therapy may have significant side effects such as diabetes, heart attack, and bone mass conditions and for some individuals does not produce a significant benefit. Some studies have found that traditional medicine has been helpful in treating some HIV-related conditions and in controlling side effects of the antiretroviral therapy, prompting some patients to turn to traditional medicine. Finally, cultural and traditional beliefs about the positive effects of traditional medicine may lead people to use it; studies have shown that almost 70–80% of people from South Africa utilize the services of a traditional healer.

M.-C. Vicol (✉)
Department of Bioethics, University of Medicine and Pharmacy "Gr. T. Popa", Iasi, Romania
e-mail: mihavicol@yahoo.com

S. Loue (ed.), *Mental Health Practitioner's Guide to HIV/AIDS*,
DOI 10.1007/978-1-4614-5283-6_10, © Springer Science+Business Media New York 2013

Use of Traditional and Alternative Medicine

At the end of the 1990s, it was estimated that over 70% of the people living in South Africa attend traditional healers and that traditional practitioners numbered around 350,000. According to the World Health Organization, in Africa, traditional medicine and self-care medication are the main healthcare resources for 80% of the people, including individuals living with HIV/AIDS. Studies conducted in Australia also found that more than half of the patients utilizing antiretroviral therapy use traditional remedies. A study conducted in Canada by Furler and colleagues found that a high proportion of HIV-positive patients used vitamins; minerals; various activities and services such as meditation, aromatherapy, reflexology, and massage; and various other products, such as ginseng and Echinacea, in their efforts to maintain their well-being.

According to the studies in the area, traditional/alternative remedies (usually made of natural plants, herbs) may contribute to the general well-being of the HIV/AIDS patient. Cited benefits include symptomatic relief, weight gain, reduced pain, cure of some HIV-related infections such as *Candida albicans*, and recovery of lost vitamins and electrolytes. Fish oil may be helpful in decreasing cholesterol, which may be increased as a side effect of some HIV medications. Whey protein may help some individuals gain weight and may also help to reduce diarrhea and increase CD4 counts. Various other remedies have been studied for their potential benefit in HIV/AIDS. For example, *Prunella vulgaris* is under research for its potential benefit as a tea infusion. The remedy called "life everlasting" made of *Gnaphalium polycephalum* is given in tea infusion to prolong life and for the high energy that it induces. Licorice root seems to produce calm and peace and improve general well-being; it is under study for its potential benefit in treating hepatitis C and hemophilia associated with HIV. Other herbs, like *Hyssopus officinalis*, are used as remedies for coughing, for the dry throat symptom associated with infections in HIV.

Some often used remedies, however, may produce adverse effects. St. John's Wort, often used as a remedy for depression, may reduce the effectiveness of some anti-HIV drugs by as much as 50%. Although garlic supplements may be used to strengthen the immune system, they may also reduce the effectiveness of anti-HIV drugs by 50%.

Ethical Issues

Traditional medicine raises important ethical controversies, the major one being patient's information. In order to be able to decide and to give consent, the patient should have complete and accurate medical information. Both traditional medicine and antiretroviral therapy have potential benefits, as well as limits. This means that when using traditional or alternative remedies, the patient must be informed of the benefits as potential benefits (according to the present research) and of the risks of this therapy (sometimes the remedies might interfere with the antiretroviral therapy). The patient should also know about antiretroviral therapy. The ethical problem of patient's information comes usually from exaggerating the benefits and minimizing the risks. The second important ethical issue is the availability of antiretroviral therapy and patient's access to it because not every country provides it as an alternative traditional medicine is offered.

Implications for Mental Health Providers

Mental health providers will want to discuss with their clients, whether HIV-positive or -negative, their use of traditional or alternative treatments. While some of these treatments and processes may provide benefits, such as reduced anxiety or improvement in mood, some may lead to unwanted ill effects, including the decreased effectiveness of medications necessary to slow the progression of HIV disease or control the symptoms of HIV and/or mental illness. Such discussions are likely done more easily if the therapeutic alliance is strong and the patient and provider a reviewed as a team.

Suggested Reading

Babb, D. A., Pemba, L., Seatlanyane, P., Charalambous, S., Churchyard, G. J., & Grant, A. D. (2007). Use of traditional medicine by HIV-infected individuals in South Africa in the era of antiretroviral therapy. *Psychology, Health, & Medicine, 12*(3), 314–320.

Bird, S. R. (2010). *The big book of soul: The ultimate guide to the African American spirit.* Charlottesville, VA: Hampton Roads Publishing Company, Inc.

Bodeker, G., & Burford, G. (Eds.). (2007). *Traditional, complementary and alternative medicine: Policy and public health perspectives.* London: Imperial College Press.

Furler, M. D., Einarson, T. R., Walmsley, S., Millson, M., & Bendayan, R. (2003). Use of complementary and alternative medicine by HIV-infected outpatients in Ontario, Canada. *AIDS Patient Care, 17*(4), 155–168.

Peltzer, K., Preez, F. N., Ramlagan, S., & Fomundam, H. (2008). Use of traditional complementary and alternative medicine for HIV patients in KwaZulu-Natal, South Africa. *BMC Public Health, 8*, 255.

Squire, C. (2007). *HIV in South Africa: Talking about the big thing.* London: Taylor and Francis.

Suggested Resources

Joint United Nations Programme on HIV/AIDS (UNAIDS). (2006a). *Collaborating with traditional healers for HIV prevention and care in sub-Saharan Africa: Suggestions for programme managers and field workers.* Geneva, Switzerland: Author. Retrieved April 30, 2012 from http://data.unaids.org/publications/IRC-pub07/jc967-tradhealers_en.pdf

Joint United Nations Programme on HIV/AIDS (UNAIDS). (2006b). *Global report: UNAIDS report on the global AIDS epidemic 2010*. Retrieved January 15, 2012 from http://www.unaids.org/documents/20101123_globalreport_em.pdf

Mayo Clinic Staff. (2011). *Alternative medicine*. Retrieved April 30, 2012 from http://www.mayoclinic.com/health/hiv-aids/DS00005/DSECTION=alternative-medicine

Antiretroviral Therapy

Todd Wagner

Antiretroviral therapy (ART) for the treatment of human immunodeficiency virus (HIV) infection has improved significantly since the first successful therapeutic trial using AZT (zidovudine) in 1986. It has greatly reduced overall morbidity and mortality in individuals with HIV, and has reduced perinatal and behavior-associated transmission. In most patients who have access to these medications, treatment initiated before the onset of advanced immunodeficiency reduces plasma HIV RNA concentrations ("viral load") to undetectable levels and results in robust and sustained gains in CD4 T-cell counts. Antiretroviral therapy is currently potent, convenient, and typically well tolerated. It is important for mental health care providers to be aware of the various antiretroviral medications that can be used to treat HIV because some may interact with various psychotropic medications and others may produce neuropsychiatric effects that must be distinguished from the symptoms of the underlying mental disorder.

Despite the success of improvements in ART, many challenges exist. ART does not fully restore health. HIV-infected individuals on optimal treatment regimens still have a shorter life expectancy than their equivalent, uninfected peers. Nor does ART cure HIV infection. It requires that multiple medications be taken for life. Although typically well tolerated, ART may cause a variety of side effects and drug–drug interactions, and requires close adherence to be effective and prevent the emergence of resistance. Many HIV-infected individuals remain unaware of their status, continue to transmit HIV to others, and when diagnosed are more likely to have advanced stage disease. Finally, approximately one-half of all HIV-infected individuals screen positive for one or more psychiatric disorders, which are associated with decreased survival, impaired quality of life, and decreased adherence to ART.

Antiretroviral drugs are classified by the viral life cycle they inhibit and, in some cases, by their chemical structure. There are currently five classes of antiretroviral

T. Wagner (✉)
University Hospitals Case Medical Center, Cleveland, OH, USA
e-mail: Todd.Wagner@case.edu

S. Loue (ed.), *Mental Health Practitioner's Guide to HIV/AIDS*,
DOI 10.1007/978-1-4614-5283-6_11,

Table 1 Classes of Antiretroviral Drugs

Nucleoside reverse transcriptase inhibitors (NRTI)	Protease inhibitors (PI)
Abacavir (ABC)	Atazanavir (ATV)
Emtricitabine (FTC)	Darunavir (DRV)
Lamivudine (3TC)	Fosamprenavir (FPV)
Tenofovir (TDF)	Indinavir (IDV)
Stavudine (d4T)	Lopinavir (LPV/r)
Zidovudine (AZT)	Nelfinavir (NFV)
Didanosine (ddI)	Ritonavir (RTV)
	Saquinavir (SQV)
	Tipranavir (TPV)
Non-nucleoside reverse transcriptase inhibitors (NNRTI)	**Integrase inhibitors**
Nevirapine (NVP)	Raltegravir (RAL)
Efavirenz (EFV)	
Rilpivirine (RPV)	Entry inhibitors
Delavirdine (DLV)	Enfuvirtide (ENV)
Etravirine (ETR)	Maraviroc (MVC)

drugs: nucleoside reverse transcriptase inhibitors (NRTI), non-nucleoside reverse transcriptase inhibitors (NNRTI), protease inhibitors (PI), integrase inhibitors, and entry inhibitors (see Table 1). Although grouped by class, these medications have unique side effect profiles, drug–drug interactions, and potency. Achieving suppression of HIV requires the use of ART regiments with at least two, and preferably three, active drugs from two or more drug classes. All currently recommended treatment regiments consist of a backbone of two NRTIs and a third antiretroviral drug, typically a NNRTI, a ritonavir-boosted protease inhibitor, or an integrase inhibitor.

An ART regiment should be tailored to each patient and take into consideration expected side effects, convenience, comorbidities, interactions with concomitant medications, and the results of baseline resistant testing. Predictors of viral suppression include high potency of ART regiment, excellent adherence to the regimen, low baseline viral loads, higher baseline CD4 count, and rapid reduction in viral load in response to treatment. Treatment should be initiated in those with a CD4 T-cell count lower than 350 cells/μL, and in those with an AIDS-defining opportunistic infection or cancer. Additional indications to initiate therapy regardless of CD4 count include pregnancy, HIV-associated nephropathy, and Hepatitis B coinfection when treatment is indicated. Present ART regimens in treatment-naïve individuals suppress plasma viral loads below detection limits of commercial assays in 90% of clinical trial participants.

Although ART is safe and well tolerated, side effects are important and may have a significant influence on adherence and long-term treatment success. Nucleoside reverse transcriptase inhibitors, as a class, have the potential to develop lactic acidosis and hepatic steatosis. Older NRTIs, still used in resource-limited settings, can develop mitochondrial toxicity, which is characterized by hepatic steatosis (fatty liver), peripheral sensory neuropathy, and lipoatrophy (fat redistribution).

Lipoatrophy can be significant enough to impair an affected individual's overall body image and quality of life. Regarding non-nucleoside reverse transcription inhibitors, the commonly used efavirenz does lead to a wide variety of neuropsychiatric effects. Individuals may experience euphoria, anxiety, or worsening mood, in addition to insomnia and disturbingly vivid dreams. These symptoms generally improve within 2–4 weeks of initiating treatment, and can be mitigated by bedtime dosing. Awareness of potential side effects of ART, and timing of onset of symptoms in relation to initiation of a medication may help distinguish whether symptoms are side effects of a new medication or an acute worsening of symptoms of underlying mental illness. Protease inhibitors are metabolized by the cytochrome P450 system and all possess some element of enzyme-inhibiting or enzyme-inducing properties. This can lead to potential drug–drug interactions when co-administered with other medication that are metabolized by the cytochrome P450 system, such as many psychotropic medications. Protease inhibitors, as a class, also have the potential to cause hepatotoxicity, insulin resistance, and hyperlipidemia (high blood cholesterol), though this is not exclusive to protease inhibitors.

HIV disease progression and response to ART is monitored by the CD4 count and HIV RNA concentration ("viral load"). The CD4 count represents the number of CD4 lymphocytes (also called T-cells) and reflects the degree of immunocompromise. The HIV viral load indicates the number of copies of HIV RNA per milliliter of plasma. This reflects the burden of HIV infection and magnitude of viral replication. The immediate goal of ART is to reduce HIV replication to a threshold below which the virus does not evolve and drug resistance does not emerge. Additional testing may include genotypic and phenotypic assays, chemokine receptor tropism evaluation, and HLA-B*5701 testing.

With continued access to treatment and excellent long-term adherence to ART, HIV is now considered a chronic illness rather than a uniformly fatal disease. Additional improvements in clinical care are expected as new medications are developed, antiretroviral therapy regiments are improved upon, and primary care is delivered to those living with HIV.

Related Topics: Adherence, protease inhibitors.

Suggested Reading

Blashill, A. J., Perry, N., & Safren, S. A. (2011). Mental health: A focus on stress, coping, and mental illness as it relates to treatment retention, adherence, and other health outcomes. *Current HIV/AIDS Report, 8*, 215–222.

Department of Health and Human Services. (2011, October 14). *Guidelines for the use of antiretroviral agents in HIV-1 infected adults and adolescents*. Washington, DC: Department of Health and Human Services. Retrieved from http://www.aidsinfo.nih.gov/guidelines/html/1/adult-and-adolescent-treatment-guidelines/0/

Volberding, P. A., & Deeks, S. G. (2010). Antiretroviral therapy and management of HIV infection. *Lancet, 376*, 49–62.

Asians and Pacific Islanders

Sana Loue

The US census uses the term "Asians and Pacific Islanders" to encompass individuals with ethnic origins in the Far East, Southeast Asia, and the Indian Subcontinent. Asians and Pacific Islanders account for approximately 5.6% of the US population, with the majority living in ten states: California, Florida, New Jersey, New York, Hawaii, Illinois, Massachusetts, Texas, Virginia, and Washington. Increasing numbers of Asians and Pacific Islanders have been settling in the states of Arkansas, Connecticut, Georgia, Nevada, and North Carolina. And, although Asians and Pacific Islanders are frequently referred to as a single group, this group actually comprises more than 50 distinct subgroups that speak more than 100 different languages and dialects. The subgroups within this larger category are quite diverse with respect to other features as well. As an example, it has been estimated that 55% of Vietnamese persons older than 5 years of age do not speak English at home, compared to 22% of Asian Indians. This diversity of language, culture, and socioeconomic conditions within the larger grouping of Asians and Pacific Islanders presents challenges in HIV/AIDS prevention efforts.

Incidence, Prevalence, and Risk Factors for HIV/AIDS

Asians and Pacific Islanders have the lowest rate of HIV transmission among all ethnic groups. The rate of AIDS diagnosis among Asians and Pacific Islanders is 3.6 per 100,000, compared to 54.1 per 100,000 for African Americans, 18.0 per 100,000 for Hispanics/Latinos, 7.4 per 100,000 for American Indians and Alaska Natives, and 5.9 per 100,000 for non-Hispanic Whites. According to a report issued by the Centers for Disease Control in 2008, Asians and Pacific Islanders accounted

S. Loue (✉)
Department of Epidemiology and Biostatistics, Case Western Reserve University, Cleveland, OH, USA
e-mail: sana.loue@case.edu

S. Loue (ed.), *Mental Health Practitioner's Guide to HIV/AIDS*,
DOI 10.1007/978-1-4614-5283-6_12, © Springer Science+Business Media New York 2013

for approximately 1.1% of the 37,331 cases of HIV/AIDS that were diagnosed during 2005 and 0.6% of the total number of individuals then living with HIV/AIDS. The majority of the Asians and Pacific Islanders given a diagnosis of HIV/AIDS are men (78%); approximately 1% are children under the age of 13 years, and the remainder, 21%, are women.

Research has found that between 1994 and 2000, Asians/Pacific Islanders had the highest rate of AIDS at the time of their initial diagnosis compared to other racial/ethnic groups, suggesting that access to care may be a significant issue. The majority of Asians/Pacific Islanders with AIDS diagnoses are resident in California, New York, and Hawaii. A significant percentage of individuals with an AIDS diagnosis were born outside the USA; more than a quarter of the individuals diagnosed with AIDS between 1999 and 2002 were born in the three countries of the Philippines, Vietnam, and India. Researchers have suggested that the more open sexual norms in the USA may have allowed immigrants to engage in sexual activities that would have been highly stigmatized in their own countries, and it is these behaviors that have increased the risk of HIV transmission.

Among men, approximately two-thirds of the cases of HIV transmission are attributable to unprotected male-to-male sexual contact, while high risk heterosexual contact accounts for an estimated 15% of all transmission. Among women, more than three-quarters (80%) of cases are attributable to high risk heterosexual intercourse, followed by injection drug use (16%). In at least one study, almost one-fifth of participating Asian/Pacific Islander women reported that they had been pressured to have sex without their consent.

There is significant stigma associated with HIV/AIDS, with homosexual identity, and with injection drug use within many Asian and Pacific Islander communities. This greatly complicates prevention efforts in that individuals may avoid discussion about HIV and, as a consequence, do not have adequate information about how to prevent transmission. As an example, research has found that in some samples, a large percentage of Asian/Pacific Islander men who have sex with men had never taken an HIV test. Anti-immigrant discrimination has been found to be associated with higher levels of unprotected intercourse with secondary partners among Asian and Pacific Islander men who identify as gay.

Implications for Mental Health Care Providers

Asians and Pacific Islanders may encounter significant barriers in addition to the stigma associated with same-sex sexual behavior and HIV in their efforts to obtain HIV/AIDS prevention education, HIV testing and counseling, and HIV care if they are HIV-seropositive. Individuals who are undocumented most often lack health care insurance and consequently may find it difficult to locate sources of care. Even when individuals are able to locate an appropriate source of care, undocumented individuals may fear that they will be reported to immigration authorities. Not infrequently, the staff of a clinic, AIDS service organization, or public health department that provides HIV-related services cannot communicate in the same language as the client. These findings suggest that competent, culturally sensitive and linguistically appropriate case management services may be particularly critical in order for HIV-infected clients to obtain adequate care for both their mental health care needs and their HIV-related care needs.

Related Topics: Access to care, case management, discrimination, HIV counseling, HIV testing, immigration, sexual orientation, stigma and stigmatization.

Suggested Reading

Chin, J. J., Kang, E., Kim, J. H., Martinez, J., & Eckholdt, H. (2006). Serving Asians and Pacific Islanders with HIV/AIDS: Challenges and lessons learned. *Journal of Health Care for the Poor and Underserved, 17*, 910–927.

Zaidi, I. F., Crepaz, N., Song, R., Wan, C. K., Lin, L. S., Hu, D. J., et al. (2005). Epidemiology of HIV/AIDS among Asians and Pacific Islanders in the United States. *AIDS Education and Prevention, 17*(5), 405–417.

Suggested Resources

Centers for Disease Control and Prevention. (2008, August). *CDC HIV/AIDS fact sheet: HIV/AIDS among Asians and Pacific Islanders*. Atlanta, GA: Author. Retrieved April 5, 2012 from http://www.cdc.gov/hiv/resources/factsheets/pdf/api.pdf

National Alliance of State & Territorial AIDS Directors, & Asian & Pacific Islander American Health Forum. (2009). *Breaking the silence: Key issues and recommendations to address HIV/AIDS among Asian Americans, Native Hawaiians, and Pacific Islanders in the United States*. Retrieved April 5, 2012 from http://www.apiahf.org/sites/default/files/HIV_Report05_2009.pdf

Bisexuality

Lisa R. Norman

A significant number of people do not fit neatly into the categories of heterosexual or homosexual because they experience sexual and emotional attractions and feelings for people of different sexes at some point during their lives. For lack of a better term, they are called "bisexuals." It is important to recognize that someone who is bisexual does not necessarily experience equal attraction to men and to women. Rather, the intensity of the attraction to one sex may be greater than to the other, but the individual may, nevertheless, identify as bisexual.

Many bisexual individuals do not reveal their sexual orientation and, as a result, bisexual people as a group are nearly invisible in society. While gay and lesbian women have come together and organized politically and community-wise, bisexual people have been much slower to come out of the closet, create community, and to form political and social networks to gain visibility and political clout.

Due to the rigid dichotomy with which our society categories sexual orientation—gay/lesbian or homosexual and straight or heterosexual—many bisexuals feel alienated and rejected by gay men and lesbian women, as well as by straight men and women. Many bisexual people complain that they feel like outsiders in both the straight and gay/lesbian worlds, and that they cannot fit in anywhere, feeling isolated and confused. Research has shown that bisexual people suffer from social isolation even more than gay men or lesbians because they lack any community where they can find acceptance and role models. Being bisexual leads to social marginalization; indeed, they may be viewed as challenging the very concept of sexuality. As a result, bisexual people must struggle to invent their own identities to correspond to their own experiences. Forming a bisexual identity helps bisexual people to structure, to make sense of, and to give meaning and definition to their reality. This situation can lead to significant mental distress.

Homophobia, stigma, and discrimination still persist in the United States and other parts of the world that negatively affect the health and well-being of bisexual

L.R. Norman (✉)
Ponce School of Medicine, Ponce, Puerto Rico
e-mail: lnorman@psm.edu

S. Loue (ed.), *Mental Health Practitioner's Guide to HIV/AIDS*,
DOI 10.1007/978-1-4614-5283-6_13, © Springer Science+Business Media New York 2013

individuals. Negative attitudes concerning bisexuality can lead to rejection by friends and family, discriminatory acts, and violence. Laws and policies may also adversely affect the lives of bisexual persons. These are social determinants that can affect physical and mental health, e.g., the availability of health care services for bisexually-identified persons and the quality of the services they receive. Such barriers to health need to be addressed at different levels of society, such as the health care setting, in order to increase opportunities for improving the health of bisexual individuals. Attention to these issues is critical: bisexuals have been found to be eight times more likely to try to commit suicide; six times more likely to report high levels of depression, three times more likely to use illegal drugs, and, three times more likely to have risky sex than heterosexuals or homosexuals.

In general, bisexuals have been ignored in HIV prevention efforts and service programs. Bisexual persons, like their homosexual and heterosexual counterparts, engage in at-risk sexual and social behaviors that place them at high risk of contracting HIV infection, including unprotected sex with men, an increased number of sexual partners, the use of injection drugs, and exposure to fluids known to transmit HIV, including vaginal secretions and semen. Three sexual activities have been labeled as particularly high risk behaviors for HIV. These include oral sex (among both male and female bisexuals), sharing sex toys (among female bisexuals), and fisting (among both male and female bisexuals).

Little research has been devoted to the study of bisexual sexual play. Sexual practices, especially among female bisexuals, include genital-to-genital rubbing, sex play with toys absent of protective barriers, stimulation of genital/anal areas with hands and mouth, and other sex play that involves fluid exchange needs further study. The relationship between what constitutes sex between women and women's risk of HIV certainly deserves more attention.

While much attention has been given to men who have sex with men (MSM) and their sexual activities, much less has been given to men who engage in sexual activities with both men and women. Many messages that target MSM do not resonate with these men because they do not self-identify themselves as MSMs and as such, they see the messages as irrelevant. This is quite common in the African-American community, which is known as having sex on the "down low." This is a term that is used to describe the behavior of men who have sex with other men as well as women and who do not self-identify themselves as gay or bisexual. While it is often associated with the African-American community, the behavior exists in other groups, including non-Hispanic Whites, Latinos, and Asians. While the down low concept has gained much attention in recent years, however, there are no data to confirm or refute publicized accounts of HIV risk behavior associated with these men. Until these men are able to "come out" and disclose their sexual behavior, their risk of HIV acquisition and transmission will continue to increase. However, the stigma associated with same-sex sexual relations not only dissuades men from disclosing this important information but also results in an increase in the mental distress associated with their efforts to maintain secrecy.

Bisexuals seeking mental health services frequently present with issues of depression, suicidal ideation, and fear of rejection. However, they may face many barriers in their efforts to obtain care. There continues to be a lack of training for mental health care providers related to bisexuality and, as a result, there is often an absence of cultural sensitivity to bisexual persons seeking mental health care.

Related Topics: Cultural sensitivity, risk behaviors, sexual orientation, stigma and stigmatization.

Suggested Reading

Storr, M. (1999). *Bisexuality: A critical reader*. London: Routledge Publishers.

Weinberg, M. S., Williams, C. J., & Pryor, D. W. (1994). *Dual attraction: Understanding bisexuality*. New York, NY: Oxford.

Wright, M., & Rosser, S. (1998). *New international directions in HIV prevention for gay and bisexual men*. New York, NY: Taylor and Francis Publishers.

Blood and Blood Disorders

Beth Faiman

Blood and HIV Transmission

Blood is the main vehicle for HIV transmission. Other frequent modes of HIV transmission occur from unprotected sexual intercourse, direct needle injection with or infusion of contaminated blood or blood products, or when using unsterilized equipment previously used by a known HIV infected person. An infected mother may transmit the virus to her unborn child or through breastfeeding.

The risk of transmission from a client with HIV to a mental health practitioner is extremely low as the virus is not airborne, foodborne, or waterborne. Usual casual contacts such as holding or shaking hands, kissing, hugging, or coughing do not result in transmission. Healthcare workers are at the highest risk to contract HIV from an infected needlestick injury but this risk remains low and is estimated at <1%. Thus it is rare to develop HIV through usual care and if the practitioner performs universal precautions.

Universal precautions are designed to prevent the spread of bloodborne diseases such as HIV and hepatitis B when healthcare is administered. Developed by the Centers for Disease Control and Prevention (CDC) in 1987, universal precautions include the practices of avoiding blood and bodily fluids by using gloves, gowns or masks when applicable. The mental health practitioner can employ universal precautions by handwashing before and after client contact, and avoidance of blood and body fluids. Universal precautions are intended for *all* clients and not just those infected with HIV.

It is imperative that the mental health practitioner understand modes of HIV transmission. The client may wish to see only the mental health practitioner and not follow with a routine medical provider. Thus the practitioner needs to work with each client to reduce possible exposures. These include avoiding both contaminated

B. Faiman (✉)
Cleveland Clinic Taussig Cancer Institute, Cleveland, OH, USA
e-mail: faimanb@ccf.org

S. Loue (ed.), *Mental Health Practitioner's Guide to HIV/AIDS*,
DOI 10.1007/978-1-4614-5283-6_14,

blood such as through sharing injection equipment if using substances and unprotected sexual relations, and exercising caution with sexual relations when the client or partner is menstruating. Although approximately 6,000 women with HIV give birth per year, the risk to the unborn child of becoming infected is as low as 1–2% when antiretroviral therapy is administered during pregnancy. It is important to emphasize this reduced risk with medication adherence and routine medical care if your client is or wishes to become or pregnant.

Blood Disorders and the Bone Marrow Environment

Blood disorders are often diagnosed on a routine test called a complete blood count (CBC). A CBC is obtained by healthcare providers (HCPs) to screen for a variety of diseases and health conditions or to investigate client concerns such as fatigue. The presence of blood disorders has been well documented since the beginning of the HIV/AIDS epidemic. If untreated, blood disorders can negatively affect ones' quality of life and lead to unwanted complications such as hospitalization, prolonged illness or death.

Human bone marrow is the major site of hematopoiesis, or the formation of new blood cells. The bone marrow of a healthy individual has the ability to produce hematopoietic stem cells which mature into various cell lines. Blood disorders can occur through a series of changes or alterations to the structure of each cell line. Through a complicated mechanism, HIV itself can infect healthy bone marrow cells. This in turn causes a series of blood abnormalities.

The bone marrow produces white blood cell (WBC) precursors, erythrocytes (red blood cell [RBC] precursors) and megakaryocytes (platelet precursors). In order to evaluate these cells a bone marrow biopsy must be performed. With this procedure a needle is gently inserted into the spongy bone marrow and a small sample is removed. A hematopathologist analyzes these cell lines under a microscope. Changes to one or more of the cell lines will not allow healthy cells to mature and proliferate and lead to the development of blood disorders. A normal bone marrow environment allows WBC, RBC, and platelets the ability to move into the blood stream and carry out their roles. The number of each can be measured by a routine complete blood count (CBC) blood draw.

Red Blood Cell Disorders: Anemia

Anemia is defined as reduced blood cell (RBC) mass or blood hemoglobin (Hb) and is a sign of an underlying disorder. Hemoglobin is a molecule responsible for carrying oxygen with the blood. Symptoms of anemia include fatigue, shortness of breath, and pale skin or mucous membranes. Anemia is diagnosed on CBC when the blood Hb is low. The normal range varies according to the age of the individual but is usually between 12 and 16 gm/dL. Symptoms of anemia are more pronounced when the anemia is more severe. Many studies have demonstrated that even mild anemia can negatively affect ones' quality of life.

Reasons for anemia in HIV/AIDS may be due to bleeding, increased RBC destruction (break down of RBC in the blood), or decreased RBC production within the bone marrow. Individuals with HIV/AIDS may develop anemia from causes such as iron deficiency, vitamin B-12 deficiency or hepatitis infection. Potent antiretroviral therapies can lead to anemia which ranges from mild to severe. G6PD deficiency is a genetic condition that may cause anemia as a result of RBC destruction after exposure to oxidant drugs.

Treatment of anemia is aimed at correcting the underlying cause. Supportive care for mild anemia may include oral iron or vitamin replacement (if deficiencies occur), encouraging the individual to limit strenuous activities, and maintain adequate hydration and rest. Transfusion of packed RBC in the setting of severe anemia (Hb <8 gm/dL) may be necessary depending on the severity of symptoms.

White Blood Cell Disorders: Leukopenia and Lymphopenia

White blood cells (WBC) or leukocytes are produced on the myeloid cell line within the bone marrow. Integral to a functioning immune system, healthy WBC and their components are responsible for protecting the individual from infection. The total WBC count is comprised of cells with unique roles. Two very important components of the WBC include neutrophils and lymphocytes. Neutrophils are key infection fighting cells and first—responders to clear bacteria from a site of infection. Neutropenia refers to low blood neutrophil counts. Lymphocytes are necessary to protect against viral illness. The total population of T-lymphocytes is low or absent in HIV/AIDS. Although total WBC counts are commonly low in HIV/AIDS, most infections occur as a result of damaged T-lymphocytes and opportunistic infections rather than due to neutropenia.

Platelet Disorders

Platelets are cells that produce a variety of blood clotting factors. When blood platelets are low (called thrombocytopenia), they place the individual at risk for spontaneous bleeding with little or no trauma. A diagnosis of thrombocytopenia is made when platelet counts fall below 150×10^9/L. The average lifespan of a platelet is 5–9 days.

The pathophysiology of platelet disorders is quite complex. However, similar to anemia, platelets can be low due to decreased bone marrow platelet production or increased platelet destruction. Idiopathic thrombocytopenia purpura (ITP) and thrombotic thrombocytopenia purpura (TTP) are two platelet disorders seen in HIV/AIDS.

The diagnosis of thrombocytopenia is first made by drawing a CBC which quantifies the blood platelet count. When thrombocytopenia is diagnosed, a hematopathologist will look at a blood smear under the microscope. This can identify if there is peripheral destruction of platelets once the cells mature and migrate out of the bone marrow. If the blood smear does not show platelet destruction, a bone marrow aspiration and biopsy will be necessary. This will evaluate if the megakaryocytes, or platelet precursors, are present or absent which may explain why healthy functioning platelets are not being produced.

The emphasis of treatment for thrombocytopenia is to determine the cause of low platelets and prevent bleeding. Immune therapies such as corticosteroids or change in medication regimen can be expected if destruction is occurring. Blood platelet transfusions may be necessary if platelet counts are critically low $<20 \times 10^9$/L when the risk of spontaneous bleeding is high.

Additional Considerations

It is important for the mental health practitioner to be aware of blood transmission, blood disorders and their manifestations. Casual contact does not result in HIV transmission, thus the practitioner should remain confident to provide the same care to an individual with HIV as they would to another. Prevention of HIV occurs through avoidance of blood and body fluids. Treatment with antiretroviral therapy during pregnancy can prevent the spread of HIV from an infected mother to her baby.

Blood disorders may occur throughout the course of the disease. Newer drugs are less likely to impact blood counts as in the past, but HIV/AIDS itself may cause blood disorders. If a client complains of feeling tired, experiences easy bruising or bleeding, referral to a medical care provider for further evaluation is warranted. Prompt recognition and treatment of anemia, leukopenia and thrombocytopenia can prevent unnecessary complications in these individuals.

Related Topics: Antiretroviral therapy, prevention strategies.

Suggested Reading

Aberg, J. A., Kaplan, J. E., Libman, H., Emmanuel, P., Anderson, J. R., Stone, V. E., et al. (2009). Primary care guidelines for the management of persons infected with human immunodeficiency virus: 2009 Update by the HIV Medicine Association of the Infectious Diseases Society of America. *Clinical Infectious Diseases, 49*(5), 651–681.

Recht, M. (2009). Thrombocytopenia and anemia in infants and children. *Emergency Medicine Clinics of North America, 27*(3), 505–523.

Stasi, R., Willis, F., Shannon, M. S., & Gordon-Smith, E. C. (2009). Infectious causes of chronic immune thrombocytopenia. *Hematology/Oncology Clinics of North America, 23*(6), 1275–1297. doi:10.1016/j.hoc.2009.08.009.

Suggested Resources

Centers for Disease Control and Prevention. (2012). Retrieved January 18, 2012 from http://www.cdc.gov/niosh/topics/bbp/universal.html

The Merck Manual of Hematology and Oncology (2012). On-line. Retrieved January 14, 2012 from http://www.merckmanuals.com/professional/hematology_and_oncology.html?qt=&sc=&alt=

Caregiving and Caregivers

Helen Land

Remarkable strides have been made in the treatment of HIV/AIDS, yet a considerable proportion of those infected with the virus may continue to require care. Those with cognitive deficits, those aging into a second decade of HIV infection, and those struggling with debilitating physical and mental symptoms may need at home caregiving. Since its inception, AIDS caregivers have provided physical, mental, and spiritual support to the infected. As AIDS was first identified the majority of caregivers were young, white, gay males who were largely unprepared to provide care for a young, terminally ill partner or friend. Today, HIV is increasingly a chronic disease of the disenfranchised: the poor, especially women and men of color, injection drug users, sex workers, the homeless, the young, and those approaching their senior years. Paralleling changes in the HIV infected are changes in the face of AIDS caregivers. Caregivers are a diverse group of people with varied perceptions and experiences of caregiving. Yet even under the best of all possible circumstances, there is one factor which binds them together: the stress of caregiving for a person with AIDS is often experienced as being burdensome at some level. Whether caregiving burden is perceived to be largely a physical burden, a psychological burden, or both and what mediates the burdensome experience depends on a number of factors. Even when the amount of burden reported differs across caregiver group, the common sequelae of caregiving for a person with AIDS are often physical health problems and depression.

Caregivers continue to provide a valuable service. As AIDS care has moved to home-based care and health care costs persistently rise, the significance of informal systems of care becomes commensurately greater. This entry examines the needs of a diversity of HIV caregivers and targets recommendations for each caregivers group on methods of increasing caregiver well-being.

H. Land (✉)
School of Social Work, University of Southern California, Los Angeles, CA, USA
e-mail: Land@usc.edu

S. Loue (ed.), *Mental Health Practitioner's Guide to HIV/AIDS*,
DOI 10.1007/978-1-4614-5283-6_15,

Differences in the Stress Process and Experience of Burden

Generally, stress is experienced both on physical and psychological levels. Objective burden is conceptualized as the strain resulting from direct negotiation of situational stressors, including the demands of the physical activities required in the caretaking process (e.g., bathing and feeding the care recipient). Subjective burden is conceptualized as the emotional/experiential appraisal of caregiving such as feeling entrapped by the tasks required, feeling anxious or depressed about what the future holds for the ill family member, and the additional conflicts between family members secondary to the strain of caretaking. Moreover, findings indicate that the cultural background of the caregiver greatly influences the appraisal of burden, in addition to stressful events, use of support, and coping behaviors. Investigations suggest that differences in the quantity of burden a caregiver reports is associated with ethnicity or racial culture. Importantly, the experience of burden varies with caregiver characteristics including relationship to the person with AIDS, residence of the care giver, the ethnic or racial and cultural background of the caregiver, religious and spiritual involvement, the number of years in providing care, age of both the caregiver and the recipient, and the physical health status of both. Recent studies suggest that caregiving is indeed experienced in diverse ways; thus we must first understand the experience if we are to provide support for diverse groups of caregivers.

A Closer Perspective of AIDS Caregivers: A Varied Group with Varied Needs

Gay Men

Most scientific information on AIDS caregiving is available on gay male caregivers as men who have sex with men were the first to receive highly active antiretroviral therapy (HAART) and move from hospital care to home. Along with this shift in care came the needs for caregiving. With HIV viral loads reduced for countless numbers, many gained a renewed life; others with HIV continued to experienced decline or debilitating side effects from medication including insulin resistance, elevated triglycerides with increased risk of heart attack, and heightened risk of bone fractures and avascular necrosis due to corticosteroid therapy. The need for hip and knee replacements became more likely. For this group, because illness associated with aging is showing up earlier than expected in peer cohorts, assistance with activities of daily living (ADLs) is often required. Other symptoms of aging with HIV include memory and cognitive deficits, and liver and kidney disease. These are conditions that may be experienced as especially burdensome for caregivers.

Caregivers for this group largely consist of aging gay men experiencing episodes of severe depression that are associated with objective burden: the direct tasks of caregiving such as bathing, toileting, managing problematic behavior, and cognitive impairments. In fact, male caregivers seem to be more vulnerable to feeling overloaded in their caregiving roles than do other groups, perhaps because they are less socialized to perform such tasks. In fact, among these caregivers vulnerability to depression rises as ecological factors such as younger caregiver age, lower income, lower educational level, and unemployment increase. Other factors impacting depression may include internalized homophobia and HIV-related stigma. Moreover, it likely that this group of caregivers has experienced sustained multiple HIV-related losses which can result in a potent prescription for depression. Yet for others with dispositional optimism who cope by viewing everyday as a gift of life to savor, resiliency to stress is more readily at hand. Other conditions which appear to buffer stress in this group of caregivers include higher feelings of self worth, stronger sense of mastery over life, and an active coping styles. Among those caregivers who are themselves HIV-positive, family support can play a cardinal role in lowering stress and depression.

Today, middle-aged and older partners and male friends of men who have sex with men continue to provide care to the HIV infected who have aged into their middle and senior years. Service providers will need to assess the specific type of burden experienced by this group of caregivers. Objective burdens often respond to increased caregiving resources such as housekeeping services and respite care. Depression treatment including medication evaluation may be necessary. Support groups in the gay community are readily available and can be quite effective in increasing sense of control and empowerment.

Women as Caregivers

Women have provided caregiving for people with AIDS since the beginning of the pandemic. Commonly, working class and poor women of color now assume the bulwark of caregiving. Such women may be wives, mothers, sisters, and in-laws of those requiring care. Even female adolescents and pre-teens provide a portion of AIDS caregiving to disabled mothers and fathers.

Female AIDS caregivers dedicate an extensive portion of their lives to all manner of caregiving: to their families including children, partners, parents, and in-laws in addition to caregiving for a person affected by HIV/AIDS. Research findings reveal that about half of these women are themselves infected and are caring for others with HIV, thus resulting in multiple caregiving responsibilities for people of all ages. Female caregivers of color are a very diverse group. The majority is Latina from diverse cultures including the Caribbean, Central and South America, or they are of African-American heritage. While HIV in Asian populations is growing, Asian female informal caregivers continue to be fewer in number in the USA and Canada. It is paramount for service providers to assess cultural values with Latin cultural groups as those whose ethnic origin is the Caribbean may hold distinct values from those of Central or South America. Migration history is important to assess and particularly recency of arrival to the USA as acculturative stress may profoundly impact the burden experienced in caregiving.

Latina Caregivers. Particularly in Latino communities where cultural gender role expectations are strong women comprise the great majority of AIDS caregiving. Especially for the newly immigrated, the caregiving experience may be more burdensome than for other groups. Latina AIDS caregivers may be coping with the stress of acculturation and they may be monolingual Spanish-speaking. Therefore, they may lack knowledge of medical and social service resources, and importantly, few may exist in their neighborhoods and even fewer with cultural values parallel to their own. Moreover, this group of caregivers likely ended their compulsory education at grade eight, and they may have arrived in the USA from rural areas where a complex bureaucratic system of medical care and associated medical regimens simply do not exist. In spite of this situation, research findings indicate that family members and caregivers themselves view outside social service support as unnecessary, intrusive, and insensitive to family needs. Hence, these caregivers may be reluctant to seek outside help or early care for their own illnesses. In addition, those who are undocumented may fear being deported. Those who are seropositive likely were infected through heterosexual contact with an injecting drug user, through use of unsterile injecting equipment used for culturally prescribed medical treatment, or more commonly, through sexual contact with a man who had unprotected sex with another man. Often their serostatus goes undetected until a prenatal appointment reveals a high viral load. For these women, being seropositive is simply one condition among other chronic illnesses including diabetes, asthma, heart disease, and hypertension, all of which may culminate in physical depletion and impair caregiving responsibilities. Often, it is common in Latina cultures to put the needs of others ahead of one's own (*simpatía*) and to be long suffering in the face of stress in imitation of the Virgin Mary (*Marianismo*). In addition, religious coping such as *mandas* (rituals of sacrifice such as hair cutting) are customary.

Literature reveals that the stress process differs for this group of caregivers. Major life events such as being forced to move from one's home also have been implicated in the stress process. Moreover, due to HIV stigma it is quite likely that many women involved in AIDS caregiving lack a confidant(e), even within the family, who is aware of the particulars of their situation including the HIV status of themselves and the care recipient. To be an effective caregiver, they must care for a sick relative, facilitate required services often within a complex urban environment, understand the care plan, and maintain adequate health to care for others in the family.

In light of these circumstances, it is not surprising that these women face a powerful stress process. Despite heavy caregiving responsibilities, few report objective burden due to direct caregiving. Instead, in combination with poor health and major life events, it is the management of cognitive difficulties with the care recipient, feeling trapped and isolated in the caregiving role, and poor self esteem which predict poorer mental health for Latina AIDS caregivers. In addition, anxiety due to low adherence behaviors in others has been frequently cited.

Implications for service call for a multipronged approach to meet both physical and mental health needs. Advances in service call for culturally appropriate service plans. Health promoters (*promotoras*) who are indigenous to the community may succeed in providing support, education, and limiting psychological burdens for this caregiver group. Moreover, they may succeed in influencing belief systems that affect stigma and guilt surrounding HIV. Because religious and spiritual coping is likely to be strong, service providers may include spiritually based interventions such as prayer and meditation, which may be efficacious as affect regulators. In addition a Spanish speaking telephone buddy who may be called on for advice and support may be useful. It is unlikely that services such as support groups which require additional time commitment and are externally based would provide needed assistance. However, a cooperative caregiving service including a church-based or community-based approach to support is likely to be effective in reducing caregiving burden.

African-American Women. African-American female AIDS caregivers are a very diverse group. They are older women caring for adult daughters with HIV, young women caring for children whose health is compromised by HIV, and women caring for partners. Others may include adolescents caring for infected parents. Both professionally and informally, African-American women have long provided care for others in this country. Literature suggests that informal caregiving is largely culturally normative among African-Americans compared to other US-born populations. These women are a strong resource in their community and often lead lives of self-sacrifice and dedication caregiving for multiple family members in more than one generation. They are often of lower socioeconomic status, have greater disease burden, and have lower life expectancies than other cohorts of HIV caregivers.

There are many interacting circumstances which make caregiving especially challenging for this group. First, drug use and increased incarceration of drug offenders in African-American communities have fueled infection rates due to HIV. Prevalence rates of HIV among African-American men who have sex with men is very high. Moreover, in many communities those who are HIV-negative may harbor homophobic reactions resulting in substantial stigmatization of HIV-positive men and their caregivers. Further, the African-American church is not seen as a resource for the HIV-infected; hence, it plays less of a central role in addressing social welfare needs of the community of infected and their caregivers. Such is the case in large part due to stigma surrounding HIV transmission methods. Thus, HIV lives underground in many African-American communities, present yet absent in acknowledgment of its damage.

Impacting caregiving is the status for whom caregivers provide care. African-American women are at high risk for disease transmission primarily due to drug use and secondarily due to unprotected sexual activity with an HIV infected partner. Importantly, disproportionate drug use and competing subsistence needs among African-Americans contribute to lower access to HIV treatment. Moreover, economic costs for HIV medical care for injection drug users are greater due to their commensurately greater use of hospital services. Drug and alcohol use may follow with the increased need to regulate emotional responses due to these realities. Not surprisingly, use of substances may result in injurious outcomes for those who are seropositive. These factors set a background against which HIV care giving plays out. In the context of little access to formal medical care, informal care needs may be especially great. The culmination of these influences compound the complexity of caregiving for African-American female caregivers.

In the majority, HIV-positive African-American women are likely to be low income single parents who are unemployed and/or receive public assistance. The need to provide care to others presents an overwhelming demand on scarce resources. Unfortunately, these are women who are at very high risk for a number of reasons. They are more likely than other HIV-positive women to be at risk for substance abuse and subsistence sex work. Other sources suggest that alcohol is used as a method for self medication among African-American women and especially in those caregivers who have access to fewer resources and great childcare and family responsibilities. Moreover, such women are more likely than men with alcohol problems to experience depression and anxiety. Considerable evidence also documents that rates of heavy drinking and drug use are higher among people living with HIV/AIDS and their caregivers and specifically higher among African-American HIV-positive women with lower incomes and lower levels of education who are caregiving than among other seropositive caregivers. In fact, study findings report that of African-American female caregivers who provide primary support of the people with AIDS, 26% were current drug users, 6% reported drinking daily, a majority were living below the poverty line (54%), and nearly a quarter of these women were HIV positive. Because alcohol use among people with HIV/AIDS is associated with behavioral issues related to the treatment and management of HIV disease, these caregivers have diminished chances of being prescribed antiretroviral treatment (HAART). For those who do receive HAART, heavy alcohol use is associated with higher HIV (RNA) levels and lower CD4 counts, indicating reduced efficacy of treatments. In addition to impacting the effectiveness of these medications, heavy drinking has been shown to amplify the toxicity of HIV medications. These findings have substantial implications both for many African-American HIV-infected female caregivers and the person for whom they provide care. Of great concern, these women often experience late diagnosis and treatment of their HIV illness. They are disproportionately impacted by histories of physical and sexual abuse, and both emotional and physical abuse in their adult intimate relationships. Depression and other mental health problems are implicated as outcomes.

There are multiple implications for caregiver services targeted for this group. Economic and structural supports such as financial help, housing, and child care are crucial. In addition, there is the clear need for advocacy in the area of medical treatment for HIV and, if needed, substance abuse treatment. Depression screening and treatment may also be required. These services should be gender-sensitive and focus on the needs of the African-American female experience. The history of caregiving among women of African-American heritage is long and strong. Programs must be designed to be relevant to these women who have cared for others across the generations.

Non-Hispanic White Women. Investigations indicate that Non-Hispanic White female AIDS caregivers differ substantially from their sisters of color. Most have attained high levels of education, have medical insurance, are HIV seronegative, and are caring for an adult partner or child with HIV. Moreover, this group of caregivers experiences fewer physical illnesses and has more years AIDS caregiving than other female caregiving groups. Major stressors associated with elevated depression center on subjective burden, such as a feeling of being captive to the caregiving role and a loss of identity to caregiving. Stronger levels of self-esteem appear to mediate this relationship. In addition, White women seek more services for depression than any other group of caregivers which may point to their knowledge of resources and willingness to reach out for help.

For this group of caregivers, efforts such as respite care and support groups may be helpful in decreasing loss of identity and role captivity and increasing social network, self esteem, and supportive psychoeducation. Depression treatment may be assessed and referrals made to appropriate facilities.

Male Primary Caregivers of Children

It is little known that the number of male primary caregivers of children with HIV is substantial in the USA. Fathers, uncles, and grandfathers have taken up where mothers and other female relatives have left off in the primary care of these children. Only about half have some support of a female caregiver.

The majority (75%) are biological fathers and adoptive fathers of the child with AIDS. It is estimated that about 10% of these men are caring for more than one HIV-infected child and about half have other children in the home for whom they provide care. A large percentage of these invisible caregivers are African-American (58%) and Latinos (23%) caring for children with AIDS between the ages of 5 and 12 years. These men of color suffer from particular issues related to gender and racial discrimination with service agencies. For example, African-American men are the bearers of many negative stereotypes, most commonly the absentee father. As a result, medical and service providers may hold prejudices concerning the father's skill level for setting limits with children, or believe that they are limited in caring for or communicating with a sick child. Fathers may face challenges in terms of custodial rights to their children, thus complicating their fathering and caregiving responsibilities. Social service agencies may investigate and evaluate these fathers in a way that mothers do not have to endure. Plans for foster care placement for these children may surface without adequate assessment of the family status. Interrogations by medical and service providers and school personnel involved in the child's life may be experienced by male primary caregivers as shaming, intrusive, hostile, and emotionally exhausting. About a quarter of all male primary caregivers are estimated to be HIV-infected themselves and thus may have diminished energy for these external demands.

Such children, many of whom are HIV-infected, grow up with significant physical, developmental, and emotional problems. Hence, parenting these children poses a compelling challenge. Most male primary caregivers live alone with one or more children and have only sporadic instrumental or emotional support from friends and relatives on which to rely. Moreover, both child and father are likely to be actively grieving from the loss of the female relationship presence in the home. Because the bereavement process itself is experienced as depressing and enervating, caregiving resilience is likely to be inhibited. In addition, because children of different ages grieve differently, the father must have a repertoire of varying responses to the emotional needs of his children during this most complicated time. Anxiety surrounding how they will raise their children in the absence of their spousal support may be present. Those men with jobs face particular challenges with caregiver-job role strain as they must negotiate whether to go to work or stay at home with a sick child, or whether to reduce their work load hours or quit their jobs. Reduced hours and unemployment inevitably have an impact as financial obligations escalate, especially during economically challenging times. Given both internal and external stress, it is easy to understand why fathers are reluctant to access services and may be hesitant to provide information about their needs to service providers. Such circumstances may culminate in a sequence of mounting needs with few supports to meet them.

It is paramount for service providers to make time to build strong rapport and a working alliance with these caregivers. One is to inquire about the father's perception of need in the assessment. Service providers succeed when a strengths model is used. An alliance between client and provider is sustained when the client's own words can be accessed and repeated back to empower, sustain, and to continue on as head of their household. Concomitantly, service providers may assist in coaching and supporting fathers with this multilayered complex situation.

Grandparents and Other Older Relatives

Grandparents have been caregivers of their grandchildren for generations prior to the AIDS pandemic. Particularly in African-American and Latino communities, grandmothers have played a vital role in the family system, supporting parents who worked several jobs, or assuming the entire responsibility for child rearing where parents were unable to do so.

In the presence of AIDS, grandparents are a foundation for many children orphaned by the disease. Here, the conjugal picture involves a family system that may be extended to the utmost as aging grandparents care for young children when they themselves may require care.

Stress for these caregivers begins to proliferate as abridged energies in this group of senior caregivers inexorably confronts the needs of children who may be sick due to HIV infection, or who have been bereaved. The manifold needs of children coupled with the needs of the caregiver must be recognized. If the child is HIV-positive, the grandparent may grow to be anxious about medication regimen and overall health maintenance issues. Such ongoing stress can be extremely compromising.

A major stressor for this group of caregivers revolves around emotional and behavioral issues of grandchildren. At times, grandparents are caring for both their own offspring and grandchild. Bereaved children present a challenging set of circumstances even under ideal conditions. It is likely that these children have had to undergo several residential relocations, they have changed schools, they have lost a major attachment with their primary caregiver, and sometimes, they are sick themselves. Disruption in stability may result in behavioral problems. Grandparents have described externalizing behaviors as major caregiving concerns. Health concerns for this group are also significant should the grandparent need to go to the hospital or become ill themselves.

Such an intricate care situation presents challenges in service provision. Caregiver needs may include both physical and psychological care associated with their stressors. As with other caregivers, depression is a frequent occurrence and should be addressed. Moreover, given the tendency of these caregivers, mostly women, to put the needs of their grandchildren ahead of their own, service providers must take special consideration to inquire about caregiver well-being and needed services. A psychoeducational approach which encompasses sensitivity and knowledge of their unique situation coupled with education about available community services is a starting place. More definitively, caregiver grandparents may benefit from telephone support groups, stress management training, and case management for the multiple needs of all family members.

Conclusion

In their daily lives, many caregivers endure continuous fatigue, chronic substantial stress and illness, lasting depression and rely on few resources. Many face poverty; nearly all face stigma. Despite these conditions, countless AIDS caregivers report a sense of gain from HIV caregiving, more so than do caregivers coping with other illnesses. Those who fare better seem to adopt an attitude of having control over the role that HIV has in life, thus putting the virus in perspective. Getting involved in HIV/AIDS work outside the immediate caregiving relationship seems to increase feelings of empowerment and altruism for some groups. Others describe heightened intimacy within the caregiving relationship. A sense of personal gain and purpose may take different expressions for varying caregiver groups. Other beneficial themes evident in the caregiving literature involve personal growth and positive personality changes, increased understanding of others and their illnesses, a sense of satisfaction and achievement, and gained perspective in life.

Each group of caregivers presents a distinctive set of conditions that necessitate service providers to, in a sense, be cognizant of all major groups affected by HIV disease. Such is the case as caregivers are representatives from these groups. They are gay men, women, single fathers, the aging, and grandparents. They are Latino/a, African-American, and Caucasian. Some are better off economically but most face poverty and the enormous odds of living in neighborhoods ravaged by drugs, violence, and stigma. Some have better capacities to access resources, others have very few resources available to meet their own needs, let alone the needs of the HIV-infected. Some caregivers are addicted, some fear leaving children or partners behind. Many are bereaved. A multitude of uncertainties lives in the lives of AIDS caregivers; one issue is definite: caregivers are prodigious in their commitment to those for whom they provide care.

Related Topics: Coping, social support.

Suggested Reading

Anderson, V. M. (1998). HIV infection in children: A medical overview. *Journal of the Child Welfare League of America, 57*, 107–114.

Aranda, M. P., & Knight, B. G. (1997). The influence of ethnicity and culture on the caregiver stress and coping process: A sociocultural view and analysis. *Gerontologist, 37*, 342–354.

Awad, A. G., & Voruganti, L. N. P. (2008). The burden of schizophrenia on caregivers: A review. *Pharmacoeconomics, 26*(2), 149–162.

Baronet, A. (1999). Factors associated with caregiver burden in mental illness: A critical review of the research literature. *Clinical Psychology Review, 19*(7), 819–841.

Beals, K. P., Wight, R. G., Aneshensel, C. S., Murphy, D., & Miller-Martinez, D. (2006). The role of family caregivers in HIV medication adherence. *AIDS Care, 18*(6), 589–596.

Billings, D. W., Folkman, S., Acree, M., & Moskowitz, J. T. (2000). Coping and physical health during care giving: The roles of positive and negative affect. *Journal of Personality and Social Psychology, 79*(1), 131–142.

Carlisle, C. (2000). The search for meaning in HIV and AIDS: The care-ers' experience. *Qualitative Health Research, 10*(6), 750–765.

Centers for Disease Control and Prevention. (2006). *CDC HIV fact sheet: HIV/AIDS among women*. Atlanta, GA: CDC. National Center for HIV, STD, and TB Prevention, Division of HIV/AIDS.

Chimwaza, A. F., & Watkins, S. C. (2004). Giving care to people with symptoms of AIDS in rural sub-Saharan Africa. *AIDS Care, 16*(7), 795–807.

Devine, D., Forehand, R., Morse, E., Simon, P., Clark, L., & Kernis, M. (2000). HIV infection in inner-city African-American women: The role of optimism in predicting depressive symptomatology. *International Journal of Rehabilitation & Health, 5*, 141–156.

Engel, M. (2008, February 5). With HIV, growing older faster. *Los Angeles, Times*, 14–15.

Fein, G., Fletcher, D. J., & Di Sclafani, V. (1998). Effect of chronic alcohol abuse on the CNS morbidity of HIV disease. *Alcoholism: Clinical and Experimental Research, 22*, 196S–200S.

Flexner, C. W., Cargill, V. A., Sinclair, J., Kresina, T. F., & Cheever, L. (2001). Alcohol use can result in enhanced drug metabolism in HIV pharmacotherapy. *AIDS Patient Care and STDs, 15*, 57–58.

Fredriksen-Goldsen, K. I. (2007). HIV/AIDS caregiving predictors of well-being and distress. *Journal of Gay and Lesbian Social Services, 18*(34), 53–73.

Jones, D. J., Beach, S. R. H., Forehand, R., & The Family Health Project Research Group. (2001). Disease status in African American single mothers with HIV: The role of depressive symptoms. *Health Psychology, 20*, 417–423.

Knowlton, A. R. (2003). Informal caregiving in a vulnerable populations: Toward a network resource framework. *Social Science and Medicine, 56*, 1307–1320.

Kung, W. W. (2003). The illness, stigma, culture, or immigration? Burdens on Chinese American caregivers of patients with schizophrenia. *Families in Society: The Journal of Contemporary Human Services, 84*(4), 547–557.

Land, H., & Hudson, S. (2002). HIV serostatus and factors related to physical and mental well-being in Latina family AIDS caregivers. *Social Science and Medicine, 54*(1), 147–159.

Land, H., & Hudson, S. (2004). Stress, coping, and depressive symptomatology in Latina and Anglo AIDS caregivers. *Psychology and Health, 19*(5), 643–666.

Land, H., Hudson, S., & Stefiel, B. (2003). Stress and depression among HIV-positive and HIV-negative gay and bisexual AIDS caregivers. *AIDS and Behavior, 7*(1), 41–53.

Linsk, N., & Mason, S. (2004). Stresses on grandparents and other relatives caring for children affected by HIV/AIDS. *Health and Social Work, 29*(2), 127–136.

Magana, S. (2007). Psychological distress among Latino family caregivers of adults with schizophrenia: The roles of burden and stigma. *Psychiatric Services, 58*(3), 378–384.

McAdoo, J. L. (1993). The roles of African-American fathers: An ecological perspective. *Families in Society, 74*, 28–35.

McCauland, J., & Pakenham, K. I. (2003). Investigation of the benefits of HIV/AIDS caregiving and relations among care giving adjustment, benefit finding, and stress and coping variables. *AIDS Care, 15*(6), 853–869.

Nabors, N., Seacat, J., & Rosenthal, M. (2002). Predictors of caregiver burden following traumatic brain injury. *Brain Injury, 16*(12), 1039–1050.

Neff, J. A., Amodei, N., Valescu, S., & Pomeroy, E. C. (2003). Psychological adaptation and distress among HIV+ Latina women: Adaptation to HIV in a Mexican American cultural context. *Social Work in Health Care, 37*, 55–74.

Oliveros, C. (2008). The Latino caregiver experience among dementia and non-dementia caregivers: Can community based care management improve caregiver health? *Dissertation Abstracts, 69*(4-B), 2275.

Ortiz, C. (2005). Disclosing concerns of Latinas living with HIV/AIDS. *Journal of Transcultural Nursing, 16*, 210–217.

Pearlin, L. I., Mullan, J. T., Aneshensel, C. S., Wardlaw, L., & Harrington, C. (1994). The structure and function of AIDS care giving relationships. *Psychosocial Rehabilitation Journal, 17*, 51–67.

Pondexter, C., Linsk, N., & Wagner, R. S. (1999). He listens and never gossips. Spiritual coping without church support among older, predominantly African American caregivers, of persons with HIV. *Review of Religious Research, 40*(3), 23–243.

Redgrave, G., Swartz, A., & Romanski, A. (2003). Alcohol misuse by women. *International Review of Psychiatry, 15*, 256–268.

Samet, J. H., Horton, N. J., Traphagen, E. T., Lyon, S. M., & Freedberg, K. A. (2003). Alcohol consumption and HIV disease progression: Are they related? *Alcoholism: Clinical and Experimental Research, 27*, 862–867.

Stetz, K. M., & Brown, M. A. (2004). Physical and psychosocial health in family care giving: A comparison of AIDS and cancer caregivers. *Public Health Nursing, 21*(6), 533–540.

Strug, D., Rabb, L., & Nanton, R. (2002). Provider views of the support service needs of male primary caretakers of HIV/AIDS-infected and affected children: A needs assessment. *Families in Society, 83*(3), 303–313.

Wight, R. G., Aneshensel, C. S., & LeBlanc, A. J. (2003). Stress buffering effects of family support in AIDS caregiving. *AIDS Care, 15*(5), 595–613.

Wohl, A. R., Lu, S., Odem, S., Sorvillo, F., Pegues, C. F., & Kerndt, P. R. (1998). Sociodemographic and behavioral characteristics of African-American women with HIV and

AIDS in Los Angeles County, 1990–1997. *Journal of Acquired Immune Deficiency Syndromes and Human Retrovirology, 19*, 412–420.

Wyatt, G., Carmona, J., Loeb, T., & Williams, J. (2005). HIV-positive Black women with histories of childhood sexual abuse: Patterns of substance use and barriers to health care. *Journal of Health Care for the Poor and Underserved, 16*, 9–23.

Case Management

M. Zane Jennings

Case management is a method of providing services that involves assisting clients in accessing resources and services from complex and fragmented health care and social service systems. The goal of case management is to improve clients' independence, health, and quality of life. Case management attempts to attain these goals by increasing access to care and resources and by tailoring needed services to individual client's needs.

Case management begins with assessment. In assessment, the case manager and client identify the client's current functioning, needs, and goals. Treatment planning follows assessment. Treatment planning is a collaborative effort between the client and the case manager that results in a plan for service. In the treatment plan, the necessary tasks to accomplish goals are identified. The case manager then assists the client in accomplishing the treatment plan goals by identifying and accessing resources and services that can help meet the client's needs. An ongoing evaluation of the plan and progress toward treatment goals by the case manager and client is necessary to insure that client needs are being addressed. While cognitive impairment or involuntary status may limit client involvement, client self-determination is the normal expectation.

The services provided by case managers can be diverse. Services can include such activities as linking to community and medical resources, advocating on the client's behalf with social services and medical providers, managing those services provided within the case manager's service site, and providing education and skill development to clients and their families. Case managers can help advocate for and provide continuity of care as clients move though social service and medical systems. Case management services can be relatively brief in nature or can be long-term and ongoing in order to support client functioning.

M.Z. Jennings (✉)
Mandel School of Applied Social Sciences, Case Western Reserve University, Cleveland, OH, USA
e-mail: Zane.Jennings@case.edu

S. Loue (ed.), *Mental Health Practitioner's Guide to HIV/AIDS*,
DOI 10.1007/978-1-4614-5283-6_16, © Springer Science+Business Media New York 2013

The resources accessed within case management are also diverse. These resources include primary care physicians, specialist physicians, child and adult protective services, home health agencies, mental health providers, substance abuse services, legal assistance, income maintenance programs, and programs providing assistance in paying for medical services and medications. The resources drawn upon by case management need not be formal services, but can include peer and family supports, self-help organizations, and religious communities. Resources are not limited to those listed above.

Case management services are especially helpful to those individuals and families who have complex needs and/or who require assistance from complex service systems. Individuals can face a bewildering number of possibilities when trying to find assistance, and by working through chance and effort alone may not find a helpful response. Those affected by HIV or other chronic health problems and those who have mental disabilities may find it especially difficult to get their needs met by the complicated and fragmented social service and medical systems they face.

Case managers may be social workers, nurses, or other social service professionals. Case managers typically have a bachelors or masters degree in an appropriate social service or medical field. Case managers need a range of skills in order to effectively assist their clients. Case managers need to be able to communicate effectively, organize their own time and paperwork, and problem-solve when clients present needs that are outside the case manager's own area of expertise. Necessary skills for case managers include empathy, clinical awareness of mental health and medical issues that may affect clients, knowledge of the range of resources available to assist clients, and persuasive negotiating abilities to navigate sometimes difficult service systems.

Case management in practice can differ, depending upon the client group needs and the history of case management with a particular population. Mental health case management and HIV case management are two examples of case management within different client populations, but there are many more. Mental health case management developed from a social work model of casework and expanded during the creation of community-based alternatives to institutionalization. Mental health case management often focuses on reducing hospitalizations, increasing independent-living skills, and providing advocacy and support to individuals and their families in order to integrate individuals with mental illness into the community.

HIV case management developed more recently in response to the emergence of AIDS in the United States. These case managers are often funded by the Ryan White Care Act. Case managers working with individuals with HIV assist clients with accessing needed medical care, medications, mental health care, and appropriate housing. Case managers often also encourage medical and medication compliance in order to increase the effectiveness of the medical interventions that clients are receiving.

Though case managers working with different groups may have somewhat different areas of focus, there is substantial overlap in needs between different client groups and overlap in membership among different client groups. It is possible that a client will be eligible for case management services from more than one case manager. These situations require effective and clear communication between the case managers and the client in order to bring most benefit to the client.

Related Topics: Access to care, coping, mental health comorbidity and HIV/AIDS, Ryan White Care Act, social support.

Suggested Reading

Frankel, A. J., & Gelman, S. R. (2004). *Case management: An introduction to concepts and skills.* Chicago, IL: Lyceum Books.

Suggested Resources

Fleisher, P., & Henrickson, M. (2002). *Towards a typology of case management.* Retrieved October 2, 2011 from ftp://ftp.hrsa.gov/hab/Typology.pdf

NASW Standards for Social Work Case Management. Washington, DC: National Association of Social Workers. Retrieved from http://www.socialworkers.org/practice/standards/sw_case_mgmt.asp

Centers for Disease Control and Prevention

Robert W. Stephens

The Centers for Disease Control and Prevention (or CDC) is a United States federal agency under the Department of Health and Human Services headquartered in Greater Atlanta, Georgia. The CDC's mission is: collaborating to create the expertise, information, and tools that people and communities need to protect their health—through health promotion, prevention of disease, injury and disability, and preparedness for new health threats. The CDC works to protect public health and safety by providing information to enhance health decisions, and it promotes health through partnerships with state health departments and other organizations. The CDC focuses national attention on developing and applying disease prevention and control, environmental health, occupational safety and health, health promotion, injury prevention and education activities designed to improve the health of the people of the United States.

The CDC was founded in 1942 during World War II as the Office of National Defense Malaria Control Activities. The new agency was a branch of the US Public Health Service, and Atlanta was chosen as the location because malaria was endemic to the Southern United States. The agency changed its name to the Communicable Disease Center in 1946. The mission of CDC expanded beyond its original focus on malaria to include sexually transmitted diseases when the Venereal Disease Division of the US Public Health Service (PHS) was transferred to the CDC in 1957. Shortly thereafter, Tuberculosis Control was transferred (in 1960) to the CDC from PHS, and then in 1963 the Immunization program was established. The organization became the National Communicable Disease Center (NCDC) effective July 1, 1967. The organization was renamed the Center for Disease Control (CDC) on June 24, 1970, and Centers for Disease Control effective October 14, 1980. Effective on October 27, 1992, an act of the United States Congress appended the words "and Prevention" to the name; however, Congress

R.W. Stephens (✉)
Rynearson, Suess, Schnurbusch & Champion, L.L.C., St. Louis, MO, USA
e-mail: rstephens@rssclaw.com

S. Loue (ed.), *Mental Health Practitioner's Guide to HIV/AIDS*,
DOI 10.1007/978-1-4614-5283-6_17,

directed that the initials CDC be retained because of its name recognition. The CDC operates under the Department of Health and Human Services umbrella.

The CDC is organized into several component organizations. These include the Office of the Director; Center for Global Health; the National Institute for Occupational Safety and Health; the Office of Infectious Disease; the Office of Noncommunicable Disease, Injury and Environmental Health; the Office of Public Health Preparedness and Response; the Office for State, Tribal, Local and Territorial Support; and the Office of Surveillance, Epidemiology, and Laboratory Services.

Under the Office of Infectious Disease are the National Center for Immunization and Respiratory Diseases; the National Center for Emerging and Zoonotic Infectious Diseases; and the National Center for HIV/AIDS, Viral Hepatitis, STD, and TB Prevention. The Office of Noncommunicable Diseases, Injury and Environmental Health is comprised of the National Center on Birth Defects and Developmental Disabilities, the National Center for Chronic Disease Prevention and Health Promotion, the National Center for Environmental Health/Agency for Toxic Substances and Disease Registry, and the National Center for Injury Prevention and Control. The Office of Surveillance, Epidemiology, and Laboratory Services contains the Laboratory Science Policy and Practice Program Office, the Public Health Information and Technology Program Office, the Public Health Informatics and Technology Program Office; the Public Health Surveillance Program Office, the Epidemiology and Analysis Program Office, the Scientific Education and the Professional Development Program Office, and the National Center for Health Statistics.

The CDC seeks to accomplish its mission by working with partners throughout the nation and the world to monitor health; detect and investigate health problems; conduct research to enhance prevention; develop and advocate sound public health policies; implement prevention strategies; promote healthy behaviors; foster safe and healthful environments and; provide leadership and training. Each of the CDC's component organizations undertake these activities in conducting specific programs.

Currently the CDC focus has broadened to include chronic diseases, disabilities, injury control, workplace hazards, environmental health threats, and terrorism preparedness. CDC combats emerging diseases and other health risks, including birth defects, West Nile virus, obesity, avian, swine, and pandemic flu, *E. coli*, and bioterrorism, to name a few. The CDC funds research and prevention programs relating to HIV/AIDS and issues periodic reports that detail the incidence and prevalence of HIV/AIDS in the United States as a whole, in specific subpopulations that are particularly impacted by the disease, and in the international arena. Mental health providers whose clients are at risk of HIV infection may find these reports helpful in providing their clients with HIV prevention information.

Related Topics: Prevention strategies.

Suggested Resources

Centers for Disease Control and Prevention (CDC). *CDC organization*. Retrieved January 20, 2012 from http://www.cdc.gov/about/organization/cio.htm

Centers for Disease Control and Prevention (CDC). *Vision, mission, core values, and pledge*. Retrieved January 30, 2012 from http://www.cdc.gov/about/organization/mission.htm

Children

Ana-Gabriela Benghiac

According to UNICEF there were 3.4 million HIV-positive children under 15 years old and 250,000 AIDS deaths were registered in children under 15 years old worldwide in 2010. In 2010, 390,000 children were infected with HIV globally. That same year, in North America there were 4,500 children under 15 years of age who were infected with HIV. Most of them were infected by vertical transmission from their mothers during pregnancy, labor, delivery or breastfeeding. Children may also become infected through certain risk behaviors such as sharing needles and other injection paraphernalia, unprotected sexual intercourse, and violent situations such as rape and sexual abuse. Infection due to blood transfusion has become relatively uncommon.

It is estimated that without treatment, approximately 50% of HIV-positive children will die before the age of 2 years old. It is important to know that all children under 2 years of age are eligible for treatment and families should be encouraged to seek medical care for their children. Preventive programs developed to halt vertical transmission are thought to be efficient and they have a positive impact on the disease, reducing the transmission rate considerably.

In 2010, the World Health Organization (WHO) revised its guidelines regarding the standard of care in HIV treatment with antiretroviral drugs in order to reduce vertical transmission of the virus. A new goal was set: to virtually eliminate mother-to-child HIV transmission by 2015. HIV pediatric care and treatment are crucial both for prolonging the life of children infected with the virus and also for offering them a better quality of life and the chance to have productive, meaningful lives through early detection of the infection, proper therapy and monitoring. HIV-infected children should benefit from social protection, in order to have access to testing, treatment to improve and increase their life span, and support for their families. Living with a chronic disease from such an early age negatively impacts these children, making them more susceptible to the development of medical,

A.-G. Benghiac (✉)
Department of Bioethics, Case Western Reserve University, Cleveland, OH, USA
e-mail: dr.gabriela_benghiac@yahoo.com

S. Loue (ed.), *Mental Health Practitioner's Guide to HIV/AIDS*,
DOI 10.1007/978-1-4614-5283-6_18, © Springer Science+Business Media New York 2013

psychological and psychiatric issues than are healthy individuals of the same age. More specifically, HIV-infected children are more likely to develop learning problems, attention disorders and cognitive deficits.

Many HIV-positive children face not only the burden of the disease but also the loss of one or both parents due to the epidemic, potentially rendering them more vulnerable to mental illness and social difficulties. Too, oftentimes the families of HIV-infected children face stigma and discrimination, which are correlated with a reluctance to seek medical advice and a lack of access to healthcare facilities. Community-targeted programs to support these children and their caregivers should focus not only on prevention and treatment but also on other factors such as environmental factors that influence the epidemic; the provision of material, social, and psychological support; and the adoption of a friendly attitude by healthcare providers.. Adequate funding allocation for these programs is an important issue for ensuring a continuity of the activities and monitoring of the patients. Efforts should be made both to eliminate health access inequities and social and financial barriers and to better assess treatment outcomes.

Adolescents are a special category of this population as they are more vulnerable to HIV infection due to risk behaviors such as unprotected sex and needle sharing for substance use. They also face the dramatic changes of the transition from pediatric to adult life and become more aware of their health status and its social implications. They may present with great emotional distress and manifest difficulties in adjusting to the diagnosis. Studies have shown that people with mental health disorders are more likely to manifest high risk behaviors for HIV; thus, children and adolescents with psychiatric illnesses should be closely monitored and advised not to engage in such behaviors. The lack of efficient monitoring and treatment of mental health problems can influence both the course of the disease and the treatment compliance.

Approximately 60% of the young people infected with HIV worldwide are female. Health education can contribute in reducing these numbers by implementing special programs in schools, religious institutions, and communities with a high prevalence of HIV; providing condoms; encouraging safe sex practices and condom use; encouraging communication; and offering counseling, information leaflets and hot lines for further support.

HIV-positive children can face stigma, discrimination, violence, trauma, and neglect from their families and communities. Healthcare providers should ensure that the HIV-infected children live in environments where their emotional stability is not affected, where they feel loved and cared for, and where they can have normal development both physically and psychologically. A genuine and supportive relationship between children and their caregivers is essential and contributes to a better understanding and control of the disease and a better social adaptation. The training of HIV pediatric specialists is critical to manage these cases and sustain supportive interventions for both children and their families. Mothers should be offered proper access to early infant diagnosis and referrals for the ongoing care of their children. Continuous screening for mental health disorders should be a part of basic care programs designed for children and adolescents.

Related Topics: Adolescents, mental health comorbidity and HIV/AIDS, orphans, stigma and stigmatization.

Suggested Reading

Armstrong, F. D., Seidel, J. F., & Swales, T. P. (1993). Pediatric HIV infection: A neuropsychological and educational challenge. *Journal of Learning Disabilities, 26*, 92–103.
Brouwers, P., Wolters, P., & Civitello, L. (1998). Central nervous system manifestations and assessment. In P. Pizzo & C. Wilfert (Eds.), *Pediatric AIDS: The challenge of HIV infection in infants, children and adolescents* (3rd ed.). Baltimore, MD: Williams & Wilkins.
Brown, L. K., Lourie, K. J., & Pao, M. (2000). Children and adolescents living with HIV and AIDS: A review. *Journal of Child Psychology and Psychiatry, 41*, 81–96.
Donenberg, G. R., & Pao, M. (2005). Youth and HIV/AIDS: Psychiatry's role in a changing epidemic. *Journal of the American Academy of Child and Adolescent Psychiatry, 44*, 728–747.
Trzepacz, A. M., Vannatta, K., Gerhardt, C. A., Ramey, C., & Noll, R. B. (2004). Emotional social and behavioral functioning of children with sickle cell disease and comparison peers. *Journal of Pediatric Hematology and Oncology, 26*, 642–648.

Suggested Resources

Joint United Nations Programme on HIV/AIDS (UNAIDS). (2010). *Children and AIDS: Fifth stocktaking report, 2010*. Retrieved March 7, 2012 from http://www.unicef.org/publications/files/Children_and_AIDS-Fifth_Stocktaking_Report_2010_EN.pdf
Working Group on Pediatric Care & Treatment, Interagency Task Team on Prevention & Treatment of HIV Infection in Pregnant Women, Mothers & Their Children. (2011). *Pediatric advocacy toolkit: For improved pediatric HIV diagnosis, care and treatment in high HIV prevalence countries and regions*. Geneva, Switzerland: World Health Organization. Retrieved March 7, 2012 from http://www.who.int/hiv/pub/pediatric_toolkit2011/en/index.html
World Health Organization, UNAIDS, & UNICEF. (2011). *Progress report 2011: Global HIV/AIDS response: Epidemic update and health sector progress towards universal access*. Geneva, Switzerland: World Health Organization. Retrieved March 7, 2012 from http://www.who.int/hiv/pub/progress_report2011/en/index.html

Christianity

Ezer Kang and David Arute

Christianity, a monotheistic religious movement diverse in form and expression and marked by a common commitment to the life and teachings of its founder Jesus of Nazareth, has informed varied faith-based responses to HIV/AIDS since the beginning of the pandemic—from early pronouncements against HIV prevention measures (e.g., condom use and needle exchange) to further marginalization of gay men living with the illness. However, recent initiatives have emerged to stem the tide of the epidemic with prevention and care programs that are aligned with orthodox Christian doctrine. Christian-based HIV programming (CBHP) gained visible momentum during the second decade of the epidemic. This is most notable among churches in urban African-American enclaves in the USA and southern African countries—both regions with disproportionate representations of persons newly infected with HIV and living with AIDS. Moreover, as a result of research identifying a strong link between rising HIV incidence and inequitable socioeconomic conditions, a response to the epidemic began to gain ground, largely influenced by the evangelical social justice movement.

Established CBHP at churches and Christian-based social service organizations have included community education about HIV transmission prevention, church leadership training, HIV-stigma reduction media campaigns, outreach to HIV high-risk groups, promotion of HIV-antibody testing and counseling, and emotional and practical support for people living with HIV (PLHIV). CBHP in the USA are often conceived of and implemented in partnership with external organizations. Collaborative partnerships between churches and public health institutions are conceptualized as faith-based or faith-placed. Faith-based interventions take into account the religious culture and beliefs of targeted individuals and communities,

E. Kang (✉)
Department of Psychology, Wheaton College, Wheaton, IL, USA
e-mail: ezer.kang@wheaton.edu

D. Arute
Wheaton College, Wheaton, IL, USA

S. Loue (ed.), *Mental Health Practitioner's Guide to HIV/AIDS*,
DOI 10.1007/978-1-4614-5283-6_19,

whereas faith-placed interventions view the religious organization as a location for delivering interventions, regardless of their religious content.

Recent scholarship on the development of CBHP has highlighted the important challenge of identifying points of integration between orthodox Christian doctrine, ecclesiastical practices, and response to HIV. For example, some have argued that scriptural teachings of transformative and unconditional compassion as modeled by Jesus Christ uniquely positions CBHP to address what may be the most challenging aspect of HIV care and prevention—namely, the stigma of living with HIV and/or belonging to a perceived HIV-risk group. Texts from the Old and New Testaments that consistently referred to the sins of oppression and admonishment of those who unjustly treat those who carry less social power, have challenged Christian institutions to apply these principles to HIV/AIDS. Others have emphasized the important pairing of upholding justice and proclaiming the atoning work of Jesus Christ—a primary task for Christians. Proponents of this approach to Christian evangelism specifically argue that propagating the life and work of Christ is inseparable from teaching the responsibilities of becoming a Christian—that is, confronting social and economic injustices. Threads of liberation theology, for example, that emphasized solidarity with exploited communities have been woven into the responses of many churches in African and South-American countries.

Within Christian subgroups that acknowledge the importance of responding to the epidemic, there are formidable challenges to implementing CBHP in the Americas and southern regions of Africa. First, limited financial and human resources are generally directed towards the needs of congregation members and target constituent groups rendering involvement in HIV programming less feasible. Second, collaborations with external HIV-organizations are frequently stifled by ideological differences about HIV prevention measures, sexual ethics, substance abuse, and harm reduction interventions. Third, there exists a lingering bias against CBHP, one that was largely formed during the first decade of epidemic against fundamentalist churches that viewed HIV/AIDS as divine retribution against homosexuals. Finally, HIV involvement potentially compromises the churches' perceived moral standing and authority within their communities and may alienate the churches from their constituents. This threat of compromised social standing is particularly felt in select African countries where many coexisting churches compete in the religious marketplace for a small group of unaffiliated individuals.

Recent scholarship has focused on how religious institutions such as Christian churches influence broader social milieus within which HIV risk behavior occurs and illness stigma proliferates. The argument follows that diverse Christian traditions play a formidable role in shaping cultural and political scripts that inform social responses to the epidemic. In the USA, this is exemplified among diverse immigrant and African-American churches that weld considerable influence over community norms and values—ones that can facilitate or undermine public health efforts in HIV prevention and treatment. The importance of preserving traditional, moral, and institutional values has rendered active involvement in HIV-related activities a challenge among many ethnic Christian churches. However, researchers have urged strategic approaches to address these institutional barriers by identifying proximal and distal points of integration between HIV prevention and treatment, doctrinal teaching, and cultural faith practices.

Related Topics: Coping, faith community, prevention strategies, religion and spirituality.

Suggested Reading

Campbell, M. K., Hudson, M. A., Resnicow, K., Blakeney, N., Paxton, A., & Baskin, M. (2007). Church-based health promotion interventions: Evidence and lessons learned. *Annual Review of Public Health, 28*, 213–234.

Chin, J., Neilands, T. B., Weiss, L., & Mantell, J. E. (2008). Paradigm shifters, professionals, and community sentinels: Immigrant community institutions' roles in shaping places and implications for stigmatized public health initiatives. *Health and Place, 14*, 866–882.

DeHaven, M. J., Hunter, I. B., Wilder, L., Walton, J. W., & Berry, J. (2004). Health programs in faith-based organizations: Are they effective? *American Journal of Public Health, 94*, 1030–1036.

Francis, S. A., & Liverpool, J. (2009). A review of faith-based HIV prevention programs. *Journal of Religion and Health, 48*, 6–15.

Kang, E., Chin, J., & Behar, E. (2011). Faith-based HIV care and prevention in Asian immigrant communities in New York City. Rhetoric or reality? *Journal of Psychology & Theology, Special Issue "Faith in Practice: Reflections on Community Psychology in Action", 39*, 268–279.

Muñoz-Laboy, M., Garcia, J., Moon-Howard, J., Wilson, P. A., & Parker, R. (2011). Religious responses to HIV and AIDS: Understanding the role of religious cultures and institutions in confronting the epidemic. *Global Public Health, 6*(S2), S127–S131.

Clinical Trials

Ana-Gabriela Benghiac

The HIV/AIDS epidemic has had a great impact on people's health worldwide. Research in this field is critical if we are to develop preventive measures and efficient and affordable therapy, thereby decreasing transmission of the infection and increasing the life span and quality of life of those who are infected. The National Institutes of Health (NIH) of the United States support the largest HIV/AIDS research program in the whole world; this research program is coordinated by the Office of AIDS Research (OAR). There are other NIH institutes that fund research in the HIV/AIDS field such as: the National Institute of Allergy and Infectious Diseases (NIAID), the National Institute of Mental Health (NIMH), the National Institute of Child Health and Human Development (NICHD), the National Institute on Drug Abuse (NIDA), the National Cancer Institute (NCI), and the National Institute of Dental and Craniofacial Research (NIDCR). The best known HIV/AIDS clinical trial networks are represented by the following: the Adult AIDS Clinical Trials Group (ACTG), the International Maternal Pediatric Adolescent AIDS Clinical Trials Group (IMPAACT), the Community Programs for Clinical Research on AIDS (CPCRA), the HIV Prevention Trials Network (HPTN), Microbiocide Trials Network (MTN), International Network for Strategic Initiatives in Global HIV Trials (INSIGHT), and the HIV Vaccine Trials Network (HVTN). ACTG, which is the largest therapeutic clinical trial group worldwide, includes low-income countries. There are currently more than 5,200 HIV studies listed on the US Clinical Trials Web page, a service of the NIH. Approximately 1,200 of these trials are open studies.

Clinical trials, also known as treatment trials, represent one of the various types of clinical research. In addition to clinical trials, these include prevention trials; diagnostic trials; screening trials; quality of life trials, which are also called supportive care trials; genetic studies; and clinical epidemiological studies.

A.-G. Benghiac (✉)
Department of Bioethics, Case Western Reserve University, Cleveland, OH, USA
e-mail: dr.gabriela_benghiac@yahoo.com

S. Loue (ed.), *Mental Health Practitioner's Guide to HIV/AIDS*,
DOI 10.1007/978-1-4614-5283-6_20, © Springer Science+Business Media New York 2013

Clinical trials must meet certain scientific and regulatory requirements and conform with enunciated ethical principles that are designed both to protect the health and safety of the participants and answer the research questions that have been posed. Research trials can be conducted only if clinical equipoise exists. Clinical equipoise means that there is a real uncertainty regarding the outcome of the experimental therapy used in that specific study.

Clinical trials have four phases that address different objectives. Prior to the commencement of a trial that involves human participants, preclinical testing is performed on animals. The purpose of animal research is to establish whether the experimental therapy has a potential benefit and to ensure the safety of its use. This stage of the research is generally done in a period of 3–4 years. After reviewing the results, the information regarding the experimental therapy is sent to the FDA for approval for use in a phase I clinical trial with human participants. Phase I studies assess the toxicity and dosage of an experimental drug or therapy. Phase II and III evaluate the clinical efficacy of the experimental treatment and phase IV studies are post-marketing surveillance research that seeks to identify adverse effects of a marketed therapy after long-time use and drug interactions.

There are certain specific elements that can be found in various phases of HIV studies. Thus, in Phase I HIV clinical trials, researchers enroll participants with the disease, unlike in other studies where healthy individuals are selected. The number of participants in this study phase is between 20 and 80 participants and the study length is up to 12 months. Phase II clinical trials are conducted with the participation of several hundred human participants and focus on the evaluation of toxicity, efficacy and dosing requirements of the experimental therapy. This study phase can last up to 2–3 years. Phase III trials usually involve a larger number of participants, around 1,000–3,000 individuals. They also last longer, up to 5 years and they are generally double-blind randomized controlled trials. This means that neither the researchers nor the participants know who is enrolled in the control (comparison) arm of the study, where the treatment can be either a placebo or a currently used drug for the disease, or who is receiving the experimental therapy. After completing the first three study phases, if the outcomes of the study show that the new therapy is considered safe and efficient, an application for approval is sent to the FDA, which will review the documents. The review period may extend from 6 to 24 months. During the post-approval period, any adverse effects that are correlated to the use of the new therapy must be reported to the FDA. In the case of HIV/AIDS treatments, accelerated approval can be provided for new therapies due to the severity of the disease. This does not mean that the safeguard of the patients is not insured or that they do not respect the current requirements. Individuals who are affected by life-threatening diseases such as HIV/AIDS may be able to benefit from investigational new drugs (IND), which can be accessed through nonrandomized clinical trials.

HIV clinical trials are addressed to individuals that can meet certain eligibility criteria or inclusion criteria. Exclusion criteria are also a part of the protocol and they are important because they target certain characteristics that may have a negative impact on the well-being of the prospective participant or they can influence the results of the study. Usually these criteria are represented by certain medical or social standards such as: age, gender, medical history, current health status and medication, laboratory exams, present or possible future pregnancy. The purpose of these criteria is not to create barriers for prospective participants and deny their right to access clinical trials, but to identify appropriate individuals and protect them. HIV/AIDS trials usually require that the prospective participants are already infected or they are part of communities exposed to certain risk factors. It is important to recruit participants of all ages in HIV/AIDS research in order to create proper targeted therapy. This is critical for pediatric HIV/AIDS therapy, since some forms of drugs used in adults cannot be used in children, thus, there is a need to develop appropriate treatment for this special high-risk population.

By participating in clinical trials, individuals can benefit personally or manifest altruistic motivations such as to contribute to the enrichment of knowledge in that specific field, thus helping other people to benefit in the future from the outcomes of the research. Participants may also have access to medication that is not available outside the study; this is especially important in severe and treatment-resistant diseases where individuals may not feel any positive impact from their current therapy. Additionally, participants in trials are more closely monitored by the research team, they may be the first to benefit from the study, and they can have access to treatments that otherwise they could not afford due to inadequate health insurance or lack of any kind of medical insurance. As an example, according to researchers from the University of North Carolina at Chapel Hill, there is a "trial effect" in the early highly antiretroviral therapy (HAART) among participants in HIV clinical trials which is correlated to better outcomes compared to clinical-based therapy. The trial effect translates as a benefit experienced by the research participants compared to patients that receive the same treatment in the context of usual clinical care.

There may also be risks associated with participation in clinical trials. Experimental therapies may have unexpected side effects or may affect the health status of the prospective participants, leading to more health issues than were experienced prior to participation in the study. Participants must be informed of both the benefits and the risks of study participation during the informed consent process. Participants must be told that they can withdraw at any time from the study without affecting their relationship with their physician if he or she is conducting the research or affecting the care they receive.

Experimental therapies are not necessarily better than the standard treatment. Trial participants should be continuously aware of the fact that they are enrolled in a research trial, not a clinical care program. Some studies have protocols that stipulate that any supplementary costs of certain procedures required by the study or side effects of the experimental therapies or associated conditions are not covered by the sponsor. In such cases, the participant must pay out of pocket money or have health insurance that can cover all of the expenses. Thus, it is important to verify what is covered by the research prior to participating in a clinical trial, what is covered by the individual's medical insurance, and if there are any extra costs that the patient must assume. Participants also have to consider also the number of study visits that they need to make in order to complete the study, since this can affect their social and professional life. Too, participants who enroll in randomized clinical trials are not allowed to choose whether they are in the control or experimental arm of the study and they cannot request that study team members assign them to a specific arm of the research study, for example, the experimental arm or the comparison arm. Most clinical trials do not offer compensation for the participants, although some studies can compensate for parking, working hours, and/or meals. The compensation that is offered to participants has to be approved by the appropriate ethics review committee, generally called an institutional review board. Further, the compensation cannot be considered as a benefit of participation in the study or an incentive meant to attract more participants, especially in higher than minimal risk research.

Prospective participants can obtain information regarding HIV clinical trials from AIDS hotlines that can direct them to organizations or government agencies that can provide further information regarding research in this field. They can also request information from their physician or search clinical trials on governmental Web sites such as www.clinicaltrials.gov.

Related Topics: Council of Organizations for Medical Sciences, Declaration of Helsinki.

Suggested Reading

Chow, S. C., & Liu, J.-P. (2003). *Design and analysis of clinical trials: Concepts and methodologies*. Hoboken, NJ: Wiley.

Loue, S., & Pike, E. C. (2007). *Case studies in ethics and HIV research*. New York, NY: Springer.

Meinert, C. L. (1986). *Clinical trials: Design, conduct and analysis*. New York, NY: Oxford University Press.

Menezes, P., Miller, W. C., Wohl, D. A., Adimora, A. A., Leone, P. A., Miller, W. C., et al. (2011). Does HAART efficacy translate to effectiveness? Evidence for a trial effect. *PLoS One, 6*(7), e21824. doi:10.1731/journal.pone.0021824. Retrieved March 7, 2012 from http://www.plosone.org/article/info:doi%2F10.1371%2Fjournal.pone.0021824.

Suggested Resources

HIV/AIDS Network Coordination (HANC). *Understanding the clinical research process and principles of clinical research, participant guide*. Retrieved March 7, 2012 from http://www.hptn.org/web%20documents/CIPDocs/CABTrainingMaterials/Participant's%20Guide.pdf

National Institute of Mental Health. *A participant's guide to mental health clinical research*. Retrieved March 7, 2012 from http://www.nimh.nih.gov/health/publications/a-participants-guide-to-mental-health-clinical-research/what-are-the-different-types-of-clinical-research.shtml

Cognitive Impairment

Laura Gheuca Solovastru

It is important that those who care for HIV/AIDS patients be able to separate normal anxiety states from signs of serious psychiatric disorder that require a doctor's care. Patients experiencing depression, for example, must be warned not to self-medicate without consulting their treating physician, who can monitor drug interactions. Monitoring is especially critical for a person who is undergoing HAART. Also, caregivers should not let their own feelings prevent them from providing the help needed. An HIV patient who is having many bouts of disturbed sleep, malaise, tearfulness, and constant fatigue may need counseling or medication for depression. One should also remember that chronic pain can be a cause of depression and anxiety, and in HIV, frequent headaches and extremity pain are not unusual.

One serious complication of HIV is delirium, which can be the result of central nervous system opportunistic infections, medication side effects, and systemic illness. Most of the time, people with delirium need to be treated in an intensive care unit because they must be monitored carefully. In those who have HIV, delirium is often the result of drug (recreational or prescribed) withdrawal, low oxygen concentration in the blood, electrolyte disorders, low blood sugar level, or low blood pressure.

AIDS-associated mania usually stems from organic HIV-associated brain disease. Mania can also arise from the anxiety of dealing with a chronic illness. Unfortunately, the gold standard for treating mania—lithium—is considered too high-risk for use by an AIDS patient, who may be dehydrated and experiencing vomiting and diarrhea. Often doctors prescribe perphenazine (Trilafon) with or without lorazepam (Ativan) to stabilize the condition, followed by valproate or carbamazepine.

Signs of psychosis in HIV patients are hallucinations, delusions, and paranoid delusions, which are usually treated with midpotency neuroleptic medicines such as

L.G. Solovastru (✉)
Department of Dermatology, University of Medicine and Pharmacy "Gr. T. Popa", Iasi, Romania
e-mail: lsolovastru13@yahoo.com

S. Loue (ed.), *Mental Health Practitioner's Guide to HIV/AIDS*,
DOI 10.1007/978-1-4614-5283-6_21,

Trilafon. Psychiatric consultation is recommended. HIV-associated organic brain disease can lie at the base of any of the psychiatric syndromes mentioned.

Patients who have organic brain disease are less responsive to caregivers and less functional, conditions that sometimes result in distancing. However, these patients still need empathy and warmth, and counseling can help caregivers get through this difficulty. In the years before progression of the disease to AIDS, few people have mental changes that are truly indicative of dementia. Being "at a loss for words" and having difficulty concentrating are very frightening to people with HIV, because they immediately associate these problems with HIV-associated dementia, which typically occurs only in the late stages of AIDS. A person who does have dementia experiences marked changes in attitude, usually characterized by extreme apathy, and changes in muscle control and mental acuity. Usually, days of sharpness alternate with days of slower mental processing of input. Also, an unsteady gait is a sign of HIV-associated dementia. The degree of impairment associated with dementia linked to AIDS varies widely: some people are affected in very minor ways, and others are hit severely.

High-dose AZT therapy can reverse impairment in some people who have cognitive impairment only, but if both mood and cognitive signs are in evidence, dextroamphetamine sulfate (dexedrine) or methylphenidate hydrochloride (Ritalin) may be required. The patient who is cognitively impaired can be cared for at home, where he or she may well experience less anxiety in the familiar setting.

Chronic anxiety can also be debilitating to some people going through drug withdrawal and/or living with HIV/AIDS. The person experiencing chronic anxiety may have difficulty in concentrating, feel exhausted and agitated, and have trouble sleeping. Some people experience very frightening panic attacks. It is important to treat panic and anxiety aggressively, and there are a number of medications that work well. Behavior modification therapy can help, too.

Related Topics: HIV-associated dementia, mental health comorbidity, and HIV/AIDS.

Suggested Reading

Leserman, J. (2008). Role of depression, stress, and trauma in HIV disease progression. *Psychosomatic Medicine, 70*, 539–545.

Whetten, K., Reif, S., Whetten, R., & Murphy-McMillan, L. K. (2008). Trauma, mental health, distrust, and stigma among HIV-positive persons: Implications for effective care. *Psychosomatic Medicine, 70*, 531–538.

Suggested Resources

Arehart-Treichel, J. (2011). Experts offer advice on managing HIV neurocognitive impairment. *Psychiatric News, 46*(5), 18. Retrieved April 24, 2012 from http://pnhw.psychiatryonline.org/content/46/5/18.1.full.

Communication

Lisa R. Norman

Communication and HIV Prevention

Communication is a component of any healthy relationship, including a sexual one. In the latter, responsibility necessitates the clear discussion of sexual values and concerns, but many people have so little experience verbalizing their thoughts and opinions about sexuality that actually having sex is easier than discussing it. And yet, prior to the act, it is vital to talk with a potential or current sex partner. The benefits of such open communication are legion and include a heightening of the experience, a significant reduction of both stress and embarrassment, the dispelling of myths and the breaking of stereotypes, and lastly, a greater likelihood that safe (r)-sex techniques and contraceptives (including condoms) will be consistently utilized. In fact, the available evidence shows that sexual partners who talk about condoms and HIV are more likely to use condoms than those who do not. It is generally held that communication between intimate partners about issues of sexuality and HIV prevention is likely to influence the safe(r)-sex practices that follow. If discussing safe(r)-sex with a potential or current partner seems too daunting, doing so with a family member and/or friend may be a good way to begin. However, the ability to talk freely about sex and sexuality with a partner might well be considered a litmus test for engaging in such an intimate, potentially risky act.

Initiating an open dialogue on sex can be the hardest part of the process, and how it is accomplished will vary considerably depending on the comfort level of the person doing the initiating. Indeed, the level of comfort displayed often signals to the potential partner whether or not the planned act is deemed "right" or even desirable. The specific context of the sexual interaction, too, introduces its own set of variables, as negotiating safe(r)-sex in a casual or one-time situation often

L.R. Norman (✉)
Ponce School of Medicine, Ponce, Puerto Rico
e-mail: lnorman@psm.edu

S. Loue (ed.), *Mental Health Practitioner's Guide to HIV/AIDS*,
DOI 10.1007/978-1-4614-5283-6_22, © Springer Science+Business Media New York 2013

requires a different approach than what is to be used in an ongoing relationship. Culturally prescribed gender roles may impact whether and the extent to which individuals are able to engage in discussions about sexuality and safer sex.

Including communication models and taking interdisciplinary approaches are essential in the study of HIV/AIDS/STD prevention because communication is the core of varied relevant cultural practices. These practices range from discerning whether a potential partner is interested in sex to putting on a condom, from asking about someone's sexual background to finding HIV/AIDS/STD information. Now that HIV is a preventable disease, communication is more important than ever in terms of protection and prevention. In order to predict whether or not a given individual will feel free to discuss safer sex with a partner, the factors associated with such a discussion—such as that individual's comfort talking about safer sex and his or her anxiety associated with condom use—must be determined.

When HIV is factored into the equation with communication and mental health, a whole array of issues arises. When a person is faced with HIV, their mental health is compromised. Mental health problems can affect anybody, but it seems that people with HIV may be more likely than the general population to experience them. The groups most affected by HIV are also more likely to have mental health problems, because of the stress association with being marginalized from much of mainstream society. Experiencing HIV-related stigma can be stressful in itself. Disclosing one's HIV status or starting a new relationship are often sources of anxiety or emotional distress. Acknowledging one's feelings is an important first step to dealing with emotional distress.

Communicating Mental Health Issues

Many individuals who are HIV-positive experience anxiety, which is a feeling of apprehension or dread that bad things may happen, causing both physical and psychological effects. Getting practical advice about how to approach these difficulties may well provide a solution. Again, psychological therapies may also prove useful. Having some form of talking therapy, such as cognitive behavioral therapy, can help provide the skills and practical techniques to understand the origins of anxiety and to manage it better.

The most common mental health problem associated with HIV is depression. Key features of depression are the loss of pleasure in activities that are usually meaningful and enjoyable, social withdrawal, and isolation. Feelings of low self-worth and inappropriate or excessive feelings of guilt are also symptoms of depression, as well as thoughts of death, self-harm, or even suicide. Communication with one's partner, a good friend, or a family member about how one feels may help and should be encouraged. While antidepressants are often prescribed to persons who experience depression, communication is an important way to deal with depression as well.

Related Topics: Disclosure, disclosure laws, partner violence, prevention strategies.

Suggested Reading

Edgar, T., Noar, S., & Freimuth, V. (2008). *Communication perspectives on HIV/AIDS for the 21st century*. New York, NY: Erlbaum.

Hernandez, A. M., Zule, W. A., Karg, R. S., Browne, F. A., & Wechsberg, W. M. (2012). Factors that influence HIV risk among Hispanic female immigrants and their implications for HIV prevention interventions. *International Journal of Family Medicine*. doi:10.1155/2012/876381.

Sales, J. M., Salazar, L. E., Wingood, G. M., DiClemente, R. J., Rose, E., & Crosby, R. A. (2008). The mediating role of partner communication skills on HIV/STD-associated risk behaviors in young African American females with a history of sexual violence. *Archives of Pediatric Medicine, 162*(5), 432–438.

Suggested Resources

Looking after your emotional and mental health. Last retrieved April 30, 2012 from http://www.aidsmap.com/Looking-after-your-emotional-and-mental-health/page/1439575/

Smart, T. (2009). *Mental health and HIV: A clinical review*. Retrieved April 30, 2012 from http://www.aidsmap.com/Mental-health-and-HIV-a-clinical-review/page/1330115/

Confidentiality Laws

Mihaela-Catalina Vicol

Introduction

Privacy refers to the fundamental rights of nonintrusion, the freedom to act in personal matters, and the protection of personal information. All of these are protected by the Fourth Amendment of the United States Constitution. The concept of confidentiality, as part of privacy, plays important roles in medicine by promoting respect for patients' privacy and intimacy and encouraging patients' honesty in revealing information to physicians. According to Vaughn, additional arguments reinforce the need for such a trust bond: the harm that the disclosed information may bring about for patients, such as discrimination, stigma, and shame, and the consequences to the doctor–patient relationship, such as a rupture in trust, patient nondisclosure of information, and inability of physicians to fulfill their obligation of beneficence.

Confidentiality Laws: Evolution

With regard to HIV and AIDS, confidentiality needs specific protection, in view of the potential consequences resulting from its violation. Though there is much information on HIV, fear and misinformation about it continue to exist, laying the foundation for deleterious social attitudes such as discrimination, stigmatization, and denial of insurance.

A brief history of the evolution of HIV legislation in the United States shows that a focus on nondiscrimination has existed consistently. The Americans with Disabilities Act (1990) is a federal law that prohibits job discrimination based on

M.-C. Vicol (✉)
Department of Bioethics, University of Medicine and Pharmacy "Gr. T. Popa", Iasi, Romania
e-mail: mihavicol@yahoo.com

S. Loue (ed.), *Mental Health Practitioner's Guide to HIV/AIDS*, 151
DOI 10.1007/978-1-4614-5283-6_23, © Springer Science+Business Media New York 2013

a disability. It expands an older law, the Rehabilitation Act of 1973, which prohibits the refusal of health care to people with disabilities. The first court case, *Bragdon v. Abbot*, confirmed that HIV may be considered to be a disability under ADA.

A few years later, in 1996, Congress enacted a very important law called Health Insurance Portability and Accountability Act of 1996 (HIPAA). This Act has a special section regarding medical confidentiality, which provides standards for protecting the confidentiality of health information. The law requires protected access to any medical information that contains identifiable information such as name, address, telephone number, social security number, and medical record number. It further stipulates that health care institutions and organizations should establish who is entitled to access these information and to what extent. Another important provision of this law requires patient's informed consent for the use or disclosure of this information. In this way, the law protects an individual's right to privacy and provides civil and criminal penalties for its violation.

Medical confidentiality is not absolute and the law provides for exceptions. One of them is sharing the medical information between health care providers involved in the management of the case from the same institution. However, the exchange of the same information between health care providers from different institutions requires the patient's consent. The second exception is represented by emergency situations, where protected health information may be disclosed, but informed consent should be sought after the emergency passed. And in the end, protected health information may be disclosed to law enforcement without the patient's consent in response to an official subpoena.

Though this law does not refer specifically to HIV patients, the confidentiality of medical information, HIV status included, is protected under the general framework of this law. However, in addition to this federal law, there are some states' laws with specific provisions regarding confidentiality in HIV/AIDS.

States' laws relating to HIV/AIDS confidentiality differ with respect to several points: the information that is considered to be confidential, the disclosure of information for the protection of a third party (the *Tarasoff* duty to warn standard) and who may disclose the information. While states' laws such as those in New Jersey or Arizona cover confidential information generally, states' law such as those of California provide for civil or criminal penalties only for the unauthorized disclosure of the HIV test results. The law in Arizona stipulates that information regarding HIV/AIDS represents "confidential communicable disease related information," and provides penalties for unauthorized disclosure. Accordingly, "no person who obtains confidential communicable disease related information in the course of providing a health service or pursuant to a release of confidential communicable disease related information may disclose or be compelled to disclose that information" (Ariz. Rev. Stat. Ann. 36–664, in Dickson, 2001).

The second issue and the most controversial provision is related to the violation of confidentiality for the protection of a third innocent party; could the Tarasoff standard be applied in HIV/AIDS? That is, is there any duty to warn others of the risk presented by a specific HIV-infected person and to which professionals does this duty to warn apply? The controversy stems from the fact that the Tarasoff exception permitting a breach of confidentiality applies to situations in which there is an imminent danger or harm to an identifiable third party. However, the medical studies do not offer a certainty that the HIV virus will definitely be transmitted in the case of needle sharing or unprotected sex, but instead indicates the level of probability. It is difficult to say whether the duty to warn is or should be extended in cases of HIV/AIDS; this difficulty is not solved by the legislation.

In case there is a duty to warn, to whom does it apply? Usually, the Tarasoff rule applies to professionals. While some states' legislation explains the term to include psychiatrists, psychologists, and physicians, others fail to define the term. As a consequence, for some professionals, such as social workers, it remains unclear whether there is a duty to protect or not or if confidentiality may be breached without patient consent.

Conclusion

Confidentiality laws in the United States of America respect and protect patient's privacy. In view of the serious adverse consequences that may result from a violation of confidentiality in cases involving HIV/AIDS patients, states have enacted specific provisions for protecting confidentiality. There is still a controversy as to whether the duty to protect others in cases of HIV/AIDS transmission is an exception to the confidentiality rule, and to which professionals should this apply.

Related Topics: Contact tracing, disclosure, disclosure laws, duty to warn, legal issues for HIV-infected clients, partner notification.

Suggested Reading

Dickson, D. T. (2001). *HIV, AIDS, and the law: Legal issues for social work practice and policy*. New York, NY: Walter de Gruyter Inc.

Gert, B., Culver, C. M., & Clouser, K. D. (1997). *Bioethics: A return to fundamentals*. New York, NY: Oxford University Press.

UNESCO. (2011). *Casebook on benefit and harm: Bioethics core curriculum casebook [Series No. 2]*. Paris: UNESCO.

Vaughn, L. (2010). *Bioethics: Principles, issues and cases*. New York, NY: Oxford University Press.

Suggested Resources

United States Department of Health and Human Services. http://www.hhs.gov/ocr/privacy/

Conspiracy Theories

Daniel J. O'Shea

In the early 1980s, what came to be known as AIDS seemed to appear suddenly and mysteriously out of nowhere, striking with an unrelenting and deadly aim that killed those infected very quickly. Not surprisingly, this phenomenon caused much fear, which, compounded by institutional mistrust in some cases, led to rampant speculation about the origins or cause of the disease. Resulting "conspiracy theories" frequently built upon or exacerbated that fear and mistrust with misconceptions surrounding the illness, how people became infected, and treatment options and effectiveness.

As the HIV/AIDS epidemic now enters its fourth decade, HIV/AIDS conspiracy theories continue to hinder prevention, treatment, and research efforts across the globe. These assorted theories imply some sort of secret collusion on the part of government or other institutions. They can roughly be grouped into categories of man-made or iatrogenic origins of HIV or AIDS; HIV/AIDS denialism; divine intervention, that AIDS is a plague sent by God to punish homosexuals and American society for tolerating homosexuality; and prevention and treatment.

By far the largest category, man-made or iatrogenic origins of AIDS, includes the following beliefs. (1) AIDS is a biological weapon manufactured by the developed world to eliminate large numbers of Blacks/Africans/African Americans and homosexuals, possibly under the auspices of the U.S. federal Special Cancer Virus Program (SCVP), possibly with the help of the U.S. Central Intelligence Agency (CIA). (2) HIV was developed by the U.S. Department of Defense or defense contractors through research seeking a new virus that would be capable of destroying the human immune system with no antidote in order to give the USA absolute military supremacy, for biowarfare, and/or for population control. (3) HIV was engineered between 1977 and 1978 at a U.S. military laboratory by splicing together two other viruses, a retrovirus that causes T-cell leukemia (HTLV-1) and a sheep virus (Visna); it was tested on prison inmate volunteers, in exchange for early

D.J. O'Shea (✉)
Public Health Service, County of San Diego, San Diego, CA, USA
e-mail: Dan.OShea@sdcounty.ca.gov

S. Loue (ed.), *Mental Health Practitioner's Guide to HIV/AIDS*,
DOI 10.1007/978-1-4614-5283-6_24,

release, from whom it spread into general population. (4) U.S. government scientists developed HIV by genetically modifying a sheep virus (Visna) and then deliberately, in conjunction with a pharmaceutical company, added it to an experimental hepatitis B vaccine given to gay and bisexual men and African Americans in New York, San Francisco, and Los Angeles from 1978 to 1981, from which it spread to other populations. (5) AIDS was triggered by the mass vaccination campaign which eradicated smallpox. One theory suggests the vaccine was deliberately laced with HIV, another that smallpox vaccinations provided some protection against HIV so that eradication of smallpox and ending the mass vaccination campaign contributed to the spread of HIV. Still another related theory is that scientists in New York engineered HIV and the World Health Organization spread it under cover of the smallpox eradication program to eliminate, or at least control, the Black population. (6) The oral polio vaccine was developed in chimpanzee tissues unintentionally contaminated with simian immunodeficiency virus (SIV), the simian precursor to HIV, and an experimental mass vaccination program in the Belgian Congo introduced the virus into humans.

Conspiracy theories based on HIV/AIDS denialism suggest that HIV is only a harmless passenger virus and AIDS is caused either by the antiretroviral treatments intended to combat HIV or by other noninfectious agents such as illegal drug use and promiscuity. In Africa, AIDS is attributed to poverty, chronic disease, malnutrition, and other environmental factors. The latter was touted by Thabo Mbeki, President of South Africa, and thousands of people with HIV were discouraged from seeking treatment. Even today the theory has several high-profile believers.

Conspiracy theories related to prevention and treatment include: (1) the government is trying to limit the Black/African/African American population by encouraging the use of condoms; (2) HIV vaccines do currently exist but are being withheld from the public by those in power; and (3) the CIA and Western drug companies are secretly promoting HIV as the cause of AIDS to increase sales of anti-HIV drugs.

While not all of these theories have been definitively disproved, all are based on supposition and speculation, rather than hard evidence. Some were investigated and disproven by reputable scientists earlier in the course of the epidemic, and continuing research has invalidated those related to the origin of HIV, the cause of AIDS, and the effectiveness of prevention and treatment. Clearly, the timeframe for several theories related to the origin of HIV is nullified by current scientific consensus that HIV originated in Africa during the 1930s from the closely related SIV.

Relatively widespread beliefs in HIV conspiracies appear across several racial and ethnic groups in the USA. A 2005 survey by the Rand Corp. indicated that one in seven African Americans believed that AIDS was created by the government to control the African American population, one in three believed HIV was produced in a government laboratory, and more than half said the cure for HIV/AIDS was being withheld from the poor. Another 2006 study in Texas found that as many as 30% of Latinos and African Americans believed that HIV is a government conspiracy to kill ethnic minorities. In that study, conspiracy beliefs were also well represented in the non-Hispanic White sample. In March 2008, U.S. President Barack Obama criticized his former pastor the Rev. Jeremiah Wright for vitriolic sermons in which Wright blamed the government for "inventing the HIV virus as a means of genocide against people of color."

African Americans have many reasons to mistrust the government and the health profession, from the history of slavery, legalized segregation, intended and unintended discrimination and racism, persistent disparities in health care and outcomes, and, most significantly, the infamous 40-year-long Tuskegee Study of Untreated Syphilis by the U.S. Public Health Service, in which 399 African American men infected with syphilis, most uneducated sharecroppers, were deprived treatment so researchers could follow the progression of the disease. Given this clear disregard for the lives of the men who participated, it should be no surprise that some African Americans today embrace assertions that HIV is a man-made virus intentionally spread throughout their communities. Conspiracy beliefs among Latinos may also have their origin in historic racism, oppression, and sterilization efforts as part of their collective consciousness. This is compounded by the recent targeting of Latin American immigrants as the perceived source of social and economic problems, resulting in anti-immigrant legislation to prohibit access to emergency rooms and limit admission to hospitals.

While understandable, pervasive conspiracy theories will continue to negatively impact efforts to address the spread and treatment of HIV within communities of color already overrepresented in the HIV epidemiology, and where the epidemic is taking a deadly toll. Those who believe the government created HIV will not be receptive to the same government's health warnings: engage in behaviors to prevent acquiring or transmitting HIV, including condom use, HIV testing, adherence to recommended treatments, or participation in clinical trials. Individuals with mental illness who ascribe to one or more of the conspiracy theories relating to HIV/AIDS may be less willing to adhere to HIV prevention recommendations and/or recommended treatment for HIV/AIDS if they are already infected with the virus. To counter such beliefs, government and public health entities need to work toward obtaining the trust of these communities by acknowledging and understanding the origin of conspiracy beliefs in the context of historical discrimination and mistrust. They must also address existing discrimination, disparities, and cultural competency within the health care system, and engage community leaders and media outlets to publicly challenge conspiracy theories.

Related Topics: African Americans, Denialism, Tuskegee Syphilis Study.

Suggested Reading

Bogart, L. M., & Thorburn, S. (2005). Are HIV/AIDS conspiracy beliefs a barrier to HIV prevention among African Americans? *Journal of Acquired Immune Deficiency Syndrome, 38*(2), 213–218.

Mackenzie, S. (2011). Dissecting the social body: Social inequality through AIDS counter-narratives. *Public Understanding of Science, 20*(4), 491–505.
Ross, M. W., Essien, E. J., & Torres, I. (2006). Conspiracy beliefs about the origin of HIV/AIDS in four racial/ethnic groups. *Journal of Acquired Immune Deficiency Syndromes, 41*(3), 342–344.
Vankin, J., & Whalen, J. (2004). *The 80 greatest conspiracies of all time*. New York, NY: Citadel Press.

Suggested Resources

AVERT—Averting HIV and AIDS—AIDS & HIV Information from AVERT.org. (2011). *The origin of AIDS and HIV and the first cases of AIDS*. Horsham, West Sussex, UK. Retrieved December 30, 2011 from http://www.avert.org/origin-aids-hiv.htm
Lapidos, J. (2008). The AIDS conspiracy handbook: Jeremiah Wright's paranoia, in context. *Slate Online Magazine, posted March 19, 2008*. Retrieved January 22, 2012 from http://www.slate.com/articles/news_and_politics/explainer/2008/03/the_aids_conspiracy_handbook.html

Contact Tracing

David Bruckman

Preventing the transmission of disease is the principal goal for public health clinicians when performing two common activities: partner notification (PN) and contact tracing (CT). While many academics consider these as equivalent activities, public health practitioners consider these to be vastly different in most respects except for the principal goal. There are vastly different logistic and substantive issues that mental health professionals should consider.

Partner notification (PN) is a process used in public health to locate and notify persons infected or potentially exposed to a sexually transmitted disease. Its primary purpose is to prevent further spread of diseases such as HIV/AIDS, syphilis, and, occasionally, Chlamydia. The Centers for Disease Control and Prevention has promulgated recommendations for partner services to leverage partner notification by expanding partner counseling and referral services for other infections having similar transmission and prevention methods (e.g., hepatitis C).

Contact tracing (CT) is a process used in public health and clinical staff to locate and notify persons infected or potentially exposed to a nonsexually transmitted communicable disease. Its primary purpose is to prevent further spread of diseases including tuberculosis, H1N1, SARS, measles, hepatitis A, meningococcal meningitis, listeria, and other diseases as determined by public health officials. A number of these infections, such as tuberculosis, are not uncommon among individuals infected with HIV, although they clearly affect individuals who are not also infected with HIV. In general, the need to limit transmission and identify who may have been exposed to the infectious agent is not affected by stigma such as that associated with sexually transmitted diseases. In addition, epidemiologists, nurses, and clinicians are more involved in identifying, contacting, and tracing potential contacts than are disease intervention specialists, whose principal training is interviewing and counseling a sexual partner.

D. Bruckman (✉)
Cleveland Department of Public Health, Cleveland, OH, USA
e-mail: DBruckman@city.cleveland.oh.us

S. Loue (ed.), *Mental Health Practitioner's Guide to HIV/AIDS*,
DOI 10.1007/978-1-4614-5283-6_25, © Springer Science+Business Media New York 2013

There are some differences in how the term contact tracing is used internationally. In the United Kingdom, Africa, and Australia/Asia, contact tracing is commonly used parallel to the term partner notification. In the United States, partner notification/partner services are regarded as specifically involving sexually transmitted diseases while contact tracing is regarded as part of case investigation for nonsexually transmitted disease. More recently, the term "sexual" is used in conjunction with contact tracing, facilitating literature searches. Unfortunately, some examples exist where the terms are used interchangeably.

Similarities Between Contact Tracing and Partner Notification

Both PN and CT generally involve screening (testing) for the suspected agent, appropriate clinical treatment, and education in reducing risk of transmission or (re-) infection. Appropriate referral for public and private services, including long-term case management, is provided for individuals with HIV/AIDS and hepatitis C, a feature that is unique to these infections.

Both PN and CT are constitutionally protected as a mandate of public health, and are guided locally by state public health laws. Additional rules or guidance at the local public health agency may exist. Rea provides an excellent review of the history of contact tracing and partner notification.

Both the PN and CT processes begin with a report of a person infected or potentially exposed to the disease. In most states, clinicians, clinical laboratories, and other health care providers are required to provide timely and informative reporting of a person diagnosed with a reportable communicable disease to local or state public health agencies.

Contact Tracing Procedures

The difference between PN and CT begins here. Nonsexual communicable diseases often must be acted upon immediately in terms of treatment and the investigation of known contacts and individuals who were potentially exposed. Reporting must often be done within the first 24 to, at most, 48 h of diagnosis. In contrast, reporting for sexually transmitted diseases often is mandated within a week, rather than hours, of diagnosis.

Contact tracing is generally considered to be part of the case investigation process. Exposure history, clinical status, signs and symptoms, risk factors, laboratory evaluation and confirmation, and contact tracing are used to determine the epidemiology of the event. The epidemiology of the event is described as the route of transmission, source of the infectious agent, profile of the index case(s), spread of the agent, identification of illness, time profile of illness in the population and evolution of this profile as the investigation, amelioration, and contact treatment proceeds.

Regardless of the level of notification, information obtained by local health agencies is shared with their state-level counterpart, such as a state department of public health, as a routine duty of surveillance and reporting. The local or public health officer notified may triage the case to a disease intervention specialist (for HIV/AIDS, syphilis), epidemiologist, or other trained official to perform the initial investigation. The initial investigation involves collection of any information pertinent to the primary contact. For CT, relevant information generally encompasses a history regarding the sphere or area of exposure; the duration of the symptoms associated with infectivity (e.g., cough, droplet dispersal, and contamination); and areas of residence, employment, and education or care (in the case of a student, child, elderly or an institutionalized individual). This information includes the medical information relating to the diagnosis and tests involved; medical services involved including the physician or reporting agency; age; sex; pregnancy status if the individual is female; and personal demographic information including phone numbers, location of residence, and the place of employment or most probable location for appropriate contact. Factors specific to the patient or contact may include information about how recently the potential exposure may have occurred. This is important in classifying respiratory or gastrointestinal infections where infectivity of others through fecal–oral contamination or droplet dispersal are exceptionally high, or where there is an elevated risk of transmission to infants, children, the elderly, or immunocompromised individuals. Other pertinent issues regard the sexual and nonsexual risk behavior suspected with exposure and transmission and sexual orientation to determine those most at risk or transmission. This information is often not elicited from the patient by clinicians or obtained at the time of screening and become part of the initial interview. Other important factors include the individual's family situation; homelessness status; whether there exists a history of domestic violence, a record of violence, or psychiatric or social issues; the individual's level of mental development; and issues regarding competency. Lastly, information regarding the individual's potential reaction, such as the anticipated level of his or her cooperation and potential embarrassment, shame, anger, and other reactions is collected and considered in preparation for the initial interview.

Once the initial investigation of background information is made, an initial interview is conducted. The purpose of this interview is to prevent further transmission of the disease through the identification of the index (initial) patient and his or her partners or contacts.

The Interview

Due to the nature of the infection and the mode of transmission, generally of a nonsexual nature, index cases and contacts in a CT investigation are less uncomfortable in speaking to these professionals about a communicable disease versus a sexually transmitted disease. Instead of sexual and marital/partner relationship issues, index cases, and those (potentially) exposed tend to be less focused on the mode of exposure than on the treatment and prognosis. In patients involved in CT, embarrassment, and shame and concern about the exposure of themselves and others tends to outweigh the shadow of stigma, shame, fear, and anger that are often observed in patients involved in PN of sexually transmitted diseases. Other issues such as sexual abuse and domestic violence, loss of sexual partners, and some legal repercussions are not generally at issue with CT as they are with PN. Consequently, mental health professionals and social workers can expect a much different spectrum of behavioral issues among persons involved with contact tracing. They should be aware of the potential responses of the index individual and those potentially exposed.

Generally, most people are cooperative with the case investigation and contact tracing regarding nonsexually transmitted diseases. Fear and nervousness are the most common emotion in patients diagnosed with nonsexually transmitted communicable diseases, whereas anger is most common in patients diagnosed with sexually transmitted diseases. Socially distanced patients are more likely to respond to medical professionals asking about symptoms and location history compared to an investigator asking about symptoms and sexual history and risk behaviors. Patients and contacts may feel overwhelmed by the process of diagnosis, treatment, and risk reduction (as with tuberculosis). Regret and embarrassment are common among index cases, who may spread the illness or put others at risk. When noncompliance is an issue, contacts may be required to comply with screening and examination recommendations. These procedures may involve screening over several months. Such pressures may manifest into refusal, anger, rejection, isolation, and lowered access to necessary medical care. Social workers and mental health specialists should be aware that, while the spectrum of emotional response is attenuated with contact tracing, it is important to maintain a high index of awareness regarding potential responses.

Reducing misconceptions and misinformation is the most important factor in contact investigations. Misunderstanding and ignorance should be ameliorated through culturally sensitive and educationally appropriate education by public health clinicians.

Patients and identified contacts must understand the importance of naming potential contacts and the serious nature of the disease. Providing clear information about the causative agent, the illness, the dangers of infection and the risk to others, treatment protocols and the need for adherence must be done at a level that the listener can understand. Moreover, the potential for additional transmission, quarantine, or isolation must be carefully explained to the individual who is the index or contact case. Each must understand the importance of exposure, transmission and illness, and the risk they may transmit to or confer on others. Such social isolation can be a great source of stress among patients and their immediate social and employment network.

The sex of the interviewer is less of an issue with contact tracing of a nonsexually transmitted disease than it would be with partner notification of a sexually transmitted infection. This is because partner notification may raise issues of stigma and morality when the sex of the interviewing individual differs from the sex of the contact individual being interviewed. In general, women tend to be more open to cooperating with investigations.

In contrast to CT, partner notification of HIV status can be emotionally devastating. Fear and anger are the most common and powerful reactions among index cases. Sexual partners notified of potential exposure to HIV endure these emotions amplified by the discomfort of being identified. Personal issues of stigma involving sexual activity and issues of sexual orientation, domestic violence, sexual and relational commitment, and the potential for extra-dyadic, extra-matrimonial sexual activity are not uncommon. These issues likely resonate with mental health professionals.

Related Topics: Partner notification, sexually transmitted infections.

Suggested Reading

Centers for Disease Control and Prevention. (2008). Recommendations for partner services programs for HIV infection, syphilis, gonorrhea, and chlamydial infection. *Morbidity and Mortality Weekly Report*, 57(RR-9), 1–63.

Clarke, J. (2001). Distressed women take contact tracing seriously. *British Medical Journal, 323* (7306), 236.

Evans, C. A., O'Connell, C. J., & American Public Health Association Special Initiative on AIDS-AIDS Working Group. (1988). *Contact tracing and partner notification.* Washington, DC: American Public Health Association.

Hogben, M., McNally, T., McPheeters, M., & Hutchinson, A. B. (2007). The effectiveness of HIV partner counseling and referral services in increasing identification of HIV-positive individuals a systematic review. *American Journal of Preventive Medicine, 33*(2 Suppl), S89–S100.

Hoxworth, T., Spencer, N. E., Peterman, T. A., Craig, T., Johnson, S., & Maher, J. E. (2003). Changes in partnerships and HIV risk behaviors after partner notification. *Sexually Transmitted Disease, 30*, 83–88.

Kampf, A. (2008). A 'little world of your own': Stigma, gender and narratives of venereal disease contact tracing. *Health: An Interdisciplinary Journal for the Social Study of Health, Illness and Medicine, 12*(2), 233–250.

Kissinger, P. J., Niccolai, L. M., Magnus, M., Farley, T. A., Maher, J. E., Richardson-Alston, G., et al. (2003). Partner notification for HIV and syphilis: Effects on sexual behaviors and relationship stability. *Sexually Transmitted Disease, 30*, 75–82.

Rea, A. J. (2003). Doing the analysis differently: Using narrative to inform understanding of patient participation in contact tracing for sexually transmissible infections. *Journal of Health Organization and Management, 17*(4), 280–326.

Rothenberg, K. H., & Paskey, S. J. (1995). The risk of domestic violence and women with HIV infection: Implications for partner notification, public policy, and the law. *American Journal of Public Health, 85*, 1569–1576.

Shrestha-Kuwahara, R., Wilce, M., DeLuca, N., & Taylor, Z. (2003). Factors associated with identifying tuberculosis contacts. *International Journal of Tuberculosis & Lung Disease, 7*(12 Suppl. 3), S510–S516.

Ward, H. (2005). Partner notification and contact-tracing. *Medicine, 33*(9), 28–30.

West, G. R., Corneli, A. L., Best, K., Kurkjian, K. M., & Cates, W., Jr. (2007). Focusing HIV prevention on those most likely to transmit the virus. *AIDS Education and Prevention, 19*(4), 275–288.

Suggested Resources

California Department of Health Services and Executive Committee of the California Tuberculosis Controllers Association (CDHA/CTCA). (1997). *Guidelines for the placement or return of tuberculosis patients into high risk housing, work, correctional, or in-patient settings.* Sacramento, CA: Authors.

California Department of Health Services and Executive Committee of the California Tuberculosis Controllers Association (CDHS/CTCA). (1998, November 12). *Contact investigation guidelines.* Retrieved October 21, 2011 from http://www.ctca.org/guidelines/IID1contactinvestigation.pdf

California Department of Health Services and Executive Committee of the California Tuberculosis Controllers Association (CDHA/CTCA). (2009, May 1). *Guidelines for the assessment o tuberculosis patient infectiousness and placement into high risk and lower risk settings.* Sacramento, CA: Authors. Retrieved November 24, 2011 from http://www.ctca.org/guidelines/ctca_infectiousness_guidelines.pdf

Centers for Disease Control and Prevention, Department of Health and Human Services, & Division of Tuberculosis Elimination. (2006). *Effective TB interviewing for contact investigation: Facilitator-led training guide.* Retrieved October 21, 2011 from http://www.cdc.gov/tb/publications/guidestoolkits/Interviewing/facilitator/pdf/facilitatorguide.pdf

New Jersey Department of Health and Senior Services (NJDHSS). (2008, June). *Listeriosis.* Retrieved October 21, 2011 from http://www.nj.gov/health/cd/documents/chapters/listeriosis_ch.pdf

Serpelloni, G., Simeoni, E., & Crestoni, L. *An analysis of contact tracing and partner notification procedures: Possible problems, quality requirements and possible solutions to the problems.* Retrieved October 21, 2011 from http://www.giovanniserpelloni.it/file/argomenti/47/1/Seconda%20parte%20ENG.pdf

Coping

Brandy L. Johnson

In life, every person experiences different situations that require assessment, evoke emotions, and result in a reaction. When we, as human beings, have such experiences and demands are made upon us, we must be able to respond and recover. The capacity to respond to, recover from, and manage the experiences, demands, crises, and/or traumas we find stressful or overwhelming is known as coping. Coping can also be defined as the ability to manage the internal and external stresses/demands placed upon a person, or traumas/crises faced by a person, when those demands, stresses, traumas, and/or crises are greater than the resources available to him or her. Thus, coping is the ability to tackle the difficulties of life and take the actions necessary to overcome them.

Individuals face numerous experiences over the course of their life that require the ability to cope, e.g., professional and personal relationships. Many people are forced to cope with medical and psychiatric conditions. Individuals with symptoms of mental illness face numerous challenges in their efforts to manage their illness and cope with the demands of everyday life. These may be heightened by efforts to prevent HIV or, if they are HIV-positive, to manage the HIV infection in addition to the mental illness. For example, an individual who is diagnosed with HIV and bipolar disorder will, more likely than not, find him- or herself in an overwhelming situation and have to find ways to cope with his or her new reality.

The process of coping involves the utilization of coping mechanisms (coping strategies), that is, remedial actions used to overcome, tolerate, reduce, and/or accept an overwhelmed persons' demands stress, and/or trauma. They can provide a sense of comfort or permit people to obtain a sense of control over a situation. Coping strategies can be psychological and/or behavioral, and, as they are heavily influenced by previous experience, are specific to each individual. Although many people may utilize the same coping mechanism, the mechanism may be

B.L. Johnson (✉)
Rynearson, Suess, Schnurbusch & Champion, L.L.C., St. Louis, MO, USA
e-mail: bjohnson@rssclaw.com

S. Loue (ed.), *Mental Health Practitioner's Guide to HIV/AIDS*,
DOI 10.1007/978-1-4614-5283-6_26,

more effective for, or more heavily relied upon by, one individual than another. Additionally, men and women tend to cope differently.

Coping mechanisms will differ by geographic area, community type, social unity, personality type, and previous experiences. Coping mechanisms can also be affected by socioeconomic factors. For example, some societies may be more accepting of alcohol consumption than others. If more accepted, the use of alcohol to reduce stress or manage demanding situations may be highly relied upon by members of those societies.

In general, there are two basic types of coping strategies: problem-solving strategies and emotion-focused strategies. The problem-solving approach to coping focuses on managing the demands of a situation. Such a strategy usually involves taking some kind of action to reduce the stresses or demands of a situation or to increase the resources available to address those stresses or demands (e.g., learning new skills). The emotion-focused approach, on the other hand, concentrates on how an individual thinks and feels about a situation. A problem-focused approach is often utilized when the person believes the situation can be affected by action. When there is no action that can alleviate the overwhelming situation, an emotion-focused strategy is more appropriate.

Although men often resort to problem solving and women are prone to an emotionally focused approach, people often employ both of these coping strategies. For example, an individual who has just learned that he has HIV may engage in a treatment regimen to control the effects of the disease. While this strategy can help the individual in coping with the situation, he will still have to come to terms emotionally with the fact that he has an incurable disease.

Coping mechanisms can be positive or negative in their overall effect. An active coping strategy permits an individual to reduce the demand/stressor/crisis/trauma or how he or she perceives it. Conversely, avoidant coping mechanisms allow an individual to eschew the stressor/demand/crisis/trauma. Active coping strategies often tend to produce effects that are longer lasting and more beneficial. Some recognized positive coping mechanisms include:

- Utilizing a support system of family and friends
- Communication
- Exercise and physical activity
- Making time for recreation and hobbies
- Meditation or prayer
- Keeping a journal
- Interaction with animals

Negative coping mechanisms, while permitting a temporary escape, can lead to unhealthy conditions and additional stressors/demands. Coping mechanisms that have been found to be negative include:

- Alcohol and drug (illegal or prescription) abuse
- Overeating
- Addictive activities (e.g., gambling, self-harming, risk-taking behaviors, etc.)

- Denial, dissociation, repression, displacement, and compartmentalization
- Anger, manipulation, and violence
- Overworking
- Isolation

Like problem-solving and emotion-focused coping strategies, the coping strategies people employ will usually include both positive and negative coping mechanisms. Individuals whose strategies include more positive mechanisms than negative ones will often be healthier and better able to cope with the difficulties and crises in their lives.

As mentioned above, individuals who discover they have contracted HIV or have AIDS will have to cope with their newly diagnosed medical conditions. In addition to coping with the physical aspects of the disease, the individual must cope with the terminal nature of the disease, the social stigma attached to it, and the financial expenses of treatment. Some positive ways of coping with the situation including: (1) learning as much as possible about the disease; (2) investigating and utilizing available resources such as clinics, social workers, counselors, and advocacy programs; (3) acknowledging any fears, but continuing to live life; (4) knowing one's legal rights and disclosing obligations; (5) meditation or prayer; (6) eating well and staying physically active; (7) communicating with family and friends, including expressions of concern and fear; (8) obtaining the information needed to anticipate what may happen medically and/or psychiatrically and putting plans into place that protect oneself and one's loved ones; (9) eliminating any unnecessary stressors; and (10) taking steps to accept the condition.

Related Topics: Faith community, Internet, religion and spirituality, social support.

Suggested Reading

Burns, K., & Maultsby, M. (1986). *Coping better . . . anytime, anywhere: The handbook of rational self-counseling* (4th ed.). Alexandria, VA: RBT Center LLC.

Clark, R., Hayes, J., & Maupin, R. (2012). *A woman's guide to living with HIV infection* (2nd ed.). Baltimore, MD: The Johns Hopkins University Press.

Critzer, T. (2004). *HIV and me: Firsthand information for coping with HIV and AIDS*. San Francisco, CA: Firsthand Books.

Johanson, P. (2007). *HIV and AIDS (coping in a changing world)*. New York, NY: Rosen Publishing Group.

Snyder, C. R. (1999a). *Coping: The psychology of what works*. New York, NY: Oxford University Press.

Snyder, C. R. (1999b). *Coping with stress: Effective people and processes*. New York, NY: Oxford University Press.

Vaillant, G. (1995). *Adaptation to life*. Cambridge, MA: Harvard University Press.

Yamada, S. (2012). *Psychological distress: Symptoms, causes, and coping*. Hauppauge, NY: Nova Science Pub Inc.

Council of International Organizations for Medical Sciences

Beatrice Gabriela Ioan

The Council for International Organizations of Medical Sciences (CIOMS) is an international, nongovernmental and nonprofit organization that was created in 1949 by the World Health Organization (WHO) and the United Nations Scientific and Cultural Organization (UNESCO). In 2010, CIOMS brought together over 55 international and national organizations from biomedical disciplines, national academies of sciences and medical research councils. Through its activities, CIOMS seeks to facilitate and promote international activities in biomedical sciences, by maintaining relations with the United Nations and its specialized agencies, especially WHO and UNESCO.

CIOMS initiates and coordinates activities that take place within long-term programs, such as: Bioethics, Health Policy, Ethics and Human Values—An International Dialogue, Drug Development and Use, International Nomenclature of Diseases. CIOMS and WHO activity on ethics in biomedical research on humans began during the late 1970s. The *Proposed International Ethical Guidelines for Biomedical Research Involving Human Subjects* was produced in 1982. This guide and its subsequent revisions were developed in order to provide details on the practical application of the provisions of the Helsinki Declaration.

Following the publication of this guide, new issues emerged, especially related to HIV/AIDS and large-scale trials for testing vaccines or treatments for this disease. The organization of clinical trials of HIV/AIDS treatment regimens on people was criticized by human rights activists on the grounds that there was insufficient involvement of local communities in countries with low and medium resources, where clinical trials were conducted and that inadequate information and/or insufficient safeguards were provided to research participants.

In order to obtain valid scientific results on vaccines and therapy for HIV/AIDS, research should be conducted on populations in which HIV incidence and the risk of

B.G. Ioan (✉)
Legal Medicine, Medical Deontology and Bioethics Department, University of Medicine and Pharmacy "Gr. T. Popa", Iasi, Romania
e-mail: ioanbml@yahoo.com

S. Loue (ed.), *Mental Health Practitioner's Guide to HIV/AIDS*,
DOI 10.1007/978-1-4614-5283-6_27,

HIV transmission are high and where therapeutic and/or preventive intervention can have maximum effect. These populations, however, often have a high degree of social vulnerability. Such populations include women and girls in sub-Saharan Africa, commercial sex workers, men who have sex with men, and injecting drug users. Because of their vulnerability, many of these people lack adequate power to protect their rights during or after the completion of the trial, which has led to the need for specific ethical rules to prevent violation of the rights of participants in research.

In this context, CIOMS, WHO Global Programme on AIDS and WHO began the revision process of the *Proposed International Ethical Guidelines for Biomedical Research Involving Human Subjects*. The result was the development of the *International Guidelines for Ethical Review of Epidemiological Studies* in 1991 (revised and further updated in 2009) and the *International Ethical Guidelines for Biomedical Research Involving Human Subjects* in 1993.

The development of the *International Ethical Guidelines for Biomedical Research Involving Human Subjects* in 1993 was followed by new challenges in research, especially related to the conduct of controlled clinical trials with external sponsors in countries with limited resources. One of the primary challenges in these studies arose because the study sponsor is required to ensure that participants in clinical trials receive the standard of care. Opinions were divided within the scientific community between those researchers who believed that the focus should be on the identification of local solutions that are affordable, even if less efficacious, and those who claimed that economic issues should not influence the ethical considerations. Many individuals in this latter group also asserted that relatively wealthier countries should provide the poor countries involved in research the optimal standard of care available at that time. In this context, a review process of the *International Ethical Guidelines for Biomedical Research Involving Human Subjects* was begun in 1998. The process was completed in 2002 with the publication of an updated version.

The International Ethical Guidelines for Biomedical Research Involving Human Subjects contains 21 rules, each with detailed explanations and comments, which relate mainly to "ethical justification and scientific validity of research; ethical review; informed consent; vulnerability of individuals, groups, communities and populations; women as research subjects; equity regarding burdens and benefits; choice of control in clinical trials; confidentiality; compensation for injury; strengthening of national or local capacity for ethical review; and obligations of sponsors to provide health-care services."

This guide contains several important provisions relating to research on HIV/AIDS in human subjects that are intended primarily to protect participants in clinical trials, to minimize risk and to ensure the equitable distribution of risks and benefits for participants. Participants in HIV/AIDS vaccine trials might agree to enroll believing that they have an immediate benefit, which might encourage them to behave in a more risky manner, thereby increasing the risk of contracting the infection. To reduce the likelihood of such situations, participants must be properly informed of the fact that they can contract HIV if they do not take the necessary precautions, even if they are enrolled in a clinical trial. Also, the participants should be advised that they are included in clinical research, and that the vaccine or medication that is provided to them is at an experimental stage.

When established effective therapy exists, placebo-controlled trials are not acceptable in severe clinical situations, such as HIV/AIDS, because the risk faced by participants in the control group who would be deprived of therapy is too great for their lives and health. In order to reduce the risks for participants in the control group, the CIOMS guide suggests using an *add-on design*, in which the test and placebo treatment are added to the standard treatment.

Concerning the fair distribution of risks and benefits, CIOMS guidelines indicate that exclusion from research due to the state of vulnerability of certain categories of people who could benefit from research should be well justified (e.g., patients with HIV/AIDS, cancer), especially when no therapy or prevention method with established efficacy exists. The exclusion of particular categories of people from clinical trials, such as the exclusion of individuals with mental illness, may lead to the lack of specific data on certain treatments or illnesses in these populations, which eventually would be detrimental to them.

The CIOMS guide admits that participation in trials concerning HIV/AIDS drugs or vaccines creates a significant risk of social discrimination of participants. Investigators should make efforts to reduce it by various methods. For example, research participants must be able to demonstrate that they were infected with HIV due to vaccination during the trial and not naturally; also, a registry of participants in the trial should exist and a record of an individual's participation should be made available to third parties upon the request of a trial participant.

In the proceedings for ethical review of research projects aimed at patients with specific diseases or impairments (such as HIV/AIDS), the guide recommends that the Research Ethics Committees consult with representatives of patients who suffer from such diseases or impairments as to whether the trial should or should not be conducted. In addition to this provision, the *International Guidelines for Ethical Review of Epidemiological Studies* suggests that when it is not feasible to obtain individual informed consent, such as the situation when working on already collected biological specimens, it is advisable to proceed to consultation with representatives of communities, different organizations (e.g., when working with information on a specific occupation), associations representing people with an increased risk of contracting a disease (such as sex workers in the case of a study of HIV infection), or patients' associations in order to determine if and to what extent people whose specimens are used would object to research should they be asked individually.

Overall, CIOMS guidelines are intended particularly for countries with limited resources, helping them to apply ethical standards to local circumstances and to properly evaluate research with human participants from an ethical perspective.

Related Topics: Declaration of Helsinki, human rights, United Nations, World Health Organization.

Suggested Reading

Council for International Organizations of Medical Sciences (CIOMS). (2002). *International ethical guidelines for biomedical research involving human subjects.* Retrieved January 4, 2012 from http://www.cioms.ch/publications/layout_guide2002.pdf

Council for International Organizations of Medical Sciences (CIOMS) & World Health Organization (WHO). *International ethical guidelines for epidemiological studies.* Retrieved January 5, 2012 from http://www.ufrgs.br/bioetica/cioms2008.pdf

Macrae, D. J. (2007). The Council for International Organizations of Medical Sciences (CIOMS) guidelines on ethics of clinical trials. *Proceedings of the American Thoracic Society, 4*, 176–179.

Rose, S. (2009). International Ethical Guidelines for Epidemiological Studies by the Council for International Organizations of Medical Sciences (CIOMS). *American Journal of Epidemiology, 170*, 1449–1452.

Suggested Resources

Council for International Organizations of Medical Sciences. http://www.cioms.ch/. Last accessed October 21, 2011.

UNAIDS. http://www.unaids.org/en/Resources/PressCentre/Featurestories/2007/December/20071203ethicalconcernsHIVtrials/. Last accessed October 21, 2011.

Cultural Sensitivity

Kristen Limbach

Cultural sensitivity is the term used most often in the psychological literature to refer to a collection of concepts developed over the past several decades by researchers endeavoring to help health care providers offer culturally relevant care to a growingly diverse clientele. These efforts have produced multiple models over the years of how best to achieve this, and the two most prevalent terms that have emerged are *cultural sensitivity* and *cultural competence*. However, these terms are not interchangeable and should not be confused. *Cultural sensitivity*, which over time has acquired a wide range of definitions, traditionally refers more to knowledge and awareness, whereas *cultural competence* is more of an umbrella term that encompasses the customary idea of cultural sensitivity with an additional emphasis on skills. Despite the prevalence of the term cultural sensitivity in the psychological literature, it has been noted that knowledge and awareness are not sufficient to provide culturally relevant care to diverse patients; rather, an increased focus on skills, particularly in communication and patient-centered interviewing, is required to achieve this goal.

In addition, knowledge of cultural beliefs and practices, as has traditionally been required to be considered culturally sensitive, has been criticized as having only limited usefulness. This is because culture is often defined as a set of characteristics shared by a group of people, including race, religion, traditions, sexual orientation, and even disabilities such as depression, but individuals are not necessarily representatives of a single cultural group. Instead, one individual may belong to an infinite number of groups, and these merge to form a culture unique to that individual. Consequently, knowledge of the values or practices of any number of the groups to which an individual may belong does not necessarily confer knowledge about that individual, and relying on such information may lead to incorrect assumptions. Thus, in more recent years the definition of cultural sensitivity has

K. Limbach (✉)
School of Medicine, Case Western Reserve University, Cleveland, OH, USA
e-mail: kel12@case.edu

S. Loue (ed.), *Mental Health Practitioner's Guide to HIV/AIDS*,
DOI 10.1007/978-1-4614-5283-6_28,

been evolving, often including the requirement of communication skills and de-emphasizing the importance of cultural knowledge.

Consequently, cultural sensitivity can be broken down into a triad of knowledge, awareness, and skills. Although greater importance is accorded to the latter two, as opposed to cultural competency, all three can be developed through a lifelong commitment to continuous self-reflection and self-critique, as well a dedication to lifelong learning and personal improvement. Self-reflection, an important practice for any provider, leads to awareness of one's own biases and cultural context in addition to recognition of the inherent imbalance of power between those providing health care and their patients. Such awareness is particularly critical for providing culturally relevant and sensitive care, as each individual, regardless of his or her background, has patterns of unintentional racism, classism, etc., which may go unnoticed without significant introspection. Furthermore, a commitment to self-critique and personal development allows the practitioner to both act on his or her observations and to have the necessary humility to admit when he or she does not have the required knowledge to provide the best possible care. This opens up opportunities to look for further resources that may be of use. Humility, in fact, is a key word here; while information regarding cultural practices and values may be of use and should not be underestimated, such knowledge cannot always be prioritized over the most accurate and relevant resource on an individual patient: the patient him- or herself.

Accordingly, the patient's view and cultural context are of particular value, and the most effective way to elicit them is through the "skills" portion of the triad, patient-focused interviewing and care. This is a manner of interaction with the patient in which substantial attention is paid to patient-initiated questions and concerns as well as the patient's perspective and expectations. Humility plays a role here as well; health care providers cannot assume that they have sufficient knowledge of the patient to provide appropriate care without first eliciting the patient's perspective and context. Only the patient is positioned to understand the convergence of the many cultural groups to which he or she belongs. Patient-centered interviewing is a helpful tool for creating a window into the patient's unique situation so that the provider can better understand their needs and concerns. Maintaining such humility may be even more difficult for those providers providing care for patients who appear to be from their own cultural group, since it is easy to assume that the patient has similar values and a shared worldview. However, regardless of the magnitude of similarity between the patient and the provider, the provider must remain focused on gleaning culturally relevant information from his or her interactions with each of the patients and remember his/her own naïveté with respect to each patient's cultural context. Thus, cultural sensitivity hinges on consistent humility, partnered with a commitment to self-reflection and improvement.

Maintaining such a commitment has been shown to produce worthwhile results. Over the past few decades, it has become clear that cultural sensitivity is not only conducive to but necessary for optimal patient outcomes, particularly when working with a diverse patient clientele. Negative consequences in its absence have been numerous and include misdiagnosis, poor treatment selection, diminished use of mental health services, and premature termination of treatment by minorities. This is in addition to more obvious but similarly undesirable outcomes, such as increased stereotyping of patients and diminished empathy, which has also been linked with decreased clinical competence. Culture is an unavoidable participant in mental health care, and practicing with cultural sensitivity can provide opportunities to better understand each patient's needs and concerns while simultaneously empowering them to participate more actively in their care.

Providing mental health services to people living with HIV/AIDS similarly requires cultural sensitivity for optimal patient outcomes, and due to HIV's unique demographics, it may be even more critical. According to the CDC, in 2008, men who have sex with men (MSM) accounted for nearly half (48%) of those living with HIV in the United States and constituted over one-half (53%) of new HIV infections that year, while injection drug users accounted for 12% of new infections. Among racial groups, African-Americans bore the greatest burden (46% of those living with HIV in the United States), and Hispanics and Latinos were also disproportionately affected (17% of those living with HIV). Although this breakdown oversimplifies a highly complex situation involving numerous interconnections, it is evident that the brunt of the impact is being borne by racial, ethnic, and sexual minorities. Factors that were once considered mere confounders, such as poverty, substance abuse, racism, homophobia, and unequal access to care, are further contributing to the unequal distribution of infection. Consequently, since many people living with HIV/AIDS culturally identify with one or more groups that have been traditionally marginalized, practicing with cultural sensitivity is of particular importance. The stigma faced by people living with HIV/AIDS can be compounded in individuals who fall into more than one high risk group, such as MSM who are also injection drug users and/or a racial or ethnic minority, and may contribute to mistrust of health care providers and reinforcement of barriers to treatment. Patient-centered interviewing to elicit and address the patient's priorities can help in more effective goal alignment and relationship building; categorization by behavior, in order to encompass a wide range of identities and avoid the appearance of holding or endorsing societal stigma, is also helpful.

In conclusion, cultural sensitivity comprises a triad of knowledge, awareness, and skills, acquired and honed through a lifelong commitment to self-reflection, self-critique, patient-centered dialog, and humility. By seeing each patient not as a member of a predefined cultural group but rather as a unique convergence of cultural identities and experiences, the provider can employ cultural sensitivity to achieve optimal outcomes among a diverse patient clientele, such as those living with HIV/AIDS.

Related Topics: African-Americans, discrimination, gender role, Latinos, sexual orientation, stigma and stigmatization.

Suggested Reading

Berthold, T., Miller, J., & Avila-Esparza, A. (Eds.). (2009). *Foundations for community health workers*. San Francisco, CA: Jossey-Bass.
Cargill, V. A., & Stone, V. E. (2005). HIV/AIDS: A minority health issue. *Medical Clinics of North America, 89*, 895–912.
Ridley, C. R., Mendoza, D. W., Kanitz, B. E., Angermeier, L., & Zenk, R. (1994). Cultural sensitivity in multicultural counseling: A perceptual schema model. *Journal of Counseling Psychology, 41*(2), 125–136.
Rowe, W. (2007). Cultural competence in HIV prevention and care: Different histories, shared future. *Social Work in Health Care, 44*(1/2), 45–54.
Tervalon, M., & Murray-Garcia, J. (1998). Cultural humility versus cultural competence: A critical distinction in defining physician training outcomes in multicultural education. *Journal of Health Care for the Poor and Underserved, 9*(2), 117–125.
Whaley, A. L. (2008). Cultural sensitivity and cultural competence: Toward clarity of definitions in cross-cultural counseling and psychotherapy. *Counseling Psychology Quarterly, 21*(3), 215–222.

Cytomegalovirus

Stefani Parrisbalogun

Human cytomegalovirus (CMV), also known as heterophil-negative mononucleosis, is a ubiquitous herpesvirus that is acquired throughout life and is common in the general population. In the United States, seroprevalence rates are 40% in adolescents and up to 60–100% in adults. The higher seroprevalence seen in adults is attributable to viral reactivation that can occur later in adult life. Increased infection develops perinatally via breast milk, in day care exposure, and then during reproductive age, related to sexual activity. Other routes of transmission include blood transfusions and organ transplantation such as bone marrow, kidney, liver, heart, and/or lung. Primary infection is usually asymptomatic in young, healthy adults but may be associated with a transient mononucleosis-like syndrome. CMV infection results in major neurologic disability, morbidity, and mortality in the setting of immunosuppression such as transplant recipients, in persons with acquired immunodeficiency syndrome, and hematologic malignant neoplasms.

Cytomegalovirus is the most common viral opportunistic infection in patients with AIDS and may be life threatening. Specifically, the severe immunodeficiency caused by infection with human immunodeficiency virus-1 (HIV-1) results in defects in cellular immunity that may involve the retina, meninges, brain, spinal cord, peripheral nerves, and muscle. It has been estimated that 21–44% of patients with AIDS acquired CMV disease in the era before the availability of highly active antiretroviral therapy (HAART) and subsequently this percentage has been reduced dramatically by the wide use of effective antiretroviral therapy. In fact with HAART, the incidence of CMV end-organ disease has decreased by more than 80%. Patients who are infected with HIV-1 in whom CD4 lymphocyte cells are decreased to fewer than 100 cells/mm^3, usually <50/mm^3, have a significantly increased risk for the development of serious CMV disease.

The most common manifestation of CMV disease in adults with AIDS is retinitis, which accounts for about 85% of cases. CMV retinitis causes a

S. Parrisbalogun (✉)
Department of Psychiatry, University Hospitals Case Medical Center, Cleveland, OH, USA
e-mail: Stefani.Parrisbalogun@UHHospitals.org

S. Loue (ed.), *Mental Health Practitioner's Guide to HIV/AIDS*,
DOI 10.1007/978-1-4614-5283-6_29, © Springer Science+Business Media New York 2013

complete-thickness infection through the retinal cells and results in progressive retinal destruction that leads to blindness within 6 months. Distinctive retinal lesions can often be seen ophthalmoscopically. Gastroenterologic manifestations of CMV infection include esophagitis, oral mucosal ulceration, sialoadenitis gastritis (an inflammation and irritation of the lining of the stomach that is associated with the inflammation of a salivary gland), hepatitis, and colitis. CNS (central nervous system) manifestations of CMV infection include encephalitis (an inflammation of the brain and spinal cord); peripheral neuropathy, which refers to damage to the peripheral nervous system that results in distortion and/or interruption of messages between the brain and the rest of the body; and polyradiculoneuritis (inflammation of multiple peripheral nerves and spinal nerve roots). Pneumonia, adrenalitis (an inflammation of one or both adrenal glands), and skin lesions are less common clinical presentations of CMV infection in adult patients with AIDS. Whether some CMV-related neurologic syndromes occur in patients with AIDS is controversial, such as myelitis-polyradiculopathy (spinal cord inflammation-nerve root thickening), encephalitis with dementia, ventriculoencephalitis, and mononeuritis multiplex (inflammation of two or more nerves, often in unrelated portions of the body, causing a loss of function of muscle tissue). However, the detection of CMV in cerebrospinal fluid using a technique known as polymerase chain reaction (PCR) has been correlated with disease. In adult patients with AIDS, the most common CNS infection caused by CMV is polyradiculopathy.

Although less frequently encountered, CMV encephalitis has several manifestations in patients with AIDS with systemic CMV infection. The most typical is a subacute, diffuse encephalopathy (brain damage, disease, or malfunction) evolving during a period of weeks that is characterized by headache, delirium, apathy, and social withdrawal. Neurologic motor findings can include hyperreflexia (exaggerated reflexes), ataxia (lack of coordination and loss of balance), and weakness. CMV ventriculitis (inflammation of ventricles in the brain) is characteristically present, and progressive ventricular enlargement may be observed. Other features may suggest brain stem encephalitis; these features include internuclear ophthalmoplegia (a type of gaze abnormality), nystagmus (rapid, rhythmic, repetitious involuntary eye movements), cranial nerve palsies, gaze paresis (weakness of gaze), ataxia, and quadriparesis (weakness of all four limbs). CMV infection manifested as a cerebral mass lesion is a rare occurrence. Other findings in these patients include cerebral infarction resulting from CMV vasculitis (inflammation of blood vessels), acute subarachnoid hemorrhage (bleeding within the space between two membranes that surround the brain), and intracerebral hemorrhage. CMV myelitis (inflammation of the spinal cord), polyradiculitis (inflammation of nerve roots), and multifocal neuritis (inflammation of multiple nerves) may also occur with CMV encephalitis. Cerebral imaging studies are of limited sensitivity and low specificity in patients with CMV encephalitis. Cerebrospinal fluid results can be variable. Treatment with ganciclovir alone or with ganciclovir and foscarnet are usually standard of care.

Related Topics: Antiretroviral therapy, cognitive impairment.

Suggested Reading

Berger, J. R., & Nath, A. (2011). Cytomegalovirus, Epstein-Barr Virus, and slow virus infections of the central nervous system. In L. Goldman & D. Ausiello (Eds.), *Cecil medicine* (24th ed.). Philadelphia, PA: Saunders Elsevier (Chap. 378).

Crumpacker, C. S., & Zhang, J. L. (2009). Cytomegalovirus. In G. L. Mandell, J. E. Bennett, & R. Dolin (Eds.), *Principles and practice of infectious diseases* (7th ed.). Philadelphia, PA: Elsevier Churchill Livingstone. Retrieved February 16, 2012 from http://www.mdconsult.com/books/page.do?eid=4-u1.0-B978-0-443-06839-3..00138-7&isbn=978-0-443-06839-3&type=bookPage&from=content&uniqId=317717572-2 (Chap. 138).

Suggested Resources

Friel, T. J. (2011, September 28). Epidemiology, clinical manifestations, and treatment of cytomegalovirus infection in immunocompetent hosts. Retrieved February 16, 2012 from Up to Date http://www.uptodate.com/contents/epidemiology-clinical-manifestations-and-treatment-of-cytomegalovirus-infection-in-immunocompetent-hosts?source=search_result&search=cytomegalovirus&selectedTitle=1%7E150

Declaration of Helsinki

Domniţa Oana Bădărău

Adopted in 1964 by the World Medical Association (WMA), the Declaration of Helsinki (DoH) was at that time the most extensive document offering ethical guidelines in conducting research with human subjects. Subsequent revisions to and interpretations of the DoH extended its application to include identifiable human material or data in research, keeping up with the advances in biomedical research and the associated ethical issues that arose. The importance of the document derives from the international dimension and substantial additional requirements and principles to follow. In comparison with the Nuremberg Code, when the guidelines were a result of the military trials, the Declaration's principles emerged from a recognized necessity to have a uniform established recommendation coming from the medical profession.

Amended six times since it was drafted, the WMA's ethical principles are applicable not only to physicians, but also to all other personnel involved in conducting research with human subjects. In addition to this, the DoH urges physicians to apply not only national ethical norms, standards, and regulations, but also all international ones that refer to conducting ethical research with humans. This makes it clear that the WMA acknowledges the dangers of having different medical research standards, which could lead researchers to conduct studies in developing countries based solely on the existence of lower standards.

Divided into three parts, from which the last two represent the core principles, the Declaration clearly states that the force of its international norms and standards should not be diminished by any regulations set at a national level or by additional legal or ethical guidelines adopted at an international level. This Article was a result of the weakening process of the Declaration after the 2000 revision that restricted the use of placebos in clinical research and recommended additional commitments to benefit the study populations in developing countries. As a response to these requirements, several countries chose to defer making references in the national

D.O. Bădărău (✉)
Institute for Biomedical Ethics, University of Basel, Basel, Switzerland
e-mail: domnita@gmail.com

S. Loue (ed.), *Mental Health Practitioner's Guide to HIV/AIDS*,
DOI 10.1007/978-1-4614-5283-6_30,

legislation to older Declaration texts and the US Food and Drug Administration eliminated references to the Helsinki Declaration altogether.

The Declaration's preamble is a moral statement about physicians' duties in relation to their patients, and a statement that this should apply in the research context as well. Populations that are more likely to be overlooked in the recruitment process and prone to additional burdens and risks are given special attention. Efforts should be made to offer access to everyone and to protect and always pursue the well-being of the participants; it is deemed imperative to continually assess all interventions, whether new or current ones.

Medical Research Principles

Reiterating the general moral standard to be pursued in research, part two of the Declaration mentions the researcher's obligation to provide research participants with protection of life and dignity, which encompass self-determination, integrity, privacy, and confidentiality of data relating to the participant. The text also addresses in general terms the accepted scientific steps that research must follow, from the literature review, to research using animals, recognizing the necessity of ensuring protection for the animals, and the need to be aware of the environmental impact. Additional Articles mandate that a study protocol describe in detail the design of the study and all information related to the study, including the funding sources, the institutions and researchers taking part in the research, the risks and benefits associated with participation, and potential conflict of interests on the part of the researchers.

Established independent ethics committees must approve protocols after careful consideration; they are given the right to require changes in the protocol. The committee may require that the researcher list all inducements, possible coercive mechanisms of recruitment, ways in which the study conforms with the DoH's requirements, and how researchers have addressed or will deal with ethical issues arising during the course of and as a result of the study. All this information must be communicated to the potential participants and researchers must ensure that the participants comprehend and voluntarily agree to participate after having weighed the risks and potential benefits. Vulnerable populations must be provided with special protections and may be invited to participate only if the research could not be conducted with other populations. The researchers may be required to provide participants with access to the study's results and proven beneficial interventions after the study ceases. At the same time, researchers must ensure the protection of subjects throughout the study and are responsible for any adverse effects, even if participants have been informed and have consented to participate.

Critiques

Since it was promulgated, the DoH has undergone many debates and several appealing critiques have been formulated. What can be seen as a significant flaw in its text is the broad and possibly unattainable high standards set in conducting research, which may undermine its wide international application and render compliance problematic. Placebo control usage and strict requirements regarding consenting competent subjects raise difficult dilemmas. Use of placebo-controlled studies is significantly restricted to situations in which there are no existing treatments or it is scientifically necessary to prove the efficacy and safety of the new intervention; a mandate to test it against the best current practiced treatment is in place. In the case of informed consent, the DoH does not leave room for conducting research with adults without informed consent, even when this is required for scientific validity and would not imply more than minimal risks.

Valuable for its goals and reduced text length, which make it more accessible while containing complex, essential ethical standards, the Declaration may lose power due to overprotective measures. Research-driven States may ignore the provisions, which may have a negative impact on the ethics of international research studies.

Related Topics: Children, clinical trials, cultural sensitivity, human rights.

Suggested Reading

Carlson, R. V., Boyd, K. M., & Webb, D. J. (2004). The revision of the Declaration of Helsinki: Past, present and future. *British Journal of Clinical Pharmacology, 57*(6), 695–713. doi:10.1111/j.1365-2125.2004.02103.x.

Carlson, R. V., van Ginneken, N. H., Pettigrew, L. M., Davies, A., Boyd, K. M., & Webb, D. J. (2007). The three official language versions of the Declaration of Helsinki: What's lost in translation? *Journal of Medical Ethics, 33*(9), 545–548. doi:10.1136/jme.2006.018168.

Puri, K. S., Suresh, K. R., Gogtay, N. J., & Thatte, U. M. (2009). Declaration of Helsinki, 2008: Implications for stakeholders in research. *Journal of Postgraduate Medicine, 55*(2), 131–134. doi:10.4103/0022-3859.52846.

Rid, A., & Schmidt, H. (2010). The 2008 Declaration of Helsinki—First among equals in research ethics? *Journal of Law, Medicine, & Ethics, 38*(1), 143–148. doi:10.1111/j.1748-720X.2010.00474.x.

Tollman, S. M., Bastian, H., Doll, R., Hirsch, L. J., & Guess, H. A. (2001). What are the effects of the fifth revision of the Declaration of Helsinki? *British Medical Journal, 323*(7326), 1417–1423.

Zion, D., Gillam, L., & Loff, B. (2000). The Declaration of Helsinki, CIOMS and the ethics of research on vulnerable populations. *Nature Medicine, 6*(6), 615–617. doi:10.1038/76174.

Denialism

Ana-Gabriela Benghiac

Denialism in science means rejecting statements and facts accepted by the scientific community. According to Diethelm and McKee, most forms of denialism share five common characteristics: conspiracy theories, fake experts, selectivity, impossible expectations of what research can deliver, and misrepresentation and logical fallacies. HIV/AIDS denialism is a public health concern as it misinforms both governments and lay people, thereby jeopardizing prevention and treatment for the infected individuals and creates confusion and distrust in the scientific community and among healthcare providers. HIV/AIDS denialism, a concept created in the late 1980s, holds that AIDS is not caused by HIV.

Denialists claim that some of the factors that are involved in AIDS pathogenesis are antiretroviral medication (ARVs), any type of intravenous drugs, depression, stress, and malnutrition. They also believe that HIV/AIDS is a conspiracy created by the pharmaceutical (Pharma) industry, researchers, physicians, governments, and certain institutions whose aim is to kill healthy individuals with toxic medication while simultaneously garnering a profit. Denialists encourage the use of vitamins, the adoption of a healthy lifestyle, and reliance on nontoxic remedies for AIDS such as acupuncture, digitopuncture, herbal medicine, music therapy, color therapy, aromatherapy, hypnosis, yoga, light therapy, and spiritual care. Among the most cited AIDS denialists are Peter Duesberg, David Rasnick, Jody Wells, Huw Christie, Michael Baumgartner, Neville Hidgkinson, Henry H. Bauer, David Crowe, Celia Farber, and 1993 Nobel Laureate for Chemistry, Kary B. Mullis.

Although scientists have demonstrated that HIV causes AIDS, denialists believe that HIV is harmless, that HIV does not exist, that HIV tests are invalid, and that AIDS is just a fabricated epidemic. They also state that HIV is not sexually transmissible. HIV/AIDS denialism has negative implications at both the governmental and individual levels. Worldwide, many children's deaths are associated

A.-G. Benghiac (✉)
Department of Bioethics, Case Western Reserve University, Cleveland, OH, USA
e-mail: dr.gabriela_benghiac@yahoo.com

S. Loue (ed.), *Mental Health Practitioner's Guide to HIV/AIDS*,
DOI 10.1007/978-1-4614-5283-6_31, © Springer Science+Business Media New York 2013

with parental HIV/AIDS denialism and their refusal to seek proper therapy for their HIV-positive offspring. The deaths of some denialists at young ages and with AIDS-like symptoms are thought to be associated with the disease itself. During their lives, several HIV denialists changed their minds and admitted that AIDS is indeed caused by HIV.

Official statements like those of the South African Health Minister Manto Tshabalala-Msimang, who recommended that AIDS be treated with alternative medicine based on garlic, beetroot, lemon, olive oil, and African potato instead of antiretroviral medications, unfortunately led to the loss of human life and vertical, mother-to-child HIV transmission that could have been prevented. The epidemic in South Africa, which was intensely studied, is mostly associated with Thabo Mbeki's government policies; the high prevalence of the disease is objective evidence of successive governments' lack of understanding, assessment, action, and denialism. Mbeki's government stated that AIDS is not caused by HIV and that the antiretroviral drugs (ARVs) are toxic. After the first two AIDS cases were identified in South Africa, the government misinformed the population by saying that the illness affects only some homosexuals and Black individuals and that there is no need for intervention, thus denying its responsibility. People were deprived of access to effective and safe treatment, not only because the government could not provide sufficient medication, but also because it was in denial. Popular beliefs, e.g., sexual intercourse with a virgin cures AIDS, AIDS is caused by voodoo curses or condoms fitted well, reflect a climate dominated by ignorance and inaction. Even though the main cause of mortality in South Africa was AIDS, Mbeki stated that the disease was not responsible for those deaths, but that crime and violence throughout the country were the cause. Denialists' theories in South Africa also promoted the idea such that AIDS has the tendency to affect more Black individuals than White people; that the disease is a punishment from God; that the spread of AIDS is limited; and that "proper Christian behavior" will protect the population from getting infected. Over time, the South African government took the counter-offensive and accused its critics of racism, even while partially acknowledging the real situation. Stanley Cohen's typology of denial applied by Pieter Fourie and Melissa Meyer in the South African AIDS context is a perfect representation of literal, interpretive, and implicatory official denial and how the government's statements and actions of denial can lead to disastrous consequences.

The Durban Declaration (2000) is a document signed by 500 scientists that affirms that AIDS is caused by HIV and emphasizes that proper medication reduces AIDS mortality by more than 80%. This represents one of the most important steps in confronting denialism by the scientific community and addressing key issues in HIV/AIDS.

HIV/AIDS denialism continues to have a voice in the media and on the Internet; these claims are often countered by AIDS activists. Some of the most renowned AIDS activists are Seth Kalichman, Martin Delaney, John Moore, and Mark Wainberg.

Related Topics: Conspiracy theories.

Suggested Reading

Chigwedere, P., & Essex, M. (2010). AIDS denialism and public health practice. *AIDS and Behavior, 14*(2), 237–247.
Cohen, S. (2001). *States of denial: Knowing about atrocities and suffering*. Oxford: Blackwell.
Diethelm, P., & McKee, M. (2009). Denialism: What is it and how should scientists respond? *European Journal of Public Health, 19*(1), 2–4.
Fourie, P., & Meyer, M. (2010). *The politics of AIDS denialism. South Africa's failure to respond*. Aldershot: Ashgate Publishing Limited.
Kalichman, S. (2009). *Denying AIDS, conspiracy theories, pseudoscience, and human tragedy*. New York, NY: Springer.
McNeill, F. G. (2009). 'Condoms cause AIDS': Poison, prevention and denial in Venda, South Africa. *African Affairs, 108*(432), 353–370.

Suggested Resources

Bergman, J. (2010). The cult of HIV denialism. *The body: The complete HIV/AIDS resource*. Retrieved February 6, 2012 from http://www.thebody.com/content/art57918.html
http://www.aidstruth.org/denialism/denialists/dead_denialists

Disability Laws

Brandy L. Johnson

Historically, the disabled, as a population, have largely been socially isolated, underserved, viewed as a burden, and either confined to their homes or institutionalized. Disabled individuals have also been frequent victims of abuse, crime, and discrimination. However, in the more recent past, societies and governments have begun taking steps to protect disabled individuals and their civil rights. The enactment and enforcement of disability laws are important measures in effecting this change.

The definition of the word "disability" will vary depending upon the purpose for which it is being used. Legislation often provides different definitions of the word "disability" for the purposes of the laws being enacted. However, in general, a disability is a physical, cognitive, emotional, developmental, sensory, or mental condition that restricts an individual's abilities. Disabilities vary in degree, severity, duration, and obviousness.

The disabled have been described as the world's largest minority. The United Nations estimated in 2006 there were 650 million individuals, or approximately 10% of the world's population, living with a disability. In the United States, there were approximately 36 million disabled individuals in 2009. As a minority population that is often misunderstood, there is a resulting stigma and discrimination against disabled individuals.

Forty-five countries had laws prohibiting discrimination against the disabled and/or other disability-specific laws in 2006. Disability laws can, and do, serve different purpose. Some legislation protects the rights of the disabled population. In the United States, the Americans with Disabilities Act (ADA) is one such piece of legislation.

The ADA is a federal law that was enacted in 1990 and amended in 2008 to protect the rights of individuals with disabilities. The ADA prohibits discrimination based on disability in employment, public accommodations, commercial facilities,

B.L. Johnson (✉)
Rynearson, Suess, Schnurbusch & Champion, L.L.C., St. Louis, MO, USA
e-mail: bjohnson@rssclaw.com

S. Loue (ed.), *Mental Health Practitioner's Guide to HIV/AIDS*,
DOI 10.1007/978-1-4614-5283-6_32, © Springer Science+Business Media New York 2013

transportation, telecommunications, and by state and local governments. To be protected under the ADA, an individual has to: (1) have a physical or mental impairment that substantially limits one or more major life activities, (2) have a record of such impairment; or (3) be regarded as having such impairment.

HIV/AIDS, both symptomatic and asymptomatic, has been recognized as a disability under the ADA. Although the courts in examining litigation brought under the ADA have tended to treat HIV/AIDS as an "impairment," the disabled individual is required to show the virus substantially limits a major life activity. Reproduction and a compromised immune system have been recognized as major life activities that are substantially impaired by HIV/AIDS.

The ADA provides the disabled individual with the ability to seek recourse for discrimination administratively through the Equal Opportunity Commission and in civil court. Despite the legal remedies provided by the ADA, the ultimate goal of the legislation is to discourage discrimination and, eventually, to eradicate it. In the United States, similar legislation has been passed by many of the states. Some states, like Florida, have even passed antidiscrimination legislation that is HIV specific.

The Fair Housing Act is another example of protective legislation. The Fair Housing Act prevents discrimination in housing based upon disability and its protections have been found to extend to individuals living with HIV/AIDS. Like the ADA, states such as California have also passed legislation at the state level that protects the housing rights of disabled individuals.

Other legislation is more prohibitive in nature and criminalizes offenses against the disabled. In the United States, a federal government study conducted in 2007 revealed the disabled were 50% more likely to be the victims of violent crimes. The most common crimes against the disabled were assault, aggravated assault, and robbery. The study further showed that disabled individuals were the victims of 1.7 million thefts, 527,000 burglaries, and 107,000 car thefts. Given that disabled persons as a population are more vulnerable and less likely to be able to defend themselves, preventive legislation is imperative to discourage such offenses and to help ensure the safety and security of the disabled.

Statutes that criminalize offenses against the disabled, in particular, will generally take one of two forms. The first type of legislation creates a distinct crime for an offense against a disabled individual. The other type of legislation enhances the penalty for an already existing crime when a disabled individual is the victim. As with protective laws for the disabled, these preventive laws are commonly found at the state and federal level.

The criminalization of the neglect of a disabled individual or the financial exploitation of a disabled individual illustrates the creation of distinct crimes for offenses against an individual with a disability. State and federal legislation creating a distinct crime for hate/bias motivated offenses against individuals with disabilities serves as yet another example. If an individual with HIV/AIDS is targeted due to a protected characteristic, such as disability or sexual orientation, he or she may be protected under the hate crime legislation.

The fact the victim of a crime is disabled can also serve to make the penalty for a crime more severe. In Illinois, for example, the crime of battery can be elevated to aggravated battery when the perpetrator knowingly, and without legal justification, commits the offense against a person with a permanent physically disabling condition. The involvement of a disabled victim takes battery from a Class A misdemeanor to a Class 3 felony.

Due to their status as a minority, disabled individuals often have little voice in effectuating change. Many of the disabled population also find themselves in the poorer segment of society, further limiting their ability as a group to effect change. However, it is precisely due to the vulnerability of the disabled population that measures must be taken to protect their civil rights, and prevent crime aimed against them.

Disability laws, though, are only one step in what must be a multistep process. The education of the public about disabilities, the promotion of an understanding of different disabilities and the disabled in general, and the provision of services that allow disabled persons to be less socially isolated are also important steps. Disability laws help disabled individuals engage in society, work, and, through these interactions, educate others and foster a greater understanding of both disabilities and the abilities of disabled individuals. Hopefully, as both tolerance and understanding increase, the need for disability laws will decrease.

Related Topics: Discrimination, hate crimes, legal issues for HIV-infected clients, stigma and stigmatization.

Suggested Reading

Bragdon v. Abbott, 524 U.S. 624, 118 S. Ct. 2196 (1998).

Breslin, M., Yee, S., & Disability Rights Education & Defense Fund. (2002). *Disability rights law and policy: International and national perspectives*. Dobbs Ferry, NY: Transnational.

Colker, R., & Milani, A. (2005). *Everyday law for individuals with disabilities*. Boulder, CO: Paradigm Publishers.

Cooper, J. (2000). *Law, rights and disability*. London: Jessica Kingsley Publishers.

Engel, D., & Munger, F. (2003). *Rights of inclusion: Law and identity in the life stories of Americans with disabilities*. Chicago, IL: University of Chicago Press.

Fleischer, D., & Zames, F. (2011). *The disability rights movement: From charity to confrontation* (2nd ed.). Philadelphia, PA: Temple University Press.

Gostin, L., & Webber, D. (2000). Discrimination based on HIV/AIDS and other conditions: "Disability" as defined under federal and state law. *Journal of Health Care Law & Policy, 3*, 266–329.

Rioux, M., Basser, L., & Jones, M. (2011). *Critical perspectives on human rights and disability law*. Leiden: Brill Academic Publishing.

Disclosure

Mihaela-Catalina Vicol

Although it might be expected that people would disclose their HIV status to family members, since family may represent an important emotional, physical, and social support, people may be afraid to do so, due to the possibility of experiencing shame, the withdrawal of financial or emotional support, and/or rejection. Disclosure of one's HIV status to family members may lead to additional discussions about the circumstances surrounding how one became HIV-positive, sexual orientation, or drug habits, all topics that are often uncomfortable, especially with family members like parents, brothers or sisters. Studies have found that nondisclosure of HIV status to family members may be due to feelings of shame, the lack of parents' education or sophistication, or parents' age or health problems.

Studies on disclosure to parents indicate a preference for disclosure to mothers rather than to fathers. However, studies are inconsistent with respect to the extent of this difference, with some reporting 23% participants disclosing to mothers and 8.1% to fathers, and others reporting a smaller difference, like 48% to mothers and 40% to fathers.

Disclosure of one's HIV status to sexual partners is often stressful; disclosure depends on the stability of the relationship and the type of the relationship. Studies have shown that usually the information is disclosed to primary partners rather than past partners, that there is a fear in long-term relationships that disclosing this information would end the relationship, and that individuals may fear violence as a result of their disclosure. Research also suggests that there is a reaction among some HIV-positive persons, called "gift givers," in which people deliberately infect others without telling them about their HIV status. Disclosure of one's HIV status to healthcare providers may arouse fears that confidentiality will be breached, which may lead to a loss of insurance or employment.

M.-C. Vicol (✉)
Department of Bioethics, University of Medicine and Pharmacy "Gr. T. Popa", Iasi, Romania
e-mail: mihavicol@yahoo.com

S. Loue (ed.), *Mental Health Practitioner's Guide to HIV/AIDS*,
DOI 10.1007/978-1-4614-5283-6_33, © Springer Science+Business Media New York 2013

Although self-disclosure of HIV status to one's sexual partners is mandated in many states in the United States and in many countries, it is not as frequently mandated for needle-sharing contacts. Nevertheless, many people do not often self-disclose, although criminal offences might apply to them.

Several reasons suggest that individuals should disclose their HIV status. First of all, people who disclose their HIV status may gain access to adequate treatment. Consider, for example, the treatment of pneumonia in a healthy patient and in an HIV immunocompromised patient; the disease has the same name, but the etiology and the treatment might be different. Also, the receipt of social support and some services, such as free treatment or care, may require disclosure of this information to social service. Disclosure of one's HIV status may also bring benefits to one's personal health. Avoidance of other, different diseases may be facilitated only if the patient tells his or her healthcare providers and partner his or her HIV status.

The second reason for disclosure would be to protect the others. Though disclosure may lead to termination of a relationship, disclosure also facilitates a responsible sexual life, family planning, and avoidance of disease transmission.

It has been suggested that as people become more and more educated, disclosure of HIV status may reduce the associated stigma and the social rejection. Last, there is the argument that disclosing the HIV status to a trustworthy person may bring psychological benefits like support, emotional freedom, and gaining positive emotions.

Disclosure of one's HIV status may arouse social, physical, and psychological prejudices. Some of the most important consequences include discrimination in hiring, employment termination, insurance, marginalization and ostracism, stigma, and the termination of relationships with partners, parents, relatives, and/or friends. These consequences may lead to adverse psychological consequences and may determine the progression of the disease or the appearance of complications. Violence against people with HIV/AIDS, domestic and nondomestic violence, eviction from houses or from the religious congregation may also occur.

The potential for such consequences determines the difficulty of disclosing the information, even though there may be criminal penalties for not fulfilling the obligation to disclose. The equilibrium between advantages and disadvantages of disclosing is very fragile and may lead the individual to experience conflict between fulfillment of a moral and legal obligation to disclose and the need for psychological, economic, and physical self-protection.

Related Topics: Confidentiality, disclosure laws, duty to warn, partner notification.

Suggested Reading

Green, K., Derlega, V. J., Yep, G. A., & Petronio, S. (2003). *Privacy and disclosure of HIV in interpersonal relationships. A sourcebook for researchers and practitioners*. Mahwah, NJ: Lawrence Erlbaum Associates Inc.

Hays, R. B., McKusick, L., Pollack, L., Hillard, R., Hoff, C., & Coates, J. J. (1993). Disclosing HIV seropositivity to significant others. *AIDS, 7*, 425–431.

Marks, G., Bundek, N., Richardson, J. L., Ruiz, M. S., Maldonado, N., & Mason, H. R. C. (1992). Self-disclosure of HIV infection: Preliminary results from a sample of Hispanic men. *Health Psychology, 11*, 300–306.

Post, S. G. (Ed.). (2004). *Encyclopedia of bioethics* (3rd ed.). MacMillan Reference: Thomson Gale.

Serovich, J. M., McDowell, T. L., & Grafsky, E. L. (2008). Women's report of regret of HIV disclosure to family, friends and sex partners. *AIDS and Behavior, 12*(2), 227–231.

Disclosure Laws

Domniţa Oana Bădărău

Disclosure of Medical and Health Information in the Health Care Context

With electronic medical records being introduced in many hospitals worldwide, the liability for data spillover is of concern to ethicists, patients, and advocacy groups. Two concepts that bear a strong value and significance in the context of health care are indissolubly linked to patient information and disclosure regulations. There cannot be a thorough discussion regarding personal health data without also addressing privacy and confidentiality rights and their exceptions. Privacy and confidentiality concepts represent the rule in attempting to avoid data misuse and discrimination and in protecting human dignity. Disclosure is the exception, regulated and accepted under specific conditions for certain cases.

Patient Information Disclosure Under HIPAA

In the United States, a recognized need to ensure protection of private information and to combat possible discrimination based on health status led to the development of privacy and disclosure laws. The Health Insurance Portability and Accountability Act (HIPAA) of 1996 represents the most comprehensive set of requirements regulating privacy standards in relation to at least three parties: the health care personnel, the patient and researchers. Part of the Act's purpose is the protection of health information, by enforcing physical and technical safeguards in addition to the medical profession's confidentiality standard. Health information is defined as a person's condition relating to his or her physical and psychological health during

D.O. Bădărău (✉)
Institute for Biomedical Ethics, University of Basel, Basel, Switzerland
e-mail: domnita@gmail.com

S. Loue (ed.), *Mental Health Practitioner's Guide to HIV/AIDS*, 197
DOI 10.1007/978-1-4614-5283-6_34, © Springer Science+Business Media New York 2013

his or her lifetime; the information registered by a health care entity, including public health authorities, employers; the educational institutions, and insurance companies; the care provided to that individual, and the financial worth of the health care provided to that individual. A particular distinction must be made regarding individually identifiable health information, which has some additional characteristics derived from the fact that it represents a fraction of the complete health information and contains demographic data, which can identify the individual or could pose the probability of identifying the individual.

Throughout the text of HIPAA, disclosure is used to signify the way in which the information is handled, used, made public, stored, copied, shared, and accessed from outside or by outside parties. Any other action resulting in information being available beyond the agent holding it must be HIPAA compliant. Electronic media, together with other physical ways of recording the information and the oral transmission of health information fall under the privacy rules. Under the Health Information Technology for Economic and Clinical Health Act (HITECH Act) of 2009, the covered entities and any associates must have established protections to prevent the disclosure of health protected information that is used by or originated from electronic records.

The standard rule is not to disclose protected health information as defined above. However, there are permissible situations, such as for victims of violence, public health and health oversight activities, and whistleblowers, as well as mandatory disclosures, as in the case of subpoenas and court orders. For research purposes, the use and disclosure is permitted if a waiver is in place or as long as an IRB approval had been obtained, along with other cases stipulated in the regulations.

Disclosure Laws and HIV/AIDS

The HIPAA's provisions contain rights and restrictions on accessing medical records by both patients and medical personnel, as well as by researchers and other parties. An additional right is given to the patient, who under the Act can require the names of the persons who accessed his or her private health information. The individual to whom the information pertains must be consulted before the disclosure and provided an opportunity to contest the disclosure, except for emergency cases when this is not feasible or for special situations specified by law, in which case disclosure is mandatory. It is permitted to use or disclose the individual's protected health information in case of treatment, for recovering financial costs, in health care operations under certain provisions, and when a valid authorization is in place, such as for psychotherapy records.

Protected health information regarding HIV or AIDS refers to any knowledge related to medical exams or tests performed in relation to HIV, the HIV status of a person, any disease associated with HIV, AIDS, the exposure to the virus, or any other additional information referring to the individual's identifiable data. Applied to health information regarding HIV infection and AIDS, HIPAA regulations restrict the disclosure of health information in situations in which there is no valid release form signed by the patient or by a legal representative. Nevertheless, in case a release exists and meets the validity conditions, the information must be kept confidential beyond the purpose and the intended beneficiaries of the release form. These regulations have to be followed not only by health care providers and their workforce and social services systems and personnel, but also by any other person that comes across information regarding or in relation to a person's HIV status or matters connected to HIV or AIDS data concerning an individual.

Other standards are set in place for the use and disclosure of de-identified data and in the case of an agreed upon restriction case. Regarding the first of these two additional standards, the de-identified information can be used and disclosed as long as no other data, code, or key that could lead to a connection between the data and the individual is disclosed. Obtaining data regarding the HIV status of a person does not require informed consent in certain limited cases. Testing for HIV is done without informed consent as part of the Comprehensive Newborn Screening, in conjunction with an autopsy to determine cause of death, for public health needs in tracking transmissible diseases, or for employees in certain public duties. The enforcement of these provisions relating to the unauthorized use and sharing of private health information may be effectuated through HIPAA's civil and criminal measures.

Partner Disclosure of HIV Status and Criminal Law

Many US states have criminal HIV disclosure laws that make it possible for HIV-infected persons or individuals with AIDS to be prosecuted for engaging in sexual activities whenever they failed to inform their partner regarding their HIV status. The severity of the sanction under the criminal law varies from state to state, so that the punishment may include a prison sentence and/or fine. In some cases, an individual may be ordered to pay a fine if there was no intent to expose the partner to infection.

Related Topics: Confidentiality laws, disclosure, HIV testing, informed consent.

Suggested Reading

DiBenedetto, D. V. (2003). HIPAA Privacy 101: Essentials for case management practice. *Lippincotts Case Management, 8*(1), 14–23.

Galletly, C. L., Difranceisco, W., & Pinkerton, S. D. (2009). HIV-positive persons' awareness and understanding of their state's criminal HIV disclosure law. *AIDS Behavior, 13*(6), 1262–1269. doi:10.1007/s10461-008-9477-y.

Gunn, P. P., Fremont, A. M., Bottrell, M., Shugarman, L. R., Galegher, J., & Bikson, T. (2004). The Health Insurance Portability and Accountability Act Privacy Rule: A practical guide for researchers. *Medical Care, 42*(4), 321–327.

HIPAA Administrative Simplification. 45 CFR Parts 160, 162, and 164, 45 CFR Parts 160, 162, and 164 C.F.R. (2006).

Schoppmann, M. J., & Sanders, D. L. (2004). HIPAA compliance: The law, reality, and recommendations. *Journal of the American College of Radiology, 1*(10), 728–733. doi:10.1016/j.jacr.2004.03.017.

Discrimination

Brandy L. Johnson

Discrimination can be defined as the oppression, unjust treatment, or unfair treatment, usually through acts and omissions, of an individual or a group of individuals. Discrimination often occurs as a result of a stigma/prejudice connected to an individual or a group of individuals. Stigma occurs due to negative beliefs, feelings, and/or attitudes toward specific individuals or a group of individuals.

In the context of HIV/AIDS, stigma and discrimination exists worldwide and can result in social isolation, abandonment, shunning, avoidance, harassment, violence, rejection, and/or gossip. Further, the stigma and discrimination that someone with HIV/AIDS experiences may be compounded by inclusion in another highly stigmatized group. For example, an individual with HIV may experience a higher level of stigma and discrimination if he or she is also a sex worker, intravenous drugs user, bisexual, or homosexual. Such individuals seem to receive less sympathy from others due to the connection made between the virus' acquisition and the individual's lifestyle.

The stigma and discrimination associated with HIV/AIDS has resulted from many factors. As the disease is fatal, fear and other strong emotions are two of these factors. Moral and religious beliefs, especially when the individual is homosexual, have led to negative attitudes, assumptions, and conclusions about people infected with the disease. Similarly, as mentioned above, other lifestyle choices or behaviors that are already frowned upon by society, such as drug use or prostitution, reinforce negative beliefs about the virus and add to the idea that its transmission resulted from personal irresponsibility. Finally, another factor in the endurance of the stigma surrounding and discrimination against those with HIV/AIDS is a lack of education and understanding of the disease. Consider the fact that in 2006, a survey in the USA showed that 37% of the public still erroneously believed HIV could be transmitted through kissing, 22% believed HIV could be transmitted through

B.L. Johnson (✉)
Rynearson, Suess, Schnurbusch & Champion, L.L.C., St. Louis, MO, USA
e-mail: bjohnson@rssclaw.com

S. Loue (ed.), *Mental Health Practitioner's Guide to HIV/AIDS*,
DOI 10.1007/978-1-4614-5283-6_35, © Springer Science+Business Media New York 2013

sharing a drinking glass, and 16% believed transmission could occur by touching a toilet seat.

Discrimination against individuals with HIV/AIDS is most commonly seen in employment, the provision of health care, the ability to acquire insurance, the freedom to travel, access to services provided through public accommodations, the ability to obtain housing, access to education, and within social networks. Discrimination can also be the result of existing laws, policies, regulations, and/or accepted practices. Unfortunately, the stigmatization of and discrimination against individuals with HIV/AIDS can result in the abandonment of the individual by family, divorce, and/or rejection by a church and other social entities.

Employment is an area where individuals with HIV/AIDS face a great deal of discrimination. The discrimination occurs in decisions involving hiring, promotion, wages, and insurance benefits. If their HIV/AIDS status becomes known, individuals may be harassed, dismissed, or pressured to resign. Discrimination can come from the employer as well as coworkers. As recently as 2006, a survey in the USA inquired into how comfortable the participants would be working with individuals with HIV. The results showed that 13% would not be too comfortable and 8% would not be comfortable at all.

Another area where individuals with HIV/AIDS face a large amount of discrimination is in the access to, and provision of, health care. This discrimination can take the form of a lesser standard of care, a refusal by health care professionals to provide care, the adoption of unnecessary infection control measures, breaches of confidentiality, the conduct of HIV testing without consent, and an inability or lessened ability to obtain medication. The People Living with HIV Stigma Index showed that in 2009, 17% of respondents in the United Kingdom reported a denial of health care. Moreover, studies in India, Indonesia, Thailand, and the Philippines have revealed that 34% of respondents experienced breaches of confidentiality by health care workers.

An individual's HIV/AIDS status may also affect his or her ability to travel. Several countries restrict the entry of people with HIV/AIDS and their ability to stay in the country. For example, until 2010, the USA barred individuals with HIV from entering the country even on a short term basis. As of 2011, UNAIDS reported that there were some sort of restrictions on the ability of people living with HIV to travel and/or remain in 47 countries, territories, and areas. Additionally, some countries' policies may violate confidentiality, require disclosure of one's HIV status, or mandate submission to HIV testing.

The ability to rent housing and eviction from it are valid concerns for individuals with HIV/AIDS. Further discrimination may take the form of harassment by neighbors, landlords, or fellow tenets. Some landlords institute policies, such as refusal to rent to individuals receiving social services, that prevent people with HIV/AIDS from renting from them.

Discrimination against individuals living with HIV/AIDS has a negative effect for both the individual and the public. Due to the fear of discrimination, people tend to be reluctant to undergo testing, disclose their HIV status, educate themselves about the disease, seek counseling, and/or obtain treatment for the disease.

The reluctance to obtain testing, education about the disease, and counseling makes such individuals more likely to infect others. They are also more likely to be diagnosed at a later stage of the disease, making treatment less effective, suffer untreated depression, and have a higher early death rate.

There are efforts being made to reduce the stigma and discrimination concerning HIV/AIDS. In 2010, UNAIDS reported that 71% of countries have laws prohibiting discrimination against individuals with HIV/AIDS. In the USA, for example, protective legislation has been passed that makes discrimination in employment, access to public accommodations, and housing actionable. Numerous organizations, charities, scientists, and foundations are making efforts to measure, understand, and reduce HIV-related stigma and discrimination.

The reduction and elimination of stigma and discrimination is of great importance. As recognized by AVERT, combating the stigma and discrimination experienced by people living with HIV/AIDS is vital to the effort to prevent and control the global HIV/AIDS epidemic. Consequently, more effort needs to be made to educate the public about the disease and combat fear, denial, negative attitudes, and erroneous beliefs. The removal of punitive laws and the strict enforcement of protective legislation, policies, and regulations would also help reduce discrimination.

Related Topics: Disability laws, hate crimes, immigration, stigma and stigmatization.

Suggested Reading

Herek, G., & Capitanio, J. (1999). AIDS stigma and sexual prejudice. *American Behavioral Scientist, 42*, 1126–1143.

Suggested Resources

AVERT. (n.d.). *HIV & AIDS stigma and discrimination*. Retrieved October 27, 2011 from http://www.avert.org/hiv-aids-stigma.htm

International Association of Physicians in AIDS Care. (2010). *AIDS Treatment for Life International Survey 2010: Stigma, isolation, and discrimination and their impact on HIV serostatus disclosure: A global survey of 2,035 patients*. Retrieved October 27, 2011 from http://www.iapac.org/ATLIS/

Lange, T., & ACLU AIDS Project. (2003). *HIV & civil rights: A report from the frontlines of the AIDS epidemic*. Retrieved October 27, 2011 from http://www.aclu.org/pdfs/hivaids/hiv_civilrights.pdf

UNAIDS. (2007). *Reducing HIV stigma and discrimination: A critical part of national AIDS programmes: A resource for national stakeholders in the HIV response*. Retrieved October 27, 2011 from http://data.unaids.org/pub/Report/2008/jc1521_stigmatisation_en.pdf

UNAIDS. (2010). *Non-discrimination in HIV responses*. Retrieved October 27, 2011 from http://data.unaids.org/pub/BaseDocument/2010/20100526_non_discrimination_in_hiv_en.pdf

Duty to Warn

Sana Loue

Social workers, psychologists, psychiatrists, and other mental health professionals have an ethical and legal responsibility to maintain client disclosures in confidence. As an example, the Code of Ethics formulated by the National Association of Social Workers states:

> Social workers should protect the confidentiality of all information obtained in the course of professional service, except for compelling professional reasons. The general expectation that social workers will keep information confidential does not apply when disclosure is necessary to prevent serious, foreseeable, and imminent harm to a client or other identifiable person. In all instances, social workers should disclose the least amount of confidential information necessary to achieve the desired purpose; only information that is directly relevant to the purpose for which the disclosure is made should be revealed (National Association of Social Workers, Code of Ethics, § 1.07(c), 2008).

This duty to warn derives from a California court case, *Tarasoff v. Regents of the University of California*, in which a psychologist's client threatened to kill and then killed his former girlfriend. Although the therapist claimed that the communication from his client was confidential and could not be disclosed by the therapist absent the client's permission, the court held that:

> when a therapist determines, or pursuant to the standards of his profession should determine, that his patient presents a serious danger of violence to another, he incurs an obligation to use reasonable care to protect the intended victim against such danger. The discharge of this duty may require the therapist to take one or more of various steps, depending upon the nature of the case. Thus it may call for him to warn the intended victim or others likely to apprise that victim of the danger, to notify the police, or to take whatever other steps are reasonably necessary under the circumstances (*Tarasoff v. Regents of the University of California*, 1976, p. 344).

S. Loue (✉)
Department of Epidemiology and Biostatistics, Case Western Reserve University, Cleveland, OH, USA
e-mail: sana.loue@case.edu

S. Loue (ed.), *Mental Health Practitioner's Guide to HIV/AIDS*,
DOI 10.1007/978-1-4614-5283-6_36,

The extent to which the duty to warn has been adopted as the standard of practice varies across states. In some states, the duty to warn is mandatory; in others, it is permissive and in still others, the state law is silent. Accordingly, it is critical that a social worker learn how his or her state has implemented this responsibility.

However, whether this duty to warn applies in situations involving the transmission of HIV by an HIV-infected person to his or her sexual or needle-sharing partner remains undecided legally, as least as it concerns non-physician mental health professionals. Although some states have promulgated legislation that allows physicians, including psychiatrists, to disclose a patient's seropositivity to his or her sexual partner and/or needle-sharing partner, such legislation does not encompass social workers, psychologists or other mental health professionals. Unlike the situation in *Tarasoff*, the transmission of HIV does not per se involve violence. And, unlike the use of a gun that can lead to death with a single shot, a single sexual contact with an HIV-infected person does not necessarily result in HIV transmission. The situation involving HIV transmission is also unlike that involved in *Tarasoff* in that the needle-sharing or sexual partner of an HIV-infected individual may bear a responsibility to protect him- or herself from the transmission of the infection, e.g., through the use of a condom during intercourse, unless other circumstances, such as cognitive impairment or violence, prevent him or her from doing so.

However, the NASW Code of Ethics does not require that a threat of violence be involved, but only that the potential harm be "serious, foreseeable, and imminent." The factors enunciated by the court in *Tarasoff* may be relevant in trying to decide whether to breach client confidentiality and warn the client's sexual or needle-sharing partner of the client's HIV seropositivity: the foreseeability of the harm, the degree of certainty that the third party suffered injury, the closeness of the connection between the client's behavior and the injury suffered by the third party, the moral blame associated with the client's conduct, the policy of preventing future harm, the extent of the burden to the third party, the consequences to the community of imposing a duty to warn and liability for a failure to do so, and the availability and cost of insurance for the risk involved.

Some states impose criminal sanctions and/or civil penalties on individuals for engaging in unprotected sexual relations and/or needle-sharing without divulging their HIV-positive status to their partner. In some jurisdictions, a mental health professional, such as a psychologist, social worker, or psychiatrist, who has advised his or her client that a client's threat will be reported to the intended victim and/or police may later be required legally to testify against the client in a criminal or civil action. This is based on the idea that, if the client has been warned that his or her threat will be communicated and then is told that it has been, the client cannot have an expectation of confidentiality with respect to the communication of the threat. Again, because the law differs across the various states, mental health providers are urged to seek legal advice regarding the standard to be followed in his or her state.

Related Topics: Confidentiality laws, disclosure, disclosure laws, legal issues for HIV-infected clients.

Suggested Reading

Johnstone, G. L. (2010). Note, A social worker's dilemma when a client has a sexually transmitted disease: The conflict between the duty of confidentiality and the duty to warn sexual partners. *University of Louisville Law Review, 49*, 111–132.

Klinka, E. (2009). Note, It's been a privilege: Advising patients of the *Tarasoff* duty and its legal consequences for the federal psychotherapist-patient privilege. *Fordham Law Review, 78*, 863–931.

Paruch, D. (2011). From trusted confident to witness for the prosecution: The case against recognition of a dangerous-patient exception to the psychotherapist-patient privilege. *University of New Hampshire Law Review, 9*, 327–407.

Suggested Resources

American Psychological Association. (2010). *Ethical principles of psychologists and code of conduct*. Retrieved December 24, 2011 from http://www.apa.org/ethics/code/index.aspx

National Association of Social Workers. (2008). *Code of ethics*. Retrieved December 24, 2011 from http://www.socialworkers.org/pubs/code/code.asp

Economic Impact

Domniţa Oana Bădărău

Health care costs are increasing every year, leading to increased expenditure percentages in the gross domestic product (GDP), both in developed and developing countries. Factors such as aging populations, increased diagnoses of cases of life threatening diseases, infectious disease rates, social disparities, and economic arrangements deepen differences in health distribution within and between countries. Scarce resources add to these factors and emphasize the central role played by a continuous and steady commitment to ensure through coherent policies access to financial means in order to prevent, treat, and promote health in a population. Despite efforts, technological progress in medicine and a rising life expectancy in the world's population are affected by increasing morbidity rates leading to burdensome costs for care without better health outcomes.

The circumstances of people's lives, from birth until death, their upbringing, morbidities, and comorbidities, as well as the living environment, level of education and political structures, public health policies and health care, all constitute determinants of health. A 2001 report of the World Health Organization's Commission for Macroeconomics and Health (CMH) concluded that substantial resource allocation for health is paramount within economic development processes. A different 2008 report of the Commission on Social Determinants of Health concluded that vast differences in the distribution of wealth and differences in economic settings are responsible for negative health outcomes, but that the root of such outcomes lies in social inequities characterizing all societies, whether developed or in low-income settings.

Economic development is intertwined with social aspects; it may be a determinant or an aggravating factor of social inequalities that include gender inequities, education, and health care allocation. A direct connection exists between health and economy, both influencing and producing significant effects on the other. It can be concluded that health impacts economy by affecting the working force and

D.O. Bădărău (✉)
Institute for Biomedical Ethics, University of Basel, Basel, Switzerland
e-mail: domnita14@gmail.com

S. Loue (ed.), *Mental Health Practitioner's Guide to HIV/AIDS*,
DOI 10.1007/978-1-4614-5283-6_37, © Springer Science+Business Media New York 2013

increasing social costs; the development of an economy lays the foundation for the efficient allocation of resources to combat disease, the containment of disease in an area, the development of prevention programs, and the availability of medical care. Therefore, there can be an economic impact defined by two opposite circumstances: an economic boom or a financial crash. In an economically prosperous situation, resources can be allocated to improve health, to support public health programs, and to reduce health disparities, whenever there is adequate political will and policies are effectively implemented. On the contrary, in a poor economic environment, scarce financial resources lead to insufficient means to provide the required health care personnel, the appropriate medical technologies, and adequate resources to tackle the public health problems that affect specific population groups. In such an environment, resources wither and important public sectors provide poorer services, particularly in the domains of education and health care. As a result, differences in health between social segments are exacerbated, causing more inequities.

Social determinants can also be a contributing factor to the economic status of individuals. Discrimination against people tested for HIV or diagnosed with this infectious virus has been a significant issue from the beginning of the epidemic and leads to medical, legal, and social challenges. The HIV/AIDS epidemic is present in many countries, including developed ones. According to the 2010 National HIV/AIDS Strategy, in the USA there are more than 1.1 million people living with HIV. Given the stigmatization and negative outcomes of disclosing a patient's positive status, the USA adopted disclosure laws and legislation against discrimination. Negative effects of a HIV-positive diagnosis extend beyond the psychological stress of being stigmatized and dealing with the symptoms. The risk of being laid off or increased health care costs not covered by health insurers add to a HIV-positive patient's burden.

Internationally, HIV is a disease associated with socioeconomic inequities, affecting a higher proportion of people living in a poor economic environment. This is also the case in the USA, where HIV infection among minority groups and people from lower socioeconomic classes is considerably higher. The economic impact of the disease is proportionally greater within ethnic and racial groups, especially those living in poor neighborhoods and without stable housing. Socioeconomic status can be a risk factor for contracting HIV and influence the health care that individuals will receive after diagnosis. The impact of lower socioeconomic status has on health patterns and health care is profoundly negative and increases health and social inequities. However, individuals with a higher socioeconomic status are likely to be burdened by the increasing health care costs after the HIV-positive diagnosis. Access to high-quality and life extending care is very expensive and unlikely to be covered or to be provided throughout the disease's course by health insurance. Additionally, from diagnosis and after the individual develops AIDS, health care costs are increasing significantly and steady. The ability of a HIV-positive person to afford the standard of care that will provide the highest quality of life possible and to extend life is closely tied to his or her employment. A positive HIV diagnosis creates vulnerability for the diagnosed individual who is at a greater risk of discrimination and stigmatization, despite federal law, many state laws, and principles of human rights prohibiting discrimination. It is acknowledged that HIV-positive people whose status is disclosed are at a greater risk of becoming unemployed and suffering marginalization. Legislation has been put in place to protect people diagnosed with HIV. Human rights regulations and international legislation exist, but the individual suffering discrimination must present his or her claims before courts. These circumstances add to the burdens suffered by a HIV-positive person and increase the economic impact. In addition to health care costs and loss of income, he or she would have to have the resources to carry through a legal claim.

A different aspect of the economic impact suffered by individuals diagnosed with HIV is represented by the illness progression. As the disease progresses, HIV can result in severe disabilities, requiring additional health care, days of hospitalization, and additional health care costs. In advanced stages of the disease, the HIV-positive individual is unlikely to be able to work normally and therefore his income will decrease. Social support is necessary to cover all costs, including housing, aliments, health care, and nursing, while the individual is less capable to care for himself, both financially and physically. This puts a severe pressure on health budgets, thereby requiring countries to develop and implement national strategies to combat HIV and AIDS.

The 2001 CMH Report, in recognition of the connection between economic development and health, encouraged supplementary resource allocations for global health research and the provision of services in areas devastated by diseases such as HIV, malaria, and TB. In a 2003 Commission report, health is reaffirmed as being a fundamental human right and a cornerstone in reducing poverty levels between countries. Public health systems worldwide are under the pressure of major diseases and mortality rates, combined with increasing morbidities that dry out resources both in the short and long terms. In addition to this, economic crises such as economies in recession affect resource allocation and deepen the financial shortage in fighting disease at a global scale.

Beginning in 2007, the financial markets took a downward trend as a result of the inflated real estate boom of the past years, impacting economies worldwide. Systemic shocks hit the markets throughout the world up until the present time. The crisis has been exacerbated in the European zone, with States like Greece and Italy experiencing severe recessions. These crises have adversely affected health and health care in various countries.

The current situation in Greece illustrates the impact of the economy on health care. A letter to *Lancet* published on October 2011 reported that, based on data collected from 2007 until 2009, there had been a significant decrease in the number of Greeks who would see a doctor for treatment of health-related problems. The proportion of people not seeing a dentist or a mental health specialist is particularly high. However, despite the initial assumption that these decreased rates were due to reduced household incomes, significant cuts in wages, and increasing unemployment rates amongst the young population, the report indicated that the negative effects on health care were more closely related to the health system's lack of capacity to meet the demand. Cuts of up to 40% in hospital budgets led to increased waiting times to see a physician, which would especially discourage people travelling from other localities for doctor's appointments to seek medical care. Additionally, a significant rise in mental health issues with overwhelmingly high suicide rates has been observed. This can be explained by the everyday stress and insecurities caused by the economic situation. Greek suicide helpline callers have routinely reported that they are overwhelmed by the pressure of loans and an inability to pay them.

A particularly worrisome health indicator for Greece is the number of new HIV infection cases, which is evidencing an increasing trend. The numbers are higher among injection drug users. The underfunding of needle-exchange programs and psychosocial therapies for drug addiction, along with higher rates of prostitution and unprotected sexual behaviors, have contributed to higher HIV transmission rates. The current economic situation is affecting health from two sides: by fostering increases in behaviors such as prostitution, drug use, and injection drug use with contaminated injection equipment and by reducing the availability of financial resources at both the individual and societal levels to cope with increasing infection rates and health problems.

Among developing countries, the populations most affected by HIV/AIDS live in African countries, where the HIV infection rates exceed 50% in some populations. Efforts have been made in developing countries to facilitate access to antiretroviral therapies through governmental programs, the work of nongovernmental organizations (NGOs), and international funding sources. These efforts face serious constraints in relation to the high price of antiretrovirals drugs (ARVs) and create a need for cheaper alternatives.

Generic drugs could represent a substitute and provide access to such HIV infection treatments, as ARV prices are increasing. Higher costs for producing newer lines of ARVs limit treatment access especially in developing countries. The implementation of the World Trade Organization's (WTO) Agreement on the trade-related aspects of intellectual property rights (TRIPS) had a negative effect and has contributed to the increased prices. Under this agreement, cheaper, generic drugs would face export restrictions and the producing companies have been compelled to respect original drug pharmaceutical companies' patents. Due to the current world economic turmoil and the impact it has on the distribution of financial resources, the capacity to offer antiretroviral treatment to meet the HIV-related health needs in developing countries seems compromised.

Developing countries that have successfully addressed the issue of providing universal access to ARV therapy have committed enormous financial resources to achieve this goal. In doing so, States like Brazil and Thailand changed the legislative provisions in order to provide population treatment coverage, build public structures capable of producing ARVs, and motivate social involvement and action to support the newly founded health system. Though older lines of ARVs are not protected by patents and make possible the nationally produced generic drugs that are less expensive, the universal coverage represents a burden on States' budgets. This model was utilized successfully by Thailand and Brazil until they were confronted with obligations under various trade laws. Negotiations with pharmaceutical companies that produce expensive, newer drugs ensured that the prices will be lower, but they remain unaffordable for universal coverage.

Years before the current economic crisis, wealthier developing countries were struggling to meet the demand of HIV patients and pay for the expensive drugs delivered by drug companies owning the ARV patents. Dramatic economic impacts on health care are to be expected both in developing and developed countries, as health budgets became increasingly strained and unable to absorb the health care costs.

Related Topics: World Trade Organization.

Suggested Reading

dos Santos Pinheiro, E., Ceva Antunes, O. A., & Fortunak, J. M. D. (2008). A survey of the syntheses of active pharmaceutical ingredients for antiretroviral drug combinations critical to access in emerging nations. *Antiviral Research. Review, 79*. doi:10.1016/j.antiviral.2008.05/001.

Ford, N., Wilson, D., Costa Chavez, G., Lotrowska, M., & Kijtiwatchakul, K. (2007). Sustaining access to antiretroviral therapy in the less-developed world: Lessons from Brazil and Thailand. *AIDS, 21*(Suppl. 4), S21–S29.

Houston, M., Day, M., de Lago, M., & Zarocostas, J. (2011). Health services across Europe face cuts as debt crisis begins to bite. *British Medical Journal, 343*, d5266. doi:10.1136/bmj.d5266

Karamanoli, E. (2011). Debt crisis strains Greece's ailing health system. *Lancet. World Report, 378*(9788), 303–304.

Kentikelenis, A., Karanikolos, M., Papanicolas, I., Basu, S., & McKee, M. (2011). Health effects of financial crisis: Omens of a Greek tragedy. *Lancet. Correspondence, 10*. doi:10.1016/S0140-6736(11)61556-0.

Marmot, M., Allen, J., & Goldblatt, P. (2011). Building of the global movement for health equity: From Santiago to Rio and beyond. *Lancet, 19*. doi:10.1016/S0140-6736(11), 61506-61507.

Triantafyllou, K., & Angeletopoulou, C. (2011). Increased suicidality amid economic crisis in Greece. *Lancet. Correspondence, 378*(9801), 1459–1460.

Suggested Resources

Crowell, V., & Leotsakos, A. (2003). *Increasing investments in health outcomes for the poor. Second Consultation on Macroeconomics and Health.* Geneva, Switzerland: World Health Organization. Retrieved December 28, 2011 from http://bvs.per.paho.org/bvsacd/milenio/salud.pdf

Faith Community

Sana Loue

"Faith community" has been defined by the AIDS National Interfaith Network to include groups that are "organized around any set of beliefs or practices that involve a belief in a higher power or order, a larger organizing principle for life and the universe, or a system or code that links our values and actions to the idea that there is a reason and purpose to our existence on Earth" (American Association for World Health, 1999). In 1993, the interfaith coalition of the Council of National Religious AIDS Networks developed an interfaith declaration in response to the AIDS epidemic. The declaration emphasized that: HIV/AIDS is not a punishment from God; all individuals, regardless of their characteristics, are entitled to compassionate and nonjudgmental care and support; there is a responsibility to work to transform public attitudes and policies; the provision of accurate information relating to HIV transmission and prevention is to be encouraged; intolerance and bigotry are to be deplored; all sectors of society are to seek ways to eliminate poverty; and all are to be committed to action.

Faith-based responses to HIV/AIDS may involve specific denominations, communities, agencies, or congregations. Their efforts may include any of a wide-ranging number of services, including food and meal services, counseling, food banks, housing, hospice care, support services, AIDS education, substance use treatment, and/or day care. Some faith-based organizations also sponsor or cosponsor HIV testing, risk assessment, and counseling and provide training and technical assistance to churches and faith leaders.

However, depending upon the perspective of a faith-based organization, there may be limitations on the extent to which HIV/AIDS-related education is provided or the form that it may take. As an example, a church that believes that extramarital intercourse is sinful may be unwilling to provide education that does not focus exclusively on abstinence. In such instances, potential remedies may be

S. Loue (✉)
Department of Epidemiology and Biostatistics, Case Western Reserve University, Cleveland, OH, USA
e-mail: sana.loue@case.edu

S. Loue (ed.), *Mental Health Practitioner's Guide to HIV/AIDS*,
DOI 10.1007/978-1-4614-5283-6_38,

collaboration with a secular partner that provides the additional information regarding prevention strategies and/or assists with the delivery of the educational program and related activities, such as condom distribution.

Related Topics: Coping, religion and spirituality, social support.

Suggested Reading

Francis, S. A., & Liverpool, J. (2009). A review of faith-based HIV prevention programs. *Journal of Religion and Health, 48*, 6–15.

Suggested Resources

American Association for World Health. (1999, December 1). *Fact sheets: The faith community & HIV/AIDS and an interfaith declaration.* Retrieved December 28, 2011 from http://www.thebody.com/content/art33118.html

Fatalism

Ana-Gabriela Benghiac

Fatalism is a perspective that views the outcome of events as uncontrollable and unchangeable by an individual; it is the belief in destiny. Fate is seen as the determinant of one's life course. In the health care setting, fatalism refers to the idea that human beings cannot prevent the emergence of an illness or manage its treatment in order to eliminate it; it is associated with pessimistic and passive attitudes regarding the prevention, treatment, and the disease itself. In the context of HIV/AIDS, fatalism represents a barrier to prevention, influences people's attitudes, and may increase the likelihood that they will engage in high risk behaviors, thus increasing their vulnerability to infection due to their rejection of interventional measures. Fatalism is linked to a lack of knowledge and understanding about the disease and can have a devastating effect on the management of HIV/AIDS patients. In communities where denialism plays also an important role, interventional efforts towards better control of the disease are harder to implement.

To assess the levels of fatalism in HIV, researchers may use a modified version of the Powe Fatalism Inventory (PFI). PFI was originally designed for cancer patients and was adapted to HIV by Rosanna Hess under the name of HIV Fatalism Scale. It evaluates an individual's fatalism score according to the answers provided to the 15 items in the scale. A multidimensional fatalism scale (Fatalismo) was created by Esparza and Wiebe and is used with Mexican immigrants.

HIV fatalistic beliefs suggest that HIV/AIDS is a punishment from God, that infection is predetermined, and that it leads to an inevitable death. These ideas merge together with the denialist beliefs that AIDS is not a real disease, but rather a condition fabricated by Western countries; that it is a curse; and that discussion is taboo. Although HIV-related fatalism has been observed most frequently among HIV-infected people and their communities, researchers have also noted fatalistic ideas among physicians too. This can have a negative impact on the quality of medical services for HIV-positive patients; some health care providers feel that

A.-G. Benghiac (✉)
Department of Bioethics, Case Western Reserve University, Cleveland, OH, USA
e-mail: dr.gabriela_benghiac@yahoo.com

S. Loue (ed.), *Mental Health Practitioner's Guide to HIV/AIDS*, 217
DOI 10.1007/978-1-4614-5283-6_39, © Springer Science+Business Media New York 2013

changes in their patients' behaviors are unlikely to occur and may consequently provide little or no preventive counseling. Wayne Steward's study shows variability regarding provider fatalism; gay, white men were the most affected by the lack of counseling.

Cultural beliefs in destiny and predetermination influence the course of HIV/AIDS epidemics, especially in African countries, where people appear to have a stronger belief in fate compared to the US population. Fatalistic attitudes are correlated with rebellion, resignation, and a lack of responsibility regarding one's health status and care. Some people believe that one's sexual behavior does not play any role in the possibility of acquiring HIV and that there is no reason for preventive measures because the individuals who will become infected have been chosen by God for that purpose. They think that they have no control over the disease and they do not see the value of either having HIV tests or adhering to the recommendations regarding medical therapy and lifestyle changes. US-based studies have found that fatalism is associated with poverty and religion. Thus, many Catholic Latinos/Latinas are less likely to use condoms due to the religious ban on contraceptive measures. Some Latinos have adopted a fatalistic belief not only with respect to HIV but also with regard to cancer and diabetes prevention and screening. African-American women from urban areas have been found to believe that AIDS is connected to the prophecies from the Book of Revelations.

Mental health and other care providers can help their clients decrease HIV risk and maintain health whether the clients are HIV-negative or -positive. This can be accomplished by openly discussing mechanisms of disease transmission and strategies for maintaining health, by refraining from the use of fatalistic language, and by helping individuals explore the consequences of their decisions and behaviors.

Related Topics: Denialism.

Suggested Reading

Esparza, O. A., & Wiebe, J. S. (2008). *The development of a Multidimensional Fatalism Scale*. San Diego, CA: Society of Behavioral Medicine.

Flaskerud, J. H., & Rush, C. E. (1989). AIDS and traditional health beliefs and practices of Black women. *Nursing Research, 38*(4), 210–215.

Hess, R. F., & McKinney, D. E. (2007). Fatalism and HIV/AIDS beliefs in rural Mali, West Africa. *Journal of Nursing Scholarship, 39*(2), 113–118.

Kissinger, P., Kovacs, S., Anderson-Smits, C., Schmidt, N., Salinas, O., Hembling, J., et al. (2011). Patterns and predictors of HIV/STI risk among Latino migrant men in a new receiving community. *AIDS Behavior*. doi:10.1007/s10461-011-9945-7.

New York State Department of AIDS Institute. (1989). *Hispanics and HIV: Strategies and tactics for education/prevention*. New York, NY: Culturelinc Corp.

Steward, W. T., Charlebois, E. D., Johnson, M. O., Remien, R. H., Goldstein, R. B., Wong, F. L., et al. (2008). Receipt of prevention services among HIV-infected men who have sex with men. *American Journal of Public Health, 98*(6), 1011–1014.

Gender Identity

Heather Wollin

Introduction

"Transgender" is an umbrella term used to describe people whose gender identity and/or expression does not conform to norms and expectations associated with the sex that they were assigned at birth. Transgender clients may identify as genderqueer, gender variant, gender non-conforming, FTM, MTF, transmasculine, transsexual, or any of the above terms.

HIV and Transgender Populations

Research on HIV infection and transgender populations has been scant, with much of the literature focusing on transgender women or MTF (male to female) transgender individuals. Transgender men (FTMs), particularly those who have sex with non-transgender men, are also at risk for HIV and STI infection; the current state of prevention and outreach is inadequate for this population, as well as for people who identify as gender non-conforming or gender variant. While trans women tend to report the highest level of HIV risk and other adverse health outcomes relative to other transgender populations and prevalence of HIV infection among transgender men is very low, it is important to recognize that their prevention needs are not being met and to think about creative ways to find solutions to this issue. Studies show that transgender women are more likely than transgender men and non-transgender men and women to engage in sex work. Risk factors for HIV and other STIs among the population of transgender people engaging in sex work include forced sex or coercion from clients, injection drug use, unprotected sex

H. Wollin (✉)
School of Social Work, University of Southern California, Los Angeles, CA, USA
e-mail: heather.wollin@gmail.com

S. Loue (ed.), *Mental Health Practitioner's Guide to HIV/AIDS*,
DOI 10.1007/978-1-4614-5283-6_40,

for financial incentives, or sharing needles when using street market hormones. Transgender women are also less likely to report 90% ART adherence and to report less confidence in their abilities to incorporate treatment regimens in their daily lives. Despite low prevalence rates among transgender men, some do engage in unprotected sex with non-transgender men, participate in sex work, and share needles while using injection drugs or hormones. There is virtually no research on HIV risk among people who identify as genderqueer or gender variant.

Mental Health Issues

Transgender people disproportionately face systemic issues like discrimination, harassment, poverty, and lack of access to medical care. Transgender people, like lesbian, gay, and bisexual people, may be at greater risk for mental health issues such as depression, anxiety, PTSD, and co-occurring substance abuse disorders. A diagnosis of HIV is also often correlated with depression and other mental health issues. It is important for providers to screen clients for these issues as they may go unseen and unnoticed.

Recommendations for Clinicians

Clinicians who are working with gender variant or transgender clients must foremost take on the responsibility of educating themselves about issues related to gender identity. Since many clinicians do not identify themselves as transgender or gender variant, and may be new to working with these clients, clinician knowledge about gender identity issues is crucial. Providers should use the preferred pronoun(s) of the client and mirror the language that clients used to describe their gender identity and their body parts, understanding that this language may change over time. Providers should make sure to be client-centered in their approach to treatment, rather than assuming, for example, that each person who identifies as transgender or gender variant is interested in taking hormones or having sex reassignment surgery. They should also note that there is no one way to be transgender and that a gender transition can look a number of different ways. It is important that mental health clinicians recognize their role in diagnosing people who are undergoing gender transitions with Gender Identity Disorder or Gender Dysphoria and understand that this is an important power dynamic in the treatment of transgender people.

Screening transgender and gender variant clients for depression, anxiety, PTSD, and substance abuse, as well as other types of psychiatric illnesses may be advisable. A holistic approach is preferred in treating clients for HIV-related concerns, with an emphasis on prevention and testing if their clients are engaging in high-risk behaviors. It will be important to clients that clinicians familiarize themselves with the community-based resources in the area that work specifically with the LGBT community so that they can refer clients to these agencies, if appropriate. Clinicians may also want to familiarize themselves with other transgender or transgender-friendly therapists so that they can develop strong professional networks.

Related Topics: Gender role, transgender.

Suggested Reading

Herbst, J. H., Jacobs, E. D., Finlayson, T. J., McKleroy, V. S., Neumann, M. S., & Crepaz, N. (2008). Estimating HIV prevalence and risk behaviors of transgender persons in the United States: A systematic review. *Journal of AIDS and Social Behavior, 12*(1), 1–17.

Lombardi, E. (2007). Public health and trans-people: Barriers to care and strategies to improve treatment. In I. H. Meyer & M. E. Northridge (Eds.), *The health of sexual minorities: Public health perspectives on lesbian, gay, bisexual, and transgender populations* (pp. 638–652). New York, NY: Springer.

Sevelius, J. (2009). There's no pamphlet for the kind of sex I have: HIV-related risk factors and protective behaviors among transgender men who have sex with non-transgender men. *Journal of the Association of Nurses in AIDS Care, 20*(5), 398–410.

Suggested Resources

Center of Excellence for Transgender Health, University of California, San Francisco. http://transhealth.ucsf.edu/trans?page=home-00-00

Keating, J., & Bockting, W. (2008). *What are male to female transgender persons' (MtF) HIV prevention needs?* University of California, San Francisco, Center for AIDS Prevention Studies. Fact Sheet 41. http://caps.ucsf.edu/factsheets/transgender-persons-mtf/

Transgender Law Center. http://transgenderlawcenter.org/cms/

World Professional Association for Transgender Health (WPATH). http://www.wpath.org/about_wpath.cfm

Gender Roles

Margaret S. Winchester

Gender roles are socially prescribed and constructed norms assigned to individuals in societies based on sex differences; these vary across time and place. Roles related to gender can encompass different types of behavior, such as familial, economic, and other societal functions. Gender roles are locally unique and historically situated. Some scholars argue that gender roles are rooted in biological and evolutionary differences between males and females. However, most contemporary scholars recognize that while there are differences between males and females, the corresponding roles for men and women are largely socially constructed. Gender roles are taught through familial, social, and educational instruction and reinforced through relationships, cultural practices, and media. In the context of HIV, culturally prescribed gender roles are important in transmission of infection, experiences of living with the illness, and patterns of help seeking and treatment.

Across the globe, there are power differences between genders which can manifest in a woman's subordinate position within a household or sexual relationship. In addition to greater social burdens of HIV due to gender roles, women are also biologically more susceptible to infection. Social limitations on condom use or a woman's decreased ability to negotiate safe sex with her partner may put women at greater risk for HIV transmission and infection in certain contexts. Infidelity may also be a consequence of these power differentials, thereby increasing the possibility of introducing HIV into a marriage. In some settings, marriage is cited as women's greatest risk for contracting HIV and infidelity of men outside of marriage is not culturally forbidden or censured.

Transactional sex is commonly embedded in unequal gender and/or age relationships. This can include prostitution or more informal sexual relationships that involve the exchange of gifts or income for the individual providing sex. In some parts of sub-Saharan Africa, transactional sex between younger women and

M.S. Winchester (✉)
Department of Bioethics, School of Medicine, Case Western Reserve University, Cleveland, OH, USA
e-mail: Margaret.Winchester@case.edu

S. Loue (ed.), *Mental Health Practitioner's Guide to HIV/AIDS*,
DOI 10.1007/978-1-4614-5283-6_41, © Springer Science+Business Media New York 2013

older, wealthier men known as "sugar-daddies," is common and attributed to the spread of HIV, due to the girls' inability to negotiate safe sex or multiple concurrent partnerships on the part of either party.

Men are often assumed to be less at risk of HIV infection through heterosexual transmission than women due to their greater decision-making power in relationships and ability to control and negotiate condom use. Nonetheless, cultural norms that allow for multiple concurrent sexual partnerships can put all involved at risk for HIV infection and transmission. Globally, men consume more alcohol than women; frequent or excessive alcohol use is associated with decreased inhibitions and more casual or unprotected sexual encounters.

Economic dependence of women in low resource settings can be an inhibiting factor in leaving a strained or even abusive marriage or relationship. Physical, sexual, emotional violence or other controlling behaviors can emerge from disparate gender roles and are exacerbated in settings with high alcohol consumption and few resources for women. These behaviors can increase vulnerability for HIV infection and inhibit help-seeking behaviors once someone is already infected.

Women frequently bear a greater burden from HIV infection as household caregivers and report more feelings of shame, stigma, discrimination, and depression than men as a result of their illness. As caregivers, women are expected to provide support for all HIV-infected family members, including young children. Due to the economic dependence mentioned above, this can lead to difficulties in allocating household resources to treat illness episodes or to access antiretroviral medication and pay for the resulting increased nutritional demands. In areas where ARVs are available at a cost and multiple household members are infected with HIV, women may be given a lower priority and frequently access care later than men.

Hetero-normative gender roles in many settings can inhibit successful prevention programs because of the conflation between sexual risk behaviors and sexual orientation. For example, men who have sex with men may not identify as homosexual or access services targeted at this population. Same-sex couples also face stigma in accessing methods of prevention and treatment, particularly in areas where there is a lack of consideration or acknowledgement of sexuality, sexual identity, and same-sex relationship gender roles in HIV programs due to either social or structural constraints.

Gender roles are highly dependent on both context and relationships. Fewer than half of countries report gender-specific budgets in their HIV programming. Historically, consideration of gender roles in HIV has led to an emphasis on women and women's vulnerability. Unequal gender roles can inhibit successful programming for those at risk for HIV or already living with the illness. Therefore, gender roles for both men and women and the local nuances of relationships should be considered at all stages of planning and response to the HIV epidemic.

Related Topics: Gender identity, transgender.

Suggested Reading

Bandali, S. (2011). Norms and practices within marriage which shape gender roles, HIV/AIDS risk and risk reduction strategies in Cabo Delgado, Mozambique. *AIDS Care, 23*(9), 1171–1176.
Campbell, C. (1995). Male gender roles and sexuality: Implications for women's AIDS risk and prevention. *Social Science and Medicine, 41*(2), 197–210.
Farmer, P., Connors, M., & Simmons, J. (Eds.). (2011). *Women, poverty, and AIDS: Sex, drugs, and structural violence* (2nd ed.). Monroe, ME: Common Courage Press.
Fernandez-Davila, P., Salazar, X., Caceres, C., Maiorana, A., Kegeles, S., Coates, T. J., & Martinez, J. (2008). Compensated sex and sexual risk: Sexual coercion, social and economic interactions between homosexually- and heterosexually-identified men of low income in two cities of Peru. *Sexuality, 11*(3), 352–374.
Hirsch, J., Wardlow, H., Smith, D. J., Phinney, H., Parikh, S., & Nathanson, C. A. (Eds.). (2009). *The secret: Love, marriage, and HIV*. Nashville, TN: Vanderbilt University Press.

Suggested Resources

Pan American Health Organization, & World Health Organization. (2005). *Gender-based violence and HIV/AIDS*. Available at http://www.paho.org/English/AD/GE/Viol-HIV_FS0705.pdf

Harm Reduction

Bettina Rausa

Harm reduction is an approach to public health issues that seeks to reduce the "harm," such as risk of disease exposure and transmission, to individuals who engage in high risk health behaviors. It employs a range of strategies that includes educating individuals about how to engage in those behaviors more safely not only for themselves but also for the community at large, as well as the provision of services. The principle tenet of harm reduction is to meet the client "where they are at" in a non-judgmental, non-coercive manner by creating a safe environment through which precautionary/safer practices targeting the risky behavior can be discussed and steps to reduce individual and community harm can be identified. That is, accepting that the behavior, such as injection drug use or engaging in high risk sexual activity, will continue, but significantly reducing harm to the individual and the community at large by controlling not the specific behavior, but the spread of disease via the behavior. Harm reduction programs operate on the philosophy that some individuals will eventually, when they are ready, cease the risky behavior(s) altogether and thus the program may also offer assistance and/or referrals to an array of services such as treatment and recovery.

One example of harm reduction is those programs targeting injection drug users (IDUs). Injection drug use and HIV are explicitly connected. According to the Centers for Disease Control and Prevention (CDC), illicit drug use is one of the riskiest behaviors that leads to the spread of HIV. IDUs are at a higher risk than the general population of contracting HIV because they often share syringes, which significantly increases a person's chance of contracting and/or transmitting the HIV virus to others. Although the same can be said of heroin use, methamphetamine use (also known as meth, crystal meth, ice, and glass) in particular has high consequences for contracting and spreading HIV, not only because of syringe sharing but also because meth use impairs decision making in other aspects of the individual's life. The CDC notes that meth use can increase sexual arousal while

B. Rausa (✉)
Salk Institute for Biological Studies, La Jolla, CA, USA
e-mail: brausa@cox.net

S. Loue (ed.), *Mental Health Practitioner's Guide to HIV/AIDS*, DOI 10.1007/978-1-4614-5283-6_42,

lowering inhibitions. Meth use increases sexual risk factors because meth users are more likely to: (1) have more sex partners; (2) forgo using condoms; (3) exchange sex for money; (4) have sex with IDUs; and (5) have a history of sexually transmitted diseases (STDs). In addition, individuals who already have HIV/AIDS may use meth to self-medicate or manage their disease symptoms.

In a clean syringe exchange program, IDUs can exchange their used syringes for new, sterile ones. The primary goal is to discourage the sharing of syringes among IDUs to lower their risk of infection with HIV and other blood-borne diseases such as hepatitis. These programs not only provide access to clean syringes but also other injecting equipment and tools to sterilize syringes. Syringe exchange programs operate in a variety of ways, including through drop-in centers, street outreach, and mobile vans that move from location to location in order to be more accessible to those who need it. Some programs even include 24-h vending machines to increase access to clean syringes when there are no other options. Studies of syringe exchange programs conducted in 1997 in 81 cities around the world found that HIV infection rates decreased by 6% in 29 cities that provided this service, whereas infection rates increased by 6% in 52 cities that did not have a clean syringe program.

Another successful harm reduction program that has positive impacts on reducing the spread of HIV/AIDS is methadone treatment, also known as maintenance therapy. Methadone is a synthetic opiate which is administered orally in a stabilized dosage to individuals who have an opiate addiction, most commonly heroin. Methadone becomes a substitute for heroin and, because methadone binds to the same receptors in the brain that heroin or other opioids bind to, it can lead to the cessation of opioid use and eliminate the need to inject the drug. This in turn leads to a drop in the spread of HIV that would occur due to syringe sharing because it can eliminate the use of syringes altogether. Another way that methadone programs help reduce the spread of HIV/AIDS is by reducing the frequency of sex-for-drugs among substance-using individuals, which often includes high HIV risk behaviors such as multiple sex partners, sex without protection such as condoms, and sex with IDUs. Methadone is administered once a day at treatment centers, and it helps relieve the craving for heroin/opiates with the ultimate goal being recovery from drug addiction.

Other harm reduction programs include: (1) safe injection facilities where IDUs can inject in a safe environment with medical supervision. At the time of this writing, there is no evidence of such facilities in the United States, but programs do exist in Australia, Canada, Germany, the Netherlands, Spain, and Switzerland; (2) safer crack cocaine smoking resources which operate much like a clean syringe exchange in that they distribute clean crack-smoking equipment such as glass stems and rubber mouthpieces to reduce sharing; (3) pharmacy sale of syringes to provide IDUs access to clean syringes without a prescription. Studies show that there is a lower HIV rate in areas that permit these sales; (4) supplying tin foil to suppress the use of syringes by boiling heroin on the foil and inhaling it instead of injecting it; (5) safe syringe disposal programs designed to eliminate the unsafe disposal of contaminated syringes in order to avoid injury to others. These include drop off points, mail-back programs using special containers, residential pick-up services, and safe syringe disposal services that can be used at home; and (6) community-based outreach programs that train IDUs and sex workers to conduct peer-outreach in the provision of clean drug use equipment, the promotion and distribution of condoms, and the sharing of information about prevention and rehabilitation services when appropriate.

Related Topics: Mental health comorbidity and HIV/AIDS, prevention strategies, substance use, syringe exchange.

Suggested Reading

Beletsky, L., Davis, C. S., Anderson, E. D., & Burris, S. (2008). The law (and politics) of safe injection facilities in the United States. *American Journal of Public Health, 98*(2), 231–237. Retrieved February 26, 2012 from http://www.ncbi.nlm.nih.gov/pmc/articles/PMC2376869/pdf/0980231.pdf.

Suggested Resources

AIDS.org. *Harm reduction and HIV*. Retrieved February 13, 2012 from http://www.aids.org/topics/harm-reduction-and-hiv/

AVERT: Averting HIV and AIDS. *Needle exchange and harm reduction/needle exchange and HIV*. Retrieved February 13, 2012 from http://www.avert.org/needle-exchange.htm

Centers for Disease Control and Prevention (CDC). *Methamphetamine use and risk for HIV/AIDS (factsheet)*. Retrieved February 20, 2012 from http://www.cdc.gov/hiv/resources/factsheets/meth.htm

Centers for Disease Control and Prevention (CDC). (2002). *Methadone maintenance treatment (factsheet)*. Retrieved February 25, 2012 from http://www.cdc.gov/idu/facts/methadonefin.pdf

Drucker E., Lurie, P., Wodak, A., & Alcabes, P. (1998). *Measuring harm reduction: The effects of needle and syringe exchange program and methadone maintenance on the ecology of HIV*. New York: Department of Epidemiology and Social Medicine, Montefiore Medical Center. PMID: 9633006. Retrieved February 20, 2012 from http://www.ncbi.nlm.nih.gov/pubmed/9633006

Harm Reduction Coalition. *Principles of harm reduction*. Retrieved February 20, 2012 from http://harmreduction.org/about-us/principles-of-harm-reduction/

Hate Crimes

Brandy L. Johnson

Hate crimes are crimes that are committed as the result of intolerance towards a certain group. The victim of such crimes are targeted because of his or her inclusion, or perceived inclusion, in a specific social group. Hate crimes occur, to varying extents, in all countries.

Hate crimes consist of two elements: a criminal offense and a prejudicial motive on behalf of the perpetrator. For there to be a hate crime, there must first be a crime committed against property or an individual. Hate crimes often manifest in the form of assault, harassment, battery, murder, rape, intimidation, damage to property, arson, burglary, robbery, larceny, and vandalism. If an act is not criminal, a hate crime has not been committed.

The second element of a hate crime requires that the crime be motivated by a bias or prejudice against another. The motive requirement differentiates hate crimes from other types of crimes. To have a hate crime, the perpetrator must have targeted the victim of the crime specifically due to the victim's membership, or presumed membership, in a group that shares a particular characteristic. Hate crimes usually occur due to a prejudice based upon characteristics like race, color, religion, sexual orientation, disability, ethnicity, national origin, age, gender, and/or gender identification.

It is worth noting the use of the word "hate" in the title "hate crime" can be misleading. Hatred is a very intense emotional state that can develop for a variety of reasons. Consequently, crimes that are based upon hatred may not necessarily be categorized as hate crimes. The crime of murder is a good illustration. Murder may result from one individual's hatred of another individual. However, unless the victim was murdered because of bias against a protected characteristic, such as race, the crime would not be a hate crime. Additionally, a hate crime can occur even when the perpetrator lacks feelings of hatred toward the victimized individual. The perpetrator may, instead, only have hostile feelings toward a group to which the

B.L. Johnson (✉)
Rynearson, Suess, Schnurbusch & Champion, L.L.C., St. Louis, MO, USA
e-mail: bjohnson@rssclaw.com

S. Loue (ed.), *Mental Health Practitioner's Guide to HIV/AIDS*,
DOI 10.1007/978-1-4614-5283-6_43,

victimized individual belongs. Similarly, the victim may simply represent an idea about which the perpetrator has strong feelings. For example, if the perpetrator holds hostile feelings about immigration or against immigrants, he or she may cause damage to a school that services immigrant children or attack a stranger solely because he or she appears to be of Mexican descent. For these reasons, hate crimes may be better described as bias motive crimes.

Although hate crimes make up a minority of the crimes committed on a daily basis, they are not especially rare. In the United Kingdom, there were 52,028 hate crimes reported in 2009. In the same year, there were 8,336 victims of hate crimes reported in the United States. Of this number, 4,793 of the reported crimes were offenses against individuals and 3,517 of the reported crimes were offenses against property. It should be noted that only reported crimes can be counted and, consequently, it is reasonable to conclude that the true number of hate crimes committed in any given year is higher than the number reflected in the relevant statistics. Further, the statistics on the issue are affected by both the fact that some of the reported offenses are erroneously not characterized as hate crimes, thereby limiting the ability to gather accurate data. Some countries also have established better statistical reporting systems than others. For instance, there were only 14,222 law enforcement agencies in the United States submitting data on hate crimes in 2009. As a result, numerous hate crimes may be unaccounted for and leave an imperfect picture of the prevalence of the problem.

Hate crimes against individuals living with HIV/AIDS can occur simply due to their serostatus. Often, however, hate crimes against individuals with HIV/AIDS occur because of their membership or presumed membership in another protected class. For example, an individual with HIV/AIDS is more likely to be a target of a hate crime due to his or her sexual orientation, race, or disability than to HIV/AIDS per se. In 2009, there were 1,482 hate crimes in the United States and 4,805 hate crimes in the United Kingdom based upon bias against the victim's sexual orientation. There were 4,057 hate crimes in the United States and 43,426 hate crimes in the United Kingdom based upon bias against the victim's race.

Legislation has been utilized to help prevent hate crimes. There are four basic types of hate crimes laws. The first type of legislation classifies bias-motivated offenses as a distinct crime and provides the punishments available. The second type of legislation enhances the punishment for established crimes when bias motivated the commission of the offense. Legislation can provide a distinct civil cause of action as a remedy for victims of hate crimes. Lastly, legislation has been passed that mandates the collection of data and statistics concerning hate crimes.

The definition of a hate crime, the types of offenses included, and the punishments that can be imposed vary from country to country and even within a country, from jurisdiction to jurisdiction. In the United States, for example, hate crime legislation has been passed by the federal government, at least 45 individual states, and the District of Columbia. However, while all of the states with hate crime statutes include offenses based on race, only 31 states have statutes that include offenses based on sexual orientation. Likewise, only 13 states criminalize offenses based on gender identity as hate crimes.

The reduction and prevention of hate crimes is especially important considering that the trauma resulting from hate crimes has been found to last longer and cause a greater amount of harm than non-hate crimes. Due to the bias motivating the crimes, attacks against hate crimes victims tend to be more vicious, violent, and harmful. Victims may also experience more severe psychological trauma, including depression and anxiety, and greater feelings of violation, isolation, and/or vulnerability. As hate crimes are based upon the hatred of a specific characteristic or characteristics, victims may experience shame, a loss of self-worth, or feel a need to change something about themselves.

Hate crimes also cause harm to the targeted community. Crimes based upon a specific characteristic, like homosexuality, inject fear into members of the targeted group. Other members of the group may fear they will be the next victim. Such crimes also serve to send a message to citizens who offer support to, or defend, members of the targeted group.

Hate crimes have the power to divide and polarize societies. They can create cycles of violence and retaliation. The damage such crimes cause makes it imperative to take the steps necessary to discourage bias-motivated offenses, reduce the prejudice that causes them, and promote both the understanding and tolerance of targeted groups.

Related Topics: Discrimination, stigma and stigmatization.

Suggested Reading

Gerstenfeld, P. (2010). *Hate crimes: Causes, controls, and controversies* (2nd ed.). Thousand Oaks, CA: Sage Publications, Inc.

Levin, J., & Mcdevitt, J. (2002). *Hate crimes revisited: America's war on those who are different*. New York, NY: Basic Books.

Perry, B. (2001). *In the name of hate: Understanding hate crimes*. London: Routledge.

Suggested Resources

BBC News. (2010, November 30). *Hate crime figures published for the first time*. Retrieved October 22, 2011 from http://www.bbc.co.uk/news/uk-11875321

Federal Bureau of Investigations. (2010). *Hate crime statistics, 2009 report*. Retrieved October 22, 2011 from http://www2.fbi.gov/ucr/hc2009/index.html

National Coalition of Anti-Violence Programs. (2011). *Hate violence against lesbian, gay, bisexual, queer and HIV-affected communities in the United States in 2010*. Retrieved October 22, 2011 from http://www.avp.org/documents/NCAVPHateViolenceReport2011Finaledjlfinaledits.pdf

OSCE Office for Democratic Institutions and Human Rights. (2009). *Hate crime laws: A practical guide*. Retrieved October 22, 2011 from http://www.osce.org/odihr/36426

HIV Counseling

Daniel J. O'Shea

HIV counseling offers an opportunity to provide information about HIV disease transmission and prevention, how to decrease behaviors that increase the risk of acquiring or transmitting HIV for persons who are HIV-infected or at increased risk for HIV infection, and available care and treatment options and partner services for those infected with HIV. Referral through counseling to access relevant medical, mental health, preventive, and psychosocial services can also reduce risk for transmitting or acquiring HIV infection. HIV counseling has been linked and integrated over the course of the HIV epidemic with HIV testing, and advances in HIV prevention and medical treatment have increased the importance of these services. HIV counseling may be particularly critical for individuals with severe mental illness (e.g., major depression, schizophrenia, and bipolar disorder) who are sexually active and/or are abusing substances. Research has found that as a group, individuals with severe mental illness are at increased risk of contracting HIV. This elevated risk may be due to difficulties in processing information, leading to an inability to identify risky situations; reduced social competence including an inability to negotiate risky situations; an increased risk of partner violence which reduces the individual's ability to negotiate the use of safer sex or safer injection practices; and/or co-occurring substance use, which can lead to impaired judgment.

At minimum HIV counseling in coordination with HIV testing includes: information, consent, prevention counseling/risk-reduction intervention, results disclosure, and referral. Pre-test counseling, a core component of the original voluntary counseling and testing, was designed to assist clients in assessing personal risks and identifying strategies to cope with their test results. Post-test counseling is required when test results are given, regardless of the result.

According to the US Centers for Disease Control and Prevention (CDC), information provided before the administration of the HIV test should comprise: a description of the test; the meaning of test results in explicit, understandable

D.J. O'Shea (✉)
Public Health Service, County of San Diego, San Diego, CA, USA
e-mail: Dan.OShea@sdcounty.ca.gov

S. Loue (ed.), *Mental Health Practitioner's Guide to HIV/AIDS*,
DOI 10.1007/978-1-4614-5283-6_44, © Springer Science+Business Media New York 2013

language; the benefits and consequences of testing; the risks of transmission; strategies that can be used to prevent HIV; the seroconversion "window" period; the importance of obtaining test results and explicit procedures to do so; referrals available for treatment and other services, including, if applicable, further HIV prevention counseling; reporting requirements; the procedure following a positive test result; and where to obtain further information. Other useful information may include descriptions or demonstrations of how to use condoms correctly; descriptions of the effectiveness of using clean needles, syringes, cotton, water, and other drug paraphernalia; and information regarding risk-free and safer sex options, other sexually transmitted and blood-borne diseases, drug treatment, and the possible effect of HIV vaccines on test results for persons participating in HIV vaccine trials. For efficiency and to allow more time to focus face-to-face interactions on prevention counseling, much of the information can be provided in the form of a handout, pamphlet, brochure, or video and should be appropriate to the client's culture, language, sex, sexual orientation, age, and developmental level.

CDC guidelines issued in 2006 describe HIV prevention counseling as "an interactive process of assessing risk, recognizing specific behaviors that increase the risk for acquiring or transmitting HIV, and developing a plan to take specific steps to reduce risks." A brief individual/couple-level risk-reduction intervention is best if it includes: an introduction; a personalized risk assessment; a "filling in" of the individual's knowledge gap; the identification of teachable moments; past successes, barriers, and self-efficacy; skill-building opportunities; a client-developed risk-reduction plan; self-efficacy for current risk-reduction plan; and implications of results.

The client-centered HIV prevention counseling model involves two brief sessions built around the HIV test. Other effective models are longer, involve more sessions, or use different formats such as large- and small-group counseling with a facilitator or video-based counseling. For the two-step client-centered model, clients are physically present in a setting for the HIV test (initial session) and then return for HIV test results (follow-up session). Each face-to-face session with a counselor might require 15–20 min for clients at increased risk for HIV, including testing and referral; only a few minutes may be needed for those at lower risk. For the first session, a personalized risk assessment encourages clients to identify, understand, and acknowledge behaviors and circumstances that put them at increased risk for acquiring HIV. The session explores prior attempts to reduce risk and identifies any successes and challenges. This in-depth exploration of risk allows the counselor to assist the client in considering ways to reduce personal risk and commit to a single, specific step. In the second session, when HIV test results are provided, the counselor discusses the results, requests the client to describe the risk-reduction step attempted, acknowledges any positive steps the client has made, helps the client to identify and to commit to additional behavioral steps, and provides appropriate referrals.

The CDC recommends the following elements for all HIV prevention counseling sessions: keep the session focused on HIV risk reduction; include an in-depth, personalized risk assessment; acknowledge and provide support for positive steps already made; clarify critical rather than general misconceptions; negotiate a concrete, achievable behavior-change step that will reduce HIV risk; seek flexibility in the prevention approach and counseling process, avoiding a "one-size-fits-all" prevention message (such as, "always use condoms"); provide skill-building opportunities; and use explicit language when providing test results. Other specialists in the field also suggest the following: ensure that the client returns to the same counselor to help the client feel secure, reduce misunderstanding, and promote the likelihood of effective risk reduction; use a written protocol to help counselors conduct effective sessions; ensure ongoing support by supervisors and administrators; avoid using counseling sessions for data collection; and avoid providing unnecessary information.

While HIV prevention counseling does not require advanced degrees or extensive experience, training is critical. According to the CDC, the following skills and characteristics have been identified by specialists in the field for effective HIV prevention counseling: completion of standard training courses in client-centered HIV prevention counseling or other risk-reduction counseling models; a belief that counseling can make a difference; a genuine interest in the counseling process; active listening skills; an ability to use open-ended rather than closed-ended questions; an ability and comfort with an interactive negotiating style rather than a persuasive approach; an ability to engender a supportive atmosphere and build trust with the client; an interest in learning new counseling and skills-building techniques; knowledge regarding specific HIV transmission risks; comfort in discussing specific HIV risk behaviors, including explicit sex or drug using behaviors; an ability to remain focused on risk-reduction goals; and support for routine, periodic, quality assurance measures.

Special training and consideration are required to disclose HIV test results to persons with newly identified HIV infection, who have both immediate and long-term needs. Some individuals may be better prepared to receive positive test results than others. The emotional impact of hearing an HIV-positive test result might prevent clients from clearly understanding information during the session in which they receive their results or cause subsequent denial of HIV infection. Counselors should offer appropriate facilitated referrals, including medical care and mental health services, and, as necessary, additional sessions. Ideally, clinical case managers or mental health counselors are co-located and available for counseling. The sudden knowledge of an HIV-positive test and/or an AIDS diagnosis can radically alter a person's sense of self and his or her future. Issues of general loss, loss of future, loss of physical function, and loss of vocation along with psychological manifestations of anxiety, depression, anger, resentment, and resignation are common. Reassessment of the meaning and purpose of one's life is often forced upon persons who, because of age, have yet to consider these issues that are more commonly addressed in one's senior years. Special considerations and training are also needed to counsel persons with a recent non-occupational HIV exposure, persons with indeterminate HIV test results, persons seeking repeat HIV testing, sex or needle-sharing partners of HIV-infected persons, health care workers after an occupational exposure, participants in HIV vaccine trials, and persons who use drugs.

Rapid HIV tests allow clients to receive their HIV test results the same day. Only those receiving preliminary positive results are scheduled for a follow-up visit to receive a confirmatory test, thereby significantly reducing the number of clients receiving two prevention counseling sessions. As a result, more attention is given to single-session prevention counseling. According to the CDC, fundamentals of HIV prevention counseling with rapid HIV tests include: keep the session focused on HIV risk reduction; include an in-depth, personalized risk assessment; acknowledge and provide support for positive steps already made; clarify critical rather than general misconceptions about HIV risk; negotiate a concrete, achievable behavior-change step that will reduce HIV risk; and use flexibility in the counseling technique and process, avoiding a "one-size-fits-all" approach. CDC has found that single-session prevention counseling is feasible and well accepted by most clients and counselors.

In health care settings, prevention counseling need not be linked explicitly to HIV testing. However, testing presents an ideal opportunity, in the context of discussion of potential risks, to provide or arrange for prevention counseling to assist with behavior changes that can reduce risks for acquiring HIV. Prevention counseling should be offered or made available through referral in all health care facilities serving patients at high risk for HIV and at facilities such as STD clinics in which information on HIV risk behaviors is routinely obtained.

The 2010 US National HIV/AIDS Strategy has three primary goals: (1) reducing the number of people who become infected with HIV, (2) increasing access to care and optimizing health outcomes for people living with HIV, and (3) reducing HIV-related health disparities. Only with focused efforts and success across in the continuum of HIV prevention and care (reducing risk for infection, identifying those with HIV, linking them to and retaining them in care, and ensuring they receive optimal treatment and prevention services) can the ultimate goals of improving health, extending lives, and preventing further HIV transmission be achieved. HIV counseling plays a critical role not just with HIV testing but also at all stages of that continuum.

Related Topics: Case management, HIV testing, prevention strategies.

Suggested Reading

Centers for Disease Control and Prevention. (2001). Revised guidelines for HIV counseling, testing, and referral. *Morbidity and Mortality Weekly Report*, 50(RR-19), 1–58.

Centers for Disease Control and Prevention. (2006). Revised recommendations for HIV testing of adults, adolescents, and pregnant women in health-care settings. *Morbidity and Mortality Weekly Report*, 55(RR-14), 1–17.

Centers for Disease Control and Prevention. (2011). Vital signs: HIV prevention through care and treatment—United States. *Morbidity and Mortality Weekly Report*, 60(47), 1618–1623.

Suggested Resources

AIDS Info, & U.S. Department of Health and Human Services. (2011). Washington, DC. Retrieved November 25, 2011 from http://www.aidsinfo.nih.gov/

The AIDS InfoNet, New Mexico AIDS Education and Training Center, & University of New Mexico School of Medicine. (2011). Albuquerque, NM. Retrieved November 25, 2011 from http://www.aidsinfonet.org/

Centers for Disease Control and Prevention. (2011). *HIV/AIDS*. Atlanta, GA. Retrieved November 25, 2011 from http://www.cdc.gov/hiv/

Centers for Disease Control and Prevention. (2009, September). *Meeting summary: Consultation on revised guidelines for HIV counseling, testing, and referral in non-health-care settings*. Atlanta, GA. Retrieved November 25, 2011 from http://www.cdc.gov/hiv/topics/testing/resources/other/pdf/consultation.pdf

United Nations Programme on HIV/AIDS (UNAIDS). (2011). Geneva. Retrieved November 25, 2011 from http://www.unaids.org/en/

HIV Testing

Daniel J. O'Shea

HIV testing is the only way to determine for certain whether someone is infected with HIV, the virus which causes AIDS. Infected individuals may not have symptoms for many years. Many individuals are not tested for HIV until they or their sex or needle-sharing partner develop an AIDS-related illness. Some HIV-positive women may not obtain a test until they seek prenatal care or give birth. HIV testing offers an opportunity for infected individuals to find out they are infected and gain access to treatment that may help to delay disease progression and significantly improve health outcomes. For infected pregnant women, it may provide a viable opportunity for treatment to prevent transmission of HIV to their child. For those who think they may have been exposed to HIV, having a test and receiving a negative result can put their mind at ease. Anyone who is sexually active or using and sharing injection equipment should get tested regularly for HIV.

A positive HIV test result alone does not mean that a person has AIDS, only that HIV infection has occurred. AIDS, the end stage of HIV disease, is caused by the infection and spread of HIV within the body. HIV destroys CD4+ T blood cells which are crucial to the normal function of the human immune system. Progression from initial HIV infection to AIDS may take 10 years or more, but varies greatly depending on many factors, including a person's health status, their health-related behaviors, and access to antiretroviral therapy (ART).

HIV testing is available in the USA and most countries at health clinics, physicians' offices, local health departments, hospitals, family planning clinics, community organizations and/or sites specifically set up for HIV counseling and testing, sometimes through mobile or storefront units. An individual seeking a test generally sees a trained counselor, doctor, nurse, or other health professional in private. The health care provider explains what the test involves and what the result means, with the opportunity for questions to be asked and answered. Informed consent must be given before taking the test. Either a blood sample (from the arm or

D.J. O'Shea (✉)
Public Health Service, County of San Diego, San Diego, CA, USA
e-mail: Dan.OShea@sdcounty.ca.gov

S. Loue (ed.), *Mental Health Practitioner's Guide to HIV/AIDS*,
DOI 10.1007/978-1-4614-5283-6_45,

finger) or an oral fluid sample is taken, depending on the type of test used at the site. Based on the test used, results can take anywhere from minutes to weeks. Testing can be anonymous with a code or number, rather than a name, assigned to the test, or confidential, where results are kept confidential within medical records and cannot be shared with others without written permission from the person tested. An individual who tests positive confidentially or receives medical services for HIV is reported to the health department (records kept confidential) and counted in statistical reports. Every person who takes an HIV test must receive counseling when their test results are given, regardless of the test result.

There are several types of HIV tests. These include the HIV antibody test, P24 antigen test, and PCR test. Some types of HIV tests are used after a person has been diagnosed to measure how quickly the virus is multiplying (CD4 test and viral load test).

The most commonly used test for routine diagnosis of HIV among adults is the *HIV antibody test*. Antibody tests are inexpensive, easy to use, and very accurate. They detect HIV antibodies, rather than HIV itself, in an individual's blood, urine, or oral fluids. Antibodies are special proteins produced by the immune system in response to HIV to fight infection. Most people develop detectable antibodies within 3 months after infection, with the average at 25 days; in rare cases, it can take up to 6 months. The time period between infection and the appearance of detectable HIV antibodies is called the window period. Because HIV antibodies may not yet be detectable, the HIV antibody test is not useful during the window period and someone testing negative may actually be positive. As a result, antibody tests are recommended 3 months after any potential exposure to HIV infection. A negative test at 3 months will almost always mean a person is not infected with HIV; a negative test at 6 months, with no risks for HIV infection in the meantime, means the individual is not infected with HIV.

Test samples taken are sent to a laboratory to be analyzed, and the results of an initial antibody test are generally available within a few days. The ELISA antibody test (enzyme-linked immunoabsorbent) or EIA (enzyme immunoassay) was the first HIV test to be widely used. ELISA tests are very sensitive and can detect very small amounts of HIV antibody; however, for that same reason, their specificity (ability to distinguish HIV antibodies from other antibodies) is slightly lowered, resulting in a very small chance (less than 0.5%) that a result is a "false positive." A false-positive result means that although a person may not be infected, his or her antibody test may come back positive. Consequently, all positive test results are followed up with a second or more confirmatory tests before the results are given to the person tested. Confirmatory tests include: the Western blot assay (also used to confirm plasma HIV RNA tests); indirect immunofluorescence assay, which utilizes a microscope to detect HIV antibodies; line immunoassay; or a second ELISA test, usually a different commercial brand with a different method of detection than the first test. The latter is more common in resource-poor areas that have relatively high prevalence rates. When two tests are combined, the chance of an inaccurate result is less than 0.1%. If both tests are positive, it means the person is infected with HIV, with three exceptions: (1) babies born to HIV-infected mothers retain their mother's antibodies for up to 18 months; in these cases, the baby can receive a PCR test after birth to determine HIV status; (2) individuals who participated in HIV vaccine trials may test positive but not be infected; and (3) pregnant women may have false or unclear test results due to changes in their immune system.

Rapid HIV tests use the same technology as ELISA tests, but results from a blood sample or oral fluids are available within 20 min. In November 2010 the US Food and Drug Administration (FDA) approved the INSTI test, which gives results within 60 s. Easy to use, rapid tests do not require laboratory facilities or highly trained staff. Positive results must be confirmed with a second laboratory test, which may take from a few days to a few weeks.

Several tests are now available that detect HIV prior to the development of antibodies. Detecting HIV at earlier stages of infection is important since the amount of virus in the body is very high immediately after infection, increasing the risk for HIV transmission at that time. Within 2 weeks of infection, a *P24 antigen test* can detect the substances (antigens) on HIV that trigger the immune response to produce antibodies. The protein P24, the most common antigen on HIV, is produced in excess early after HIV infection and detectable in blood serum, although it ultimately fades to undetectable levels after HIV is fully established. Limitations for this test include a very low sensitivity and short timeframe for use before antibodies begin to be produced. As a result, rather than using it alone for general HIV diagnostic purposes, P24 antigen tests have been combined with standard antibody tests to create *fourth generation tests* which allow earlier and more accurate detection of HIV. The FDA approved the first fourth generation antigen/antibody combination test in June 2010 in the USA.

A *PCR* (polymerase chain reaction) *test*, also known as a *viral load test*, *plasma HIV RNA* (ribonucleic acid), and *HIV NAAT* (nucleic acid amplification test) detect the actual genetic material of HIV rather than the antibodies to the virus or the antigen, and thus can identify HIV in the blood as early as 1 week after infection. This test, however, is very expensive and more complicated to administer and interpret than a standard antibody test. The PCR test is recommended when recent infection is very likely, and the individual also has flu-like symptoms. Results are available in a few days to a few weeks. The viral load test is also used to measure the amount of HIV in the blood at any stage of HIV infection.

HIV home sampling and *HIV home testing* are available in some countries. *Home sampling* allows an individual to take a sample of their own blood or oral fluids, send it to a laboratory for testing, and receive the results by telephone a few days later. If positive, a professional counselor schedules a follow-up blood test at a clinic and provides emotional support and referrals. Only one US company offers an FDA-approved HIV home sampling kit, but many not approved by the FDA are marketed on the Internet. *Home testing* is a self-administered rapid antibody HIV test that provides results within minutes, using either a blood or saliva sample. As with home sampling, a preliminary positive result requires confirmation through a blood test at a clinic. In many countries, including the USA, it is illegal to sell HIV test kits to the public. Internet purchases do not come with any guarantee that the test kit is genuine or will provide accurate results.

In the USA in 2009, approximately 45% of persons aged 18–64 years reported ever testing for HIV. However, nearly one-third of diagnoses still occur late in the progression of HIV and an estimated 21% (240,000) of those infected are unaware of their status. Increased testing efforts are needed, particularly among populations most at risk for HIV infection. Knowledge of HIV status and access to treatment are important considerations, not only for maintaining and improving health but also for reducing the spread of HIV. In addition to suppressed individual and community viral load with ART, thus reducing the amount of virus available for forward transmission, studies have demonstrated that many infected persons do decrease behaviors that facilitate HIV transmission to sex or needle-sharing partners once they are aware of their status. US national efforts are now focused on ensuring that more people know their HIV status and are linked to HIV treatment. In September 2006, the US Centers for Disease Control and Prevention (CDC) recommended routine HIV screening of adults, adolescents, and pregnant women in health care settings and reducing barriers to HIV testing, and in 2007 established the Expanded Testing Initiative to significantly increase the number of persons tested in jurisdictions with a high rate of HIV among disproportionately affected populations and to support implementation of the 2006 recommendations for routine testing in all health care settings.

Related Topics: AIDS service organizations, case management, HIV counseling, prevention strategies.

Suggested Readings

Centers for Disease Control and Prevention (2006). Revised recommendations for HIV testing of adults, adolescents, and pregnant women in health-care settings. *Morbidity and Mortality Weekly Report*, *55*(RR-14), 1–17. Atlanta, GA: US Department of Health and Human Services.

Suggested Resources

AIDS Info, U.S. Department of Health and Human Services (2011). Washington, D.C. Retrieved November 25, 2011 from http://www.aidsinfo.nih.gov/

The AIDS InfoNet, New Mexico AIDS Education and Training Center, University of New Mexico School of Medicine (2011). Albuquerque, NM. Retrieved November 25, 2011 from http://www.aidsinfonet.org/

AVERT—Averting HIV and AIDS—AIDS & HIV Information from AVERT.org (2011). *HIV Testing. Horsham, West Sussex, UK*. Retrieved December 30, 2011 from http://www.avert.org/testing.htm

Centers for Disease Control and Prevention (2011). *Expanded testing program overview*. Atlanta, GA (August 22, 2011). Retrieved November 25, 2011 from http://www.cdc.gov/hiv/resources/factsheets/PDF/HIV-ETP.pdf

Centers for Disease Control and Prevention (2011). HIV/AIDS. Atlanta, GA. Retrieved November 25, 2011 from http://www.cdc.gov/hiv/

United Nations Programme on HIV/AIDS (UNAIDS) (2008). *Fast facts about HIV testing and counselling. Geneva*. Retrieved November 25, 2011 from http://data.unaids.org/pub/FactSheet/2008/20080527_fastfacts_testing_en.pdf

HIV-Associated Dementia

Brittany Daugherty-Brownrigg

HIV/AIDS has been known to cause many complications within the immune system as well as within other systems in the human body. HIV/AIDS complications that affect the neurological system in particular are known to be quite severe and have been associated with a high risk of mortality. HIV/AIDS often targets the brain because it has the necessary receptors that allow HIV to enter cells known as CD4+ and CD8+ cells. These particular cells are white blood cells that play a special role in the immune system; CD4+ cells are known to fight against infections while CD8+ cells kill cancerous or virus-infected cells.

The terms AIDS dementia complex and HIV-1-associated dementia are used to describe the various neurological and psychiatric symptoms that result from HIV infection. These symptoms include neurocognitive impairments such as a decline in concentration and memory, leg weakness, gait difficulties, and depression. Behavioral symptoms, such as social withdrawal, apathy, and strong personality changes may also be present.

HIV enters the central nervous system early on in the infection. The infection can cause neurological impairment and behavioral symptoms even in the absence of opportunistic infections. HIV infects CD4+ and monocyte cells, blood cells that travel through the brains membrane, crossing what is known as the blood-brain barrier. HIV then damages the basal ganglia by inflammation. The basal ganglia plays a key role in many movement disorders such as Parkinsons, Tourette's, and even Huntington's disease. It consists of a set of nuclei in the forebrain with various components responsible for receiving information from various brain areas and sending output information to other areas of the basal ganglia. Damage to this area can affect one's ability to control speech, movement, and memory function.

Diagnosis of HIV-associated dementia (HAD) prior to the initiation of retroviral medicine was associated with high viral loads and occurrence of opportunistic infections. Although significant improvements have been made with medicinal

B. Daugherty-Brownrigg (✉)
John Carroll University, South Euclid, OH, USA
e-mail: bdaugherty10@jcu.edu

S. Loue (ed.), *Mental Health Practitioner's Guide to HIV/AIDS*, 245
DOI 10.1007/978-1-4614-5283-6_46, © Springer Science+Business Media New York 2013

therapy, HAD still poses a public health concern among those with HIV/AIDS. Neurological complications had been found to exist in about 30% of those with HIV infection and 50% of those with AIDS. Since 1995, highly active retroviral therapy (HARRT) has been the most common treatment approach. This therapy consists of at least three drugs that block viral replication; these drugs help to restore immune function and improve CNS-related symptoms. The introduction of HAART has lowered the prevalence of HAD from 30 to 10% in the infected population. The cognitive decline in AIDS-related dementia is often treated with antidepressants, anticonvulsants, and antipsychotic drugs. Even though HIV/AIDS-related dementia has proven to be one of the most serious neurological complications of AIDS, advances in medicinal therapies and research efforts are promising.

Related Topics: Cognitive impairment, mental health comorbidity and HIV/AIDS.

Suggested Readings

Ghafouri, M., Amini, S., Khalili, K. & Sawaya, B.E. (2006). HIV-I associated dementia: symptoms and causes. *Retrovirology 3:28.* Retrieved Dec 13, 2011 from http://www.biomedcentral.com/1742-4690/3/28

Woods, S. P., Moore, D. J., Weber, E., & Grant, I. (2009). Cognitive neuropsychology of HIV associated neurocognitive disorders. *Neuropsychology Review, 19*, 152–168.

Suggested Resources

Basal Ganglia Dysfunction. www.nlm.nih.gov/medlineplus/ency/article/001069.htm

The Body. The Complete HIV/AIDS Resource. www.thebody.com

HIV-Related Cancers

Aiswarya Lekshmi Pillai Chandran Pillai

The burden of HIV-related illnesses and deaths has been increasing ever since its discovery in 1981. HIV-infected patients are at an increased risk for cancers due to the immunosuppression associated with it. They may experience significant mental trauma due to both the illness and the social stigma attached to it.

Cancers Associated with HIV

Cancer may occur as the direct result of HIV infection or may be incidental to it. In either case, HIV-infected patients have an increased risk of mortality and morbidity. The risk of cancer in HIV patients is two to three times greater than the general population. It is estimated that 30–40% of HIV-positive patients develop a malignancy during their lifetimes. Cancers affecting HIV-positive/AIDS patients are categorized as AIDS-defining cancers and non-AIDS-defining cancers.

AIDS-Defining Cancers

When HIV-positive patients get certain specific types of cancers, it indicates that they have progressed to AIDS. These cancers are known as AIDS-defining cancers.

Kaposi's sarcoma (KS): Kaposi's sarcoma is 100–300 times more likely in HIV-positive patients than in the general population. Kaposi's sarcoma is associated with human herpes virus 8 (HHV-8) infections. Low CD4 T cell counts increase the risk

A.L.P. Chandran Pillai (✉)
Department of Epidemiology and Biostatistics, School of Medicine, Case Western Reserve University, Cleveland, OH, USA
e-mail: axc434@case.edu

S. Loue (ed.), *Mental Health Practitioner's Guide to HIV/AIDS*,
DOI 10.1007/978-1-4614-5283-6_47,

and severity of KS. However, the incidence and deaths from Kaposi's sarcoma has decreased since the introduction of highly active antiretroviral therapy (HAART)

Non-Hodgkin's lymphoma (NHL): The risk of NHL or AIDS-related lymphoma is about 40–400 times that of the general population, depending on the specific study and the type of NHL. The prevalence of high-grade lymphoma is greater than that of low-grade lymphoma in HIV/AIDS patients. Like KS, the risk of NHL increases with low CD4 T cell counts. The types of NHL in HIV patients include systemic NHL, primary central nervous system NHL (PCNSL, primary brain lymphoma or cerebral lymphoma), and primary effusion lymphoma (PEL) or body cavity-based lymphoma. However, unlike KS, the risk of NHL in HIV/AIDS patients has not decreased with the introduction of HAART.

Invasive cervical cancer (ICC): The association between HIV and ICC is inconsistent though it is an AIDS-defining condition. Some studies report an approximate 5–9 times increased incidence of ICC in HIV-positive women compared to sero-negative women. HIV-infected women are likely to be co-infected with human papillomavirus (HPV) which causes cervical intraepithelial neoplasia (CIN) and squamous intraepithelial lesions (SIL). CIN and SIL are precursors to ICC. Decreased CD4 T cell count increases the risk of contracting HPV infection. The impact of the introduction of HAART on the risk of ICC is inconsistent.

Non-AIDS-Defining Cancers

Hodgkin's disease (HD): HIV/AIDS patients are 7.6–11.5 times more likely to get HD compared to the general population. Association studies of low CD4 T cell count and HD show inconsistent results. There has been no change in the risk of HD reported with the introduction of HAART.

Anal cancer: HIV/AIDS patients are 30–50 times more likely to have anal cancer than the general population with rates as high as 60-fold in HIV-positive bisexual or homosexual men. Like cervical cancer, anal cancer is associated with HPV infection which causes SIL and anal intraepithelial neoplasia (AIN). Studies on the association of low CD4 T cell count and anal cancer give inconsistent results. No change has been noted in the risk of anal cancer with the introduction of HAART.

Lung cancer: HIV/AIDS patients are 2.5–7.5 times more likely to develop lung cancer compared to the general population. Immunosuppression increases the rate of lung cancer. The association between smoking and lung cancer in HIV/AIDS patients is inconsistent. An increased incidence of lung cancer has been noted following the introduction of HAART, perhaps due to prevention of early deaths from HIV/AIDS.

Testicular germ cell tumors (GCT): HIV-positive men are 1.4–8.2 times more likely to develop testicular cancer than HIV-negative men. HPV, Epstein–Barr virus

(EBV), and human endogenous retrovirus K10 are associated with testicular cancer. Studies on the impact of immunosuppression on the incidence of GCT give inconsistent results. HAART does not seem to have had an impact on the incidence of GCT.

Other cancers with increased risk in HIV/AIDS patients are leukemia, multiple myeloma, skin cancer, cancer of the vulva/vagina and penis, leiomyosarcoma, cancer of the lip, larynx, pharynx, tongue, esophagus, stomach, pancreas, liver, kidney, brain and central nervous system (CNS), and angiosarcoma.

Mental and Emotional Issues

People are often devastated when they learn about an HIV/AIDS diagnosis. They go through various stages of the Kübler-Ross grief reaction: denial, anger, bargaining, depression, and finally acceptance. The stigma attached to HIV/AIDS often causes a sense of shame, social isolation, and rejection of the patients. Substance abuse, which is highly prevalent among some subgroups of HIV-positive patients, may cause cognitive impairment independent of the HIV infection. In people who have a preexisting mental illness, their ability to cope with the HIV disease process, adhere to treatment plans, and utilize support networks and care systems may be impeded, leading to a poorer quality of life. HIV directly affects the brain as well. The resulting inflammation damages the brain and spinal cord, causing confusion, forgetfulness, cognitive motor impairment, and behavioral changes. HIV infection can also alter the size of certain brain structures involved in learning and information processing. Dementia produced by the effect of medications, often known as "AIDS dementia complex," is known to derail the cognition of patients. Among cancers, CNS lymphomas directly cause mental deterioration and speech disturbances.

Just as with HIV/AIDS diagnosis, people are often shocked at a diagnosis of cancer. Cancer patients also experience the classical grief reaction stages besides the fear of being a burden on their family and a fear of impending death. Both the cancer and its treatment regimens, chemotherapy and radiation, may cause cognitive impairment. Patients in remission often report having to live the rest of their life in fear of cancer recurrence.

The mental and emotional turmoil of patients with HIV/AIDS often worsens when the individuals are diagnosed with cancer. These patients would have already gone through the different stages of grief reaction at the diagnosis of HIV. With the new diagnosis of cancer, they often feel that they are back to square one. In addition to the stigmatization and stress of being an HIV patient, the fear that death would beckon sooner may lead to deeper depression and despair. Suicidal tendencies, agoraphobia, and social phobia are greater in HIV/AIDS patients with cancer. Physical pain associated with cancer and the need to undergo surgery, chemotherapy, and/or radiation further weaken the morale of the patients.

How Can We Address These Issues?

The collaboration of professionals working in different intervention settings (e.g., primary prevention and clinical care) is needed to tackle the issues of cancer and emotional distress in HIV patients. Because HIV-infected patients are at higher risk, they should be regularly screened for cancer. This would help in the early diagnosis and management of the disease. Social support in addition to radiation and chemotherapy should be offered to HIV-positive patients with cancer. Communities can help to address the mental health issues of HIV/AIDS patients with cancer by establishing behavioral and group interventions that improve coping skills; providing and enhancing social support and peer support systems; maintaining a 24-h help desk or phone line; teaching relaxation techniques; providing and encouraging fitness training; maintaining suicide prevention services; providing counseling services; providing rehabilitation facilities; and enhancing access to and awareness about substance use treatment centers and palliative care units. Health care providers can help to address the needs of HIV-infected individuals with cancer through improved pain management, conducting screening and providing treatment for coexisting mental disorders, and increasing public awareness to alleviate the stigma attached to HIV/AIDS.

Related Topics: Antiretroviral therapy, cognitive impairment, coping, social support.

Suggested Readings

Brown, L., Macintyre, K., & Trujillo, L. (2003). Interventions to reduce HIV/AIDS stigma: What have we learned? *AIDS Education and Prevention, 15*, 49–69.

Frisch, M., Biggar, R. J., Engels, E. A., & Goedert, J. J. (2001). Association of cancer with AIDS-related immunosuppression in adults. *Journal of the American Medical Association, 285*, 1736–1745.

Sherman, A. C., Mosier, J., Leszcz, M., Burlingame, G. M., Ulman, K. H., Cleary, T., et al. (2004). Group interventions for patients with cancer and HIV disease: Part I: Effects on psychosocial and functional outcomes at different phases of illness. *International Journal of Group Psychotherapy, 54*, 29–82.

Suggested Resources

Cancer.net. (2010, April). *Depression and anxiety* (2010). Retrieved December 27, 2011 from http://www.cancer.net/patient/Coping/Emotional+and+Physical+Matters/Depression+and+Anxiety

Fayed, L. (2010, Nov 8). AIDS-related cancer: The causes, symptoms, types, and treatment of AIDS-related cancer. Retrieved December 27, 2011 from http://cancer.about.com/od/cancerlistaz/a/AIDS_related.htm.

HIV-InSite: Comprehensive, up-to-date information on HIV/AIDS treatment, prevention, and policy from the University of California San Francisco. Retrieved December 27, 2011 from http://hivinsite.ucsf.edu/

Newcomb-Fernandez, J. (2003). *Cancer in the HIV-infected population.* Retrieved December 27, 2011 from TheBody.com. http://www.thebody.com/content/art16834.html.

Housing and Homelessness

Vanessa A. Forro

More than 33 million people are living with HIV/AIDS worldwide. Half of new infections are among people 25 years old and younger. The United Nations Declaration of Human Rights states that housing in addition to food, clothing, and medical care are basic human rights. HIV/AIDS is unique because it deprives families, communities, and entire nations of their young and most productive people. Risk factors such as gender, stigma, and homophobia impact both housing stability and HIV/AIDS contraction. Fifty-eight percent of the world's HIV/AIDS cases are among women, who represent the majority of the world's poor and suffer disproportionately from inadequate housing. In addition, men who have sex with men (MSM) are the group most at-risk of HIV infection across the globe. Homelessness and unstable housing are strongly associated with greater HIV risk, inadequate health care, poor health outcomes, and early death. Studies have indicated that stable housing eases the burden of care and support and optimizes health outcomes for people living with HIV/AIDS (PLWHA) and their families.

The Centers for Disease Control and Prevention estimate that there are approximately 1.1 million people living with HIV/AIDS in the United States, and one in five people are unaware of their status. Housing status has been identified as a key factor affecting access to treatment, health care services, and behavior among PLWHA. Research has shown that public investment in housing not only improves health outcomes but also actually saves taxpayer money. In response to the increasing need for housing assistance among PLWHA, the Housing Opportunities for Persons with AIDS (HOPWA) program was established in 1992. HOPWA is managed by the Department of Housing and Urban Development (HUD) Office of HIV/AIDS. It is the only federally funded program dedicated to address the housing needs of PLWHA and their families and offers short- and long-term housing assistance. The 2010 HOPWA fiscal year report found a significant goal achievement for the over 25,000 households receiving housing assistance.

V.A. Forro (✉)
Neurological Outcomes Center, Case Western Reserve University, Cleveland, OH, USA
e-mail: Vanessa.Forro@case.edu

S. Loue (ed.), *Mental Health Practitioner's Guide to HIV/AIDS*,
DOI 10.1007/978-1-4614-5283-6_48, © Springer Science+Business Media New York 2013

Ninety-six percent achieved housing stability (rental-assistance based) and 94% achieved permanent housing in community residences.

Half of all people living with HIV/AIDS are at-risk of becoming homeless. Some statistics reveal approximately a quarter of the homeless population are HIV-infected. There is a high morbidity and mortality rate among homeless PLWHA. In addition homeless PLWHA have high comorbidities such as substance abuse, mental illness, and are at-risk for contracting other highly infectious diseases such as tuberculosis. The United States government has recognized the fact that adequate housing is a barrier to effective HIV prevention, treatment, and care.

In the early 1990s, Dr. Sam Tsemberis, a professor of psychiatry at NYU School of Medicine, pioneered the Housing First program. The Housing First model centers on providing chronically homeless people with housing quickly and then providing support services, case management, and health care, as needed. The goal of Housing First is to reduce the time people experience homelessness and prevent further episodes of homelessness. It embraces a harm reduction approach where people do not have to remain substance-free or linked to services in order to receive housing. In 1999, Congress directed HUD to spend 30% of its funding on Housing First programs. Research has shown that Housing First initiative in cities such as Seattle, Washington and Chicago, Illinois reduce the costs of emergency department visits, detox visits, and incarcerations among homeless populations. Housing First programs are proven to decrease morbidity and mortality, increase health care access and anti-retroviral treatment, address substance abuse and mental health issues, and improve the overall health of PLWHA.

Inadequate housing and homelessness are major risk factors for the contraction of HIV/AIDS globally. Social determinants of HIV acquisition include gender, stigma, and homophobia. In order to address the needs of people living with HIV/AIDS countries must address the larger inequalities that affect their societies as well as the world. PLWHA can live a long, productive, and contributory life if they are afforded the basic human rights and support.

A major consequence of HIV infection is difficulty in securing or maintaining steady employment, and PLWHA who disclose their status to their employer run the risk of being terminated due to stigma and fear. Oftentimes people are kicked out of their homes when their HIV-positive status is revealed. In Bolivia, it is common that homeless shelters discriminate against PLWHA. In Panama the Ministry of Housing provides grants for emergencies, eradicating poverty and hunger, and subsidized housing for indigenous populations, but no housing programs exist specifically for PLWHA.

Gender inequalities and stigma are strongly associated with the spread of HIV/AIDS. Ninety percent of women living with HIV/AIDS in India are infected by their husbands or intimate sexual partners. The Indian government issues below poverty line (BPL) cards to PLWHA to ensure access to nutrition assistance and housing resources, as well as a monthly stipend for those on anti-retroviral treatment. Female property rights are insecure or nonexistent in many developing countries, and even more so in the context of HIV/AIDS. Therefore, when husbands die the women are either forced to leave the marital home or have sex with other male in-laws in order to keep a roof over their heads. In Kenya, widows who have lost their husbands to HIV/AIDS are often blamed for the illness and harassed by in-laws until they leave the marital home. A major issue in Kenya is women's rights, as they bear the greatest burden of the HIV/AIDS epidemic, and reformed legislation must be a top priority in order to see a decrease in HIV incidence rates.

Nigeria has the second highest rate of HIV/AIDS in the world (2.95 million PLWHA in 2008) after South Africa. One out of every three PLWHA in Nigeria resides in slums; and the challenges of overcrowding and inadequate infrastructure and poor public services lead to poor health among PLWHA. Most people in slum communities cannot afford adequate housing because of AIDS-related consequences and maintaining adequate income is difficult or impossible for PLWHA because of the stigma associated with the disease.

PLWHA in the developed world face less extreme housing situations than persons living with the disease in developing countries and have more housing resources and rights. In Sydney, Australia, 1–3% of PLWHA are either homeless or in unstable housing. Currently, there are no institutions that solely exist to address housing vulnerability for PLWHA. And as people are living longer with the disease they are expected more and more to be able to provide for themselves, which has been seen in the governmental funding shifts since the 1990s, which reduce funding resources that support PLWHA. Almost half of PLWHA in the province of Ontario, Canada, have problems with housing. In November 2010, the Homeless Partnering Strategy (NPS) in Canada was renewed for another 3 years, which was started in 2007 in order to address the needs of low income Canadians, those at-risk of homelessness, and the homeless.

Related Topics: Access to care, survival sex, stigma and stigmatization.

Suggested Readings

Larimer, M. E., Malone, D. K., Garner, M. D., Atkins, D. C., Burlingham, B., Lonczak, H. S., Tanzer, K., Ginzler, J., Clifasefi, S. L., Hobson, W. G., & Marlatt, G. A. (2009). Health care and public service use and costs before and after provision of housing for chronically homeless persons with severe alcohol problems. *Journal of the American Medical Association, 301*(13), 1349–1357.

Schwarcz, S. K., Hsu, L. C., Vittinghoff, E., Vu, A., Bamberger, J. D., & Katz, M. H. (2009). Impact of housing on the survival of persons with AIDS. *BMC Public Health, 9*, 220.

Wolitski, R. J., Kidder, D. P., & Fenton, K. A. (2007). HIV, homelessness, and public health: critical issues and a call for increased action. *AIDS Behavior, 11*(Suppl 6), 167–171.

Wolitski, R. J., Kidder, D. P., Pals, S. L., Royal, S., Aidala, A., Stall, R., Holtgrave, D. R., Harre, D., Courtenay-Quirk, C., & Housing and Health Study Team. (2010). Randomized trial of the effects of housing assistance on the health and risk behaviors of homeless and unstably housed people living with HIV. *AIDS Behavior*, 14(3), 493–503.

Suggested Resources

Barrett, J. (2008, March 6). Homeless Study Looks at "Housing First": Shifting policies to get chronically ill in homes. *Wall Street Journal*. Retrieved from http://www.aidschicago.org/pdf/2008/home_wall_street_journal.pdf.

International HIV/AIDS Alliance: http://www.aidsalliance.org/homepagedetails.aspx?id=1

Menchaca, M., Martinez, L., Stewart, J., Treherne, L., Vicic, W., Audain, G., & Post, P. (2008). *Adapting your practice: Treatment and recommendations for homeless patients with HIV/AIDS*. Nashville, TN: Health Care for the Homeless Clinicians' Network, National Health Care for the Homeless Council, Inc. Retrieved from http://www.nhchc.org/HIVguide2008.pdf.

National AIDS Housing Coalition, Inc. (2010). *More than just a roof over my head: Housing for people living with HIV/AIDS around the world.* Retrieved from http://www.nationalaidshousing.org/PDF/More%20Than%20Just%20a%20Roof.pdf.

National Coalition for the Homeless: http://www.nationalhomeless.org

Human Rights

Simona Irina Damian

Human rights are innate and equally important to individuals, stretching across all areas of life: civil activity, personal values, political freedom, social needs, economic well-being, cultural pursuits, and environmental quality. They are recognized as universal legal guarantees protecting individuals and groups against actions and omissions that could alter fundamental freedoms, entitlements, and human dignity.

As a vital response to the World War II atrocities, the international community agreed to the UN Charter (1946) and the Universal Declaration of Human Rights (1948) which marked a starting point in the ongoing development of all international human rights law. Ever since, governments, communities, and organizations have been going through a comprehensive evolution in understanding that human rights are not simply utopian ends or goals to which we all aspire, but benchmarks of a just and equitable society, thus leading to become increasingly well defined in recent years. Codified in international, regional, and national legal systems, human rights enact a set of performance standards against which governments as well as duty bearers at all levels of society can be held accountable.

In establishing a global legal framework there are two main sources of binding international human rights law: customary international law and conventions/treaties between nations. In some countries, international law is automatically part of national law and enforceable in their national courts—a legal system called "monism." In most countries, however, domestic legislation must be enacted to integrate international law, in a system called "dualism." In either case, national legislation and policies must detail how the State's human rights obligations will be discharged at national, provincial, and local levels, and the extent to which individuals, companies, local government units, nongovernmental organizations (NGOs), or other organs of society will directly assume the responsibility for implementation. Altogether, the fulfillment of commitments under international

S.I. Damian (✉)
University of Medicine and Pharmacy Gr. T. Popa, Iasi, Romania
e-mail: si_damian@yahoo.com

S. Loue (ed.), *Mental Health Practitioner's Guide to HIV/AIDS*,
DOI 10.1007/978-1-4614-5283-6_49,

human rights treaties is monitored by independent expert committees called "treaty bodies," which also help to clarify the meaning of particular human rights.

Public health and human rights are meant to share a common goal, that of promoting and protecting the well-being of all individuals. Ever since the first global AIDS strategy was developed in 1987, it has been reaffirmed that human rights are fundamental to any response to HIV/AIDS.

Endorsing human rights in the context of HIV/AIDS is not only an imperative of justice to overcome existing forms of discrimination and intolerance but also a tool to prevent the further spread of the epidemic, as human rights action can help to empower individuals and communities to respond to HIV/AIDS, to reduce vulnerability to HIV infection, and to lessen the impact of HIV/AIDS on those infected and affected.

Within the United Nations system, a subsidiary intergovernmental body of the General Assembly, which plays an active part in addressing and promoting human rights in the context of HIV/AIDS, is The United Nations Human Rights Council (formerly known as the United Nations Commission on Human Rights), by adopting resolutions and carrying out special procedures in this particular field of expertise.

Established in 1994 by a resolution of the UN Economic and Social Council and launched in January 1996, The Joint United Nations Programme on HIV and AIDS (UNAIDS) is the main advocate for accelerated, comprehensive, and coordinated global action on the HIV/AIDS epidemic. This is an innovative joint programme that has brought together a number of co-sponsoring UN organizations, laid strong foundations of partnerships with individuals and organizations from all sectors of society, and steadily developed strategies and initiatives to help contain AIDS. In response to a request made by the Commission on Human Rights which underscored the need and the imperative to provide guidance for Governments and others on how to take concrete steps to best promote, protect, and fulfill human rights in the context of the HIV epidemic, the United Nations Centre for Human Rights and the Joint United Nations Programme on HIV/AIDS (UNAIDS) convened the Second International Consultation on HIV/AIDS and Human Rights in Geneva, from 23 to 25 September 1996. The result was the International Guidelines on HIV/AIDS and Human Rights, adopted in annex I from the report of the Secretary-General to the Commission on Human Rights in document E/CN.4/1997/37, later on published in 1998 by the Office of the High Commissioner for Human Rights (OHCHR) and UNAIDS.

In June 2001, heads of State and representatives of governments met at the United Nations General Assembly Special Session dedicated to HIV/AIDS and issued the Declaration of Commitment on HIV/AIDS. The Commission on Human Rights adopted a resolution in which it stated that the right to the highest attainable standard of health includes access to antiretroviral therapy for HIV. Following this, in 2002, OHCHR and UNAIDS sponsored the Third International Consultation on HIV/AIDS and Human Rights in order to revise Guideline 6 to reflect the human rights dimensions of access to HIV prevention, treatment, care, and support.

In 2006 UN Member States met to review progress achieved in realizing the targets set out in 2001. They also reaffirmed the Millennium Development Goals (MDGs of 2000), in particular, the goal to halt and begin to reverse the spread of AIDS by 2015.

Worldwide efforts to sustain the human rights of those coping with HIV/AIDS marked significant developments concerning the right to health and access to HIV-related prevention, treatment, care, and support, including advances in the availability of diagnostic tests and HIV-related treatments, such as antiretroviral therapies. There have been increased commitments at the international, regional, and domestic levels towards the full realization of all human rights related to HIV, as well as improved access to health services for people living with HIV.

Related Topics: Council of International Organizations for Medical Sciences, Declaration of Helsinki, United Nations.

Suggested Readings

Burris, S., Lazzarini, Z., & Gostin, L. O. (2002). Symposium: Health, law, and human rights: Exploring the connections. *Journal of Law, Medicine & Ethics, 30*(4), 485–754.

Suggested Resources

Gruskin, S., Tarantola, D. (2002). Human rights and HIV/AIDS. HIV InSite Knowledge Base Chapter, April 2002. Retrieved April 2, 2012 from http://hivinsite.ucsf.edu/InSite?page=kb-08-01-07

http://data.unaids.org/Publications/IRC-pub07/jc1252-internguidelines_en.pdf

http://www.ohchr.org/Documents/Publications/FAQen.pdf

http://www.ohchr.org/Documents/Publications/HandbookHIV_NHRIsAug2007.pdf

http://data.unaids.org/pub/Report/2008/JC1579_First_10_years_en.pdf

Human Trafficking

Domniţa Oana Bădărău

Institutional organized events on human rights and fights against international criminality have led to an increased focus on the issues surrounding human trafficking. The 2008 Vienna Forum generated significant discussions and frameworks of action to tackle this growing phenomenon. Recognizing it as a global problem, the United Nations had previously developed a Protocol meant to prevent, suppress, and punish trafficking in persons, noting that special categories, such as children and women, are more likely to become victims and need special protection. Under this Act, human trafficking is defined as incorporating all manner of the use of force, coercion, abduction, incentives, and/or misrepresentation that would convince someone to submit himself or herself to the recruitment, transport, transfer, procurement, and receipt by another person for exploitation purposes. It is important to emphasize that the acts of gathering people for such purposes could be done by committing acts of violence against them or by altering their mental state so that they agree to do something that they would not have agreed to if not for the external coercive influence. These actions, which constitute criminal acts and violations of fundamental human rights, facilitate the victims' exploitation in the form of sexual favors, prostitution, commoditization, enslavement, and the harvesting of their organs for illegal sale.

Transnational criminality is closely linked to human trafficking; persons are mostly recruited from developing countries, impoverished populations, and low socioeconomic classes and are frequently forced to perform as sexual slaves in Western countries. This is a new form of slavery that affects society at large, infringes upon human dignity, and discriminates against those who are weaker and find themselves facing severe hardships. In 2006, the United Nations Office on Drugs and Crime (UNODC) tried to identify worldwide human trafficking patterns; the resulting report acknowledged the inefficiency and disorganization in combating this phenomenon up to that point.

D.O. Bădărău (✉)
Institute for Biomedical Ethics, University of Basel, Basel, Switzerland
e-mail: domnita@gmail.com

S. Loue (ed.), *Mental Health Practitioner's Guide to HIV/AIDS*,
DOI 10.1007/978-1-4614-5283-6_50,

International Legislation: A Means of Combating Human Trafficking

The 1949 United Nations Convention for the Suppression of the Traffic in Persons and of the Exploitation of the Prostitution of Others was an expression of political will to combat the growing phenomenon. Since then, the number of trafficked persons, the geographic areas where trafficking occurs, and the financial gains and criminal acts committed in relation to it have increased, while the conviction, punishment, and annihilation of such networks seems to have decreased and has not kept up with this ever-growing plague. The 2000 Protocol offered strong recommendations for the design and implementation of strong measures to fight against human trafficking. It pled for a collaboration between all actors, whether national, international, public, or private, to become involved in gathering more data; conducting more research so as to understand trafficking better; identifying both the populations targeted for trafficking and the population of consumers; developing and establishing transnational communication channels and border security systems; and promulgating national laws that criminalize these offences. Another important component consists of measures to ensure victims' protection, including the establishment of shelters, counseling services, and the provision of assistance upon reintegration to society. Cross-border criminal acts must receive adequate punishment and legislation should be in place to ensure that all such acts are prosecuted, regardless of the territory in which they were committed.

Health Implications of Sexual Exploitation

Among all types of exploitation, sexual exploitation predominates, followed by forced labor. According to the 2009 UNODC *Global Report on Trafficking in Persons*, this difference could be influenced by the fact that forced prostitution is one of the most commonly reported forms of exploitation. Trafficking people for such purposes has severe negative effects on the well-being and health of those persons who are enslaved as well as on the consumers of sexual services. It is not uncommon for victims of trafficking to be forced into drug consumption or to become addicts as a way of coping with the drama they are living. Victims of sexual exploitation are exposed to a high risk of infectious disease and women commonly become pregnant, an issue that is a matter of public health.

HIV infection is highly prevalent among these groups; in some cases children are more likely to be preferred for sexual exploitation because they are perceived to be a lower risk of transmission. Incomplete information exists regarding the number of trafficked people and the number of sexual slaves, especially children. However, data suggest that this number is huge. At the same time, there are inadequate data regarding the health status of this victimized population, due to the fact that they have no access to health care, they are moved around and unaccounted for, and insufficient funds have been allocated to permit comprehensive studies. However, it is acknowledged that the morbidity and mortality rates vary significantly from region to region, depending on sexual behaviors and awareness of infection risks, and the extent to which needed care can be accessed.

Sex workers are at increased risk of contracting HIV, but children face additional ones, as they are less likely to have the ability to seek treatment or to protect themselves by using condoms. Once they have contracted other sexually transmitted diseases, they are at increased risk of HIV infection. The offspring of sexually trafficked persons may also suffer severe health effects from trafficking, including sexually transmitted disease and drug addiction due to in utero exposure, as well as primary and secondary trauma. Ignoring these issues and the socioeconomic factors that facilitate and lead to this situation is a neglect of human rights and public health safety.

Related Topics: Children, Human rights, Sex work and sex workers, United Nations, Women

Suggested Readings

Anti-Human Trafficking Unit of the United Nations Office on Drugs and Crime. (2006). *Trafficking in persons: Global patterns* (pp. 127). New York: Author.

Kjellgren, C., Priebe, G., Svedin, C. G., & Langstrom, N. (2010). Sexually coercive behavior in male youth: population survey of general and specific risk factors. *Archives of Sexual Behavior, 39*(5), 1161–1169. doi:10.1007/s10508-009-9572-9.

United Nations Office on Drugs and Crime. (2009). *Global report on trafficking in persons* (pp. 292). New York: Author.

United States Department of State. (2011). *Trafficking in persons report.* Washington, D.C.: Author.

Willis, B. M., & Levy, B. S. (2002). Child prostitution: global health burden, research needs, and interventions. *Lancet, 359*(9315), 1417–1422. doi:10.1016/s0140-6736(02)08355-1.

Suggested Resources

United Nations Convention Against Transnational Organized Crime and the Protocol to Prevent, Suppress and Punish Trafficking in Persons, Especially Women and Children (2004).

Immigration

Sana Loue

Immigration and the Medical Examination

All non-US citizens who wish to obtain permanent resident status, that is, a green card or "mica," whether through an application for a visa at an embassy or consulate of the USA or through an application for adjustment of status in the USA, must undergo a medical examination to determine whether they may be legally admitted to the USA or whether they are inadmissible because of a medical issue. Some nonimmigrants, such as fiancé(e)s, are also required to have this medical examination. The examination can only be conducted by a physician in the USA who has been authorized to conduct this examination for immigration purposes by the US government (civil surgeon) or a physician outside of the USA who has been authorized to do so by the US Department of States (panel physician).

The medical examination is designed to determine whether the individual seeking admission has a Class A condition, that is, a physical or mental condition or communicable disease of public health significance that would render him or her inadmissible, or if he or she possesses a Class B condition. A Class B condition is a physical or mental disorder that, although not constituting a specific excludable condition, represents a departure from normal health or well-being that is significant enough to possibly interfere with the person's ability to care for himself or herself, or to attend school or work, or that may require extensive medical treatment or institutionalization in the future (Centers for Disease Control and Prevention, 2010a, b). Class B conditions will not result in inadmissibility that is premised on a medical condition.

S. Loue (✉)
Department of Epidemiology and Biostatistics, Case Western Reserve University, Cleveland, OH, USA
e-mail: Sana.Loue@case.edu

S. Loue (ed.), *Mental Health Practitioner's Guide to HIV/AIDS*,
DOI 10.1007/978-1-4614-5283-6_51, © Springer Science+Business Media New York 2013

Mental Illness, HIV, and Immigration

An individual seeking legal admission to the USA who is required to undergo this examination because of the nature of his or her visa, e.g., permanent residence, may be found inadmissible and denied legal entry into the USA if he or she is found

1. To have a physical or mental disorder and behavior associated with the disorder that may pose, or has posed, a threat to the property, safety, or welfare of the alien or others
2. To have had a physical or mental disorder and a history of behavior associated with the disorder, which behavior has posed a threat to the property, safety, or welfare of the alien or others and which behavior is likely to recur or lead to other harmful behavior.

The Centers for Disease Control and Prevention, based in Atlanta, Georgia, issued revised Technical Instructions governing the medical examination for physical and mental disorders for both civil surgeons and panel physicians in 2010. According to the CDC, these revisions are consistent with the current version of the *Diagnostic and Statistical Manual for Mental Disorders*.

The civil surgeon or panel physician must determine

- Whether the individual has a mental disorder
- Whether the mental disorder is associated with any harmful behavior
- Whether a previously diagnosed condition is now in remission
- Whether any harmful behavior associated with the mental disorder is likely to occur

The diagnosis of a mental disorder made by a civil surgeon or panel physician must be consistent with the provisions of the *Diagnostic and Statistical Manual for Mental Disorders*. A finding of "harmful behavior" must be consistent with the revised definition: serious psychological or physical injury to the applicant or to others, such as a suicide attempt or pedophilia; a serious threat to the health or safety of oneself or others, such as driving while intoxicated to verbally threatening to kill someone; or major property damage. Harmful behavior in the absence of an association with a mental or physical disorder is not a ground of inadmissibility and a diagnosis of a mental disorder without associated harmful behavior is not a basis for inadmissibility.

According to the Technical Instructions, the mental disorder will be considered to be in remission if there is a favorable prognosis, the condition is under control, and at least 12 months have elapsed since the last occurrence of harmful behavior. The following factors are to be considered in determining the likelihood that the applicant's disorder will remain in remission:

- The availability of effective treatment;
- The applicant's adherence to previous treatment, his or her willingness to remain on treatment, and the extent of his or her insight into the disorder
- The natural history of the disorder

- The number of and the interval between episodes of the illness
- Any trend toward increasing severity of episodes of the illness or emergence of treatment-resistant symptoms
- The likelihood that specific life events that precipitated previous episodes of the illness will recur
- The likelihood that severe life stresses will occur that might precipitate further episodes of illness
- Unusual circumstances that precipitated a single episode of the illness that are judged unlikely to recur

Until 2010, non-US citizens wishing to enter the USA could be denied legal entry if they were found to be HIV-positive, because HIV was deemed to be a "communicable disease of public health significance." HIV was removed from the list of such diseases on January 4, 2010. Even though individuals will still be tested for HIV during the course of their medical examination, they cannot be denied legal entry to the USA on that basis alone.

Public Charge

However, a separate ground of inadmissibility, known as public charge, provides that individuals seeking admission to the USA can be excluded if they are likely to become a public charge. This means that at the time of the interview for admission to the USA, the interviewing officer can question the individual about his or her assets to determine if the individual has sufficient assets or a source of income to pay for the cost of his or her medical care. Individuals with a past or current diagnosis of mental illness may require ongoing therapy or medication management to maintain their mental health. And, although HIV seropositivity is no longer a ground of inadmissibility, the individual will still have to demonstrate that he or she has sufficient resources or health care insurance to cover the costs associated with the treatment for the illness. It is important in these situations that the client be able to provide evidence of family income; medical insurance; the ability to cover any and all health care related expenses, including prescription and travel costs; and the availability of public health services and hospitalizations for which no patient fees are expected.

Implications for Mental Health Professionals

These issues may arise in a variety of contexts. First, some clients may themselves be seeking legal status in the USA and may ask their therapist for a letter documenting their ability to work and be self-supporting and/or the nature of their mental illness and the absence of any threat of harm to themselves or anyone else. In such situations, it is also common for the client to be experiencing severe stress and anxiety due to the uncertainty of their legal status and, perhaps, the potential separation from their family in the USA

In some circumstances, a client may be romantically involved with someone who is having immigration difficulties and may be depressed at the thought that his or her partner will be forced to leave the USA due to an unresolvable immigration situation. This is not an uncommon situation among same-sex couples, since the federal government does not recognize same-sex marriages. As a consequence of this policy, legal remedies potentially available to heterosexual married couples are not available to same-sex couples, even if they have been legally married in a state or foreign country that recognizes same-sex marriages.

Suggested Readings

Loue, S. (2011). Illness, inadmissibility, waivers, and other health-related issues. In I. Scharf (Ed.), *The waivers book: Advanced issues in immigration law practice* (pp. 183–215). Washington, D.C.: American Immigration Lawyers Association.

Loue, S., Hornik, P., & Walker, R. (2011). Developments in medical grounds of inadmissibility. In *2011–2012 Immigration and Nationality Law Handbook* Washington, D.C.: American Immigration Lawyers Association.

Suggested Resources

Centers for Disease Control and Prevention. (2010, June 1). *CDC requirements: Technical instructions for physical or mental disorders with associated harmful behaviors and substance-related disorders*. Retrieved November 8, 2010 from http://www.cdc.gov/imigrantrefugeehealth/pdf/mental-health-cs-ti.pdf;

Centers for Disease Control and Prevention. (2010, June 1). *CDC immigration requirements: Technical instructions for physical or mental disorders with associated harmful behaviors and substance-related disorders*. Retrieved November 8, 2010 from http://www.cdc.gov/immigrantrefugeehealth/pdf/mental-health-pp-ti.pdf.

Centers for Disease Control and Prevention. (2010). *Technical instructions for medical examination of aliens in the United States*. Retrieved November 8, 2010 from http://www.cdc.gov/immigrantrefugeehealth/exams/ti/civil/technical-instructions/ civil-surgeons/medical-history-physical-examination.html.

Informed Consent

Domniţa Oana Bădărău

Medical profession's deontology is aligned to human rights values through several principles that have been enforced in the twentieth century by international and national guidelines. Highly controversial research studies and shocking abuses of subjects during the WWII led to a shift from what had been until that time a paternalistic approach in medicine. Patient autonomy and research subjects' right to be informed and to consent began to be the center of medical practice and research. Respect for persons requires that patients have the right to act as autonomous agents and both physicians and researchers should encourage such actions. Nevertheless, informed consent issues arise in both the clinical and research settings when dealing with vulnerable populations, and with prospective research participants with different education levels, culture, and socioeconomic levels. At the core of providing legitimacy to research with human beings and making the distinction between medical intervention and battery or assault lies informed consent, a complex concept rather than a signed document.

Defining Informed Consent: A Process

The Nuremberg Code enunciates the elements that must be included in an informed consent process; these elements are deemed to be essential in conducting research with human research volunteers. Informed consent is defined by the respect and acknowledgement that at least three criteria are met: information, comprehensiveness, voluntariness. The 1947 Code did not overlook the problem of requesting consent from specific groups of subjects and stated that potential human participants should have the legal capacity to exercise their right to participate in research or decline the invitation. On the other hand, the World Medical

D.O. Bădărău (✉)
Institute for Biomedical Ethics, University of Basel, Basel, Switzerland
e-mail: domnita14@gmail.com

S. Loue (ed.), *Mental Health Practitioner's Guide to HIV/AIDS*,
DOI 10.1007/978-1-4614-5283-6_52,

Association covers informed consent in the context of clinical care combined with research, as well as in all the other medical studies.

The Declaration of Helsinki as amended in 2008 mentions that even though there might be recognized cases in which relatives or community representatives can be invited to participate in the decision making process, in the case of competent individuals, the research can be carried out only when those individuals are free of any influence agree to participate. Importantly, the researchers must provide to the prospective participants adequate information in relation to all aspects and phases of the research study, including funding and conflict of interests. This guideline may be interpreted and is relatively subjective, but the Declaration's text offers some additional guidance in emphasizing that different potential subjects might require more or different information than others. An explanation could be found in existing differences in education, age, culture. Moreover, investigators should pay attention to the manner in which all information is related and communicated.

The Belmont Report, which identifies the basic principles for the ethical conduct of research with human volunteers, covers informed consent under the element of respect for persons. This comprises several ethical precepts, including autonomy and additional protection for persons who have limited autonomy. Autonomy is defined as the person's capacity to give considerable thought to acts and consequences in taking decisions and then to act according to those judgments in pursuing his or her own subjective wishes and aims. At the same time, this right has to be promoted by offering to a person all potentially necessary information and accepting the individual's decision whenever there is no compelling reason to deny that person's right to manifest as an autonomous agent.

A more comprehensive and extensive process of defining the notion of informed consent took place along with the development of the *International Ethical Guidelines for Biomedical Research Involving Human Subjects* by the Council of International Organizations for Medical sciences (CIOMS). Constructed as an exhaustive set of guidelines, the international document elaborates and offers commentaries to the established requirements for conducting ethical research studies. The fourth guideline sets the framework for informed consent, stating that it must be provided for the individual invited to participate in the research by a next of kin who is legally authorized to decide should the prospective participant lack capacity. In limited, special cases, informed consent can be waived, but in all such cases, the waiver may not be taken lightly and must be approved by the ethical review committee, so as to ensure that the risks for the subjects do not outweigh the benefits and that there is not a unjustified burden for the subject.

Whether nationally, internationally, or professionally defined, informed consent implies a process that requires both the participation of several agents and a predetermined structure. Starting with the recruitment phase, the process of obtaining consent for participation has to be free from any coercive elements. Therefore, in the study design, the investigator has to take into consideration the characteristics of the population or group from which the recruitment will take place, the most appropriate methods of recruiting and the personnel in charge of the recruitment. Such measures will ensure that the person asked to participate is suited for the study and could potentially benefit from it, and that he or she will be provided with information which he or she is capable of understanding and upon which a decision can be made. Moreover, informed consent is not implicitly a positive answer to participation, as the prospective research participant can decide based on the received information not to be part of the study. This can be the result of conducting a proper informed consent that empowers the individual to exercise his or her autonomy free from any coercion.

Another requirement in the informed consent process is the provision of information to the participants on an ongoing basis for the entire duration of the study; accordingly, the researcher must provide further explanations as well as reveal new developments and findings. Research participants must be guaranteed the right to ask questions and have them answered during the research. Every effort should be made to ensure that there is no doubt and that the individual agreed to participate after thoughtful consideration, consultations with other parties being allowed. Whenever language, literacy, or cultural barriers arise, these must be approached with consideration for the dignity and respect for the participant.

Essential to the respect for persons is the right of the individual to withdraw his or her consent to participate at any given time during the study. Such a decision must not be contested or questioned and should terminate the participation of the individual from that moment forward, providing that there is no threat of inflicting harm to the individual as the result of his or her sudden withdrawal from a therapy.

Vulnerable Populations

Informed consent can pose additional issues when the study requires the recruitment of vulnerable populations, that is, persons who do not have the capacity for self-determination, are exposed to additional risks due to external factors and who require special protection. In this category are usually included children, prisoners, pregnant women, persons not capable of self-determination due to an illness, and persons with a mental illness. At the same time, it is important to acknowledge that some diseases might expose individuals or groups of individuals who decide to participate in research to additional risks, such as stigmatization.

In relation to HIV status or AIDS, persons can be considered a vulnerable population, due to the historical mistreatment of patients diagnosed as HIV-positive and the social repercussions that might follow if a person's serostatus is disclosed. He or she may suffer discrimination in the workplace or rejection from family members and may be the target of stigma, especially in certain cultures where the virus transmission is associated with sexual behavior or homosexuality. Additionally, in research settings, due to the above mentioned reasons, prospective participants may be considered a vulnerable population. Recruitment, including seeking informed consent, has to be very carefully planned in order to respect the privacy and confidentiality of all persons.

With the increased number of research studies conducted in developing countries, several new issues have arisen, especially regarding access to results and possible benefits. It is acknowledged that a significant number of HIV studies take place in very poor resource settings in Africa and are conducted by investigators from developed countries. The scenario may deepen worries regarding the exploitation and the use of subjects in research who belong to a population in which HIV prevalence is very high and they are vulnerable due to their socio-economic status and/or educational level. Given the level of poverty, the burden of being HIV positive, and the knowledge gap between researchers and subjects, recruiting among such a population can be opportunistic. Potential research volunteers might be more open to participating in studies if they are to receive compensation for their investment of time and if they are provided with access to free care. These are issues that need to be addressed whenever recruitment takes place among individuals with lower income levels or populations in developing countries. The informed consent process has to provide accurate and all relevant facts to these volunteers, avoid and overcome undue inducements, and offer a realistic image in relation to current benefits and risks and future probable benefits and risks.

A main issue that arises in conducting HIV research in such settings is related to the way in which the subjects might benefit from the study and therefore how the benefits are presented. In the late 1990s HIV research conducted in developing countries spurred sustained controversy over the placebo randomized controlled trials in pregnant African women. Conducted in several African countries, the study sought to assess the efficacy of short-course AZT (zidovudine) in reducing HIV transmission during pregnancy. The study participants were randomized into two groups; one received placebo and the other a shorter course of AZT. However, it had already been demonstrated that a full course of AZT could reduce significantly the transmission rate. Accordingly, the informed consent may not have been adequate and may have suffered severe flaws. Much controversy was raised around the informed consent process and whether the study was ethically conducted. Alternative treatment should have been mentioned in the informed consent in order not to infringe upon the Declaration of Helsinki's guideline which states that information about other existing treatments must be conveyed to the participants and, in case of disease, the best standard of care known must be offered.

The study was conducted on a vulnerable population and information regarding the previous knowledge about AZT regimens and the protection in pregnancy is assumed not to have been disclosed. At the same time, informed consent is a process and researchers have a duty to protect participants from harm, even to the detriment of knowledge and science. This means that even when the individual agrees to participate in research, the investigators should not allow it if there is a belief that, despite the provision of complete information and the informed consent process, there is a misunderstanding. Comprehension plays an important role in achieving an unbiased and adequate informed consent process.

Therapeutic Misconception

In obtaining informed consent, the researchers must exercise due diligence process in disclosing the potential risks and benefits of research participation and in avoiding coercion, undue inducement or deception. However, providing information and ensuring voluntariness is not enough, if there is no clear comprehension. Such a phenomenon was first observed and defined by Appelbaum and Lidz in the context of psychiatric research. Called therapeutic misconception, the concept refers to a participant's unrealistic belief that research procedures are aligned with their care needs and that in randomized trials they will be placed in the study arm which offers the best treatment for their condition. At the same time, exaggerating the chances of future medical benefits and failing to recognize that their health care may deteriorate by participating falls under the concept of therapeutic misconception.

In the AZT studies in Africa, there are many factors that increase the probability that therapeutic misconception may exist among the recruited participants. An impoverished population, in which illiteracy is significantly high could easily be operating under a therapeutic misconception if the informed consent process is not carried out with due diligence. Recruitment in a setting where language barriers exist, individuals are not able to write and sign an informed consent form, and where poverty restricts health care and access to treatment can prove to be burdensome. Researchers should acknowledge and deal with the ethical problems that may arise, in order to obtain voluntary and ethically sound informed consent. In the AZT case, the population could have agreed to participate motivated by the proffered health care and new therapy, disregarding the likelihood of being assigned to the placebo study arm. When HIV prevalence is so high and there is no or little access to health care due to financial reasons and/or inadequate public health actions, Western researchers may be perceived as the only hope for treatment.

Existing guidelines state that researchers have an obligation to protect research participants from harm at all times. As a result, researchers must balance the risks and benefits during the course of the study and exclude the participant from the research or stop the study in case of increased harm, even when a valid informed consent is in place. This burden must not rest on the research volunteer who has agreed to participate. Therefore, researchers must take steps to identify instances of therapeutic misconception and address them properly. The persistence of such a strong misrepresentation of research goals is a clear reason for excluding individuals from research.

Related Topics: Clinical trials, Council of Organizations for Medical Sciences, Declaration of Helsinki

Suggested Readings

Appelbaum, P. S., Roth, L. H., & Lidz, C. (1982). The therapeutic misconception: Informed consent in psychiatric research. *International Journal of Law and Psychiatry, 5*, 319–329.

Corneli, A. L., Sorenson, J. R., Bentley, M. E., Henderson, G. E., Bowling, M. J., Nkhoma, J., & van der Horst, C. (2011). Improving participant understanding of informed consent in an HIV-prevention clinical trial: A comparison of methods. *AIDS Behavior*. doi:10.1007/s10461-011-9977-z.

Housri, N., Coombs, M., Orandi, B. J., Pawlik, M., & Koniaris, L. G. (2011). Ethics and the law: Is there common ground on informed consent for disparities in hospital outcomes? *Annals of Internal Medicine, 155*(4), 260–264. doi:10.1059/0003-4819-155-4-201108160-00010.

Kass, N. E., Chaisson, L., Taylor, H. A., & Lohse, J. (2011). Length and Ccomplexity of US and international HIV consent forms from federal HIV network trials. *Journal of General Internal Medicine*. doi:10.1007/s11606-011-1778-6.

Lurie, P., & Wolfe, S. M. (1997). Unethical trials of interventions to reduce perinatal transmission of the human immunodeficiency virus in developing countries. *New England Journal of Medicine, 337*(12), 853–856. doi:10.1056/nejm199709183371212.

Moreno, J., Caplan, A. L., & Wolpe, P. R. (1998). Updating protections for human subjects involved in research. Project on informed consent, human research ethics group. *Journal of the American Medical Association, 280*(22), 1951–1958.

Suggested Resources

The Nuremberg Code. (1949). Washington D.C.: Reprinted by U.S. Government Printing Office.

World Medical Association. (1964). Declaration of Helsinki. Ethical Principles for Medical Research Involving Human Subjects.

Internet

Sana Loue

The Internet has become a major vehicle for the dissemination of information generally, with approximately 100 million Americans using the Internet to seek information, play games or movies, and/or communicate with others. It has been estimated that 90% of all youths aged 15–24 years have utilized the Internet. Eighty percent of all adult users have used the World Wide Web to find health-related information, with the vast majority seeking information relating to specific diseases and almost one-half seeking information about available medical treatments for specific conditions.

In the context of HIV health, Internet utilization falls into various categories: (1) searches for sexual and romantic partners; (2) searches for health-related information; (3) utilization of social support and coping resources, such as chat rooms; and (4) Internet-based prevention efforts. Each is discussed further below.

Searching for Sex and Love

Use of the Internet to find sexual partners has been found to be relatively common among men who have sex with men, but much less so among heterosexual men and women. It has been estimated that more than one-third of men who have sex with men (MSM) seek sexual partners online and a smaller proportion of MSM seek sexual partners only online. A study conducted by Robert Garofalo and colleagues with young men who have sex with men in Chicago found that being non-Hispanic White, having a history of unprotected anal intercourse, having multiple anal intercourse partners, and engaging in sexual relations in a bathhouse or sex club were associated with meeting sexual partners through the Internet. Individuals were

S. Loue (✉)
Department of Epidemiology and Biostatistics, Case Western Reserve University, Cleveland, OH, USA
e-mail: Sana.Loue@case.edu

S. Loue (ed.), *Mental Health Practitioner's Guide to HIV/AIDS*,
DOI 10.1007/978-1-4614-5283-6_53,

found to be more likely to engage in unprotected anal intercourse with sexual partners met through the Internet if they had a history of unprotected anal intercourse. Other studies have reported similar results and have also found that MSM meeting their partners over the Internet are more likely to have had sex with more male partners during the preceding 6 months and to have higher rates of unprotected insertive and receptive anal intercourse. This suggests that the use of the Internet to find sexual partners is associated with an increased likelihood that individuals will engage in risky sexual behaviors.

This possibility is strengthened by other research findings. HIV-positive men who have sex with men who seek sexual partners through the Internet have been found to be less likely to disclose their HIV serostatus to prospective sexual partners, more likely to misrepresent their HIV serostatus to partners who they meet over the Internet, more likely to use methamphetamine, and less inclined to utilize a condom during sexual relations.

Regardless of a client's HIV serostatus, it may be important for mental health care providers to discuss with their clients the risks associated with the use of the Internet to meet sexual partners. Clients may be unaware of or deny the possibility that others may misrepresent their HIV serostatus or may not know their HIV serostatus. Either scenario, however, increases the risk of HIV transmission.

Clients who are already HIV-seropositive may feel that there is no need to disclose their serostatus because they are already HIV-positive. However, they may be susceptible to infection with additional strains of the virus and with other sexually transmitted infections. Additionally, there may be legal, as well as moral, implications to engaging in sexual relations with other individuals without truthfully disclosing one's HIV serostatus. HIV-positive clients may feel uncomfortable disclosing their serostatus to others, and fearful that they will lose prospective partners. The mental health care provider can encourage his or her client to rehearse with the provider how this information might be disclosed and how to handle feelings of rejection should that become necessary.

Searching for Health-Related Information

There are more than 200,000 Web sites devoted to the provision of information related to medicine and health. Research suggests that approximately one-third of HIV-positive individuals who use the Internet engage in searches for health-related information. Individuals who are non-Hispanic White, who are men, and who have higher levels of education and greater income have been found particularly likely to do so, while individuals who inject drugs are less likely to do so. Researchers have found that HIV-positive individuals who use the Internet for health-related functions are more likely to engage in healthful behaviors compared to those who do not, and are more likely to use active coping strategies. Many HIV-positive individuals use the Internet, as well, to find information about ongoing clinical trials and to communicate with their physicians about the information that they have found online.

Despite the helpfulness of the Internet in providing information, there are also potential challenges associated with its use. Individuals may feel overwhelmed by the amount of information available and may find it difficult to assess the credibility of the information provided on various sites. Research suggests that individuals with less education, lower incomes, and an avoidant coping style may be more likely to have difficulty in assessing the credibility of the information that they find. These findings suggest that it may be important for mental health care providers to work with their clients to develop the skills necessary to critically evaluate the content and source of information retrieved online.

Using the Internet for Social Support and Outreach

Research indicates that autobiographical narrative is one of the primary uses of Internet by individuals living with HIV/AIDS. Individuals may use the Internet to recount their experiences with the goal of helping others deal with the challenges associated with living with the disease. Chat rooms may also serve as a venue for communicating individuals' experiences.

Other individuals make use of the Internet to publicize specific activities in which they are engaged, such as songs that they have composed or books that they have written. While some of these sites established by persons living with HIV/AIDS are for the purpose of self-promotion, many are designed to provide viewers with information and advice about HIV.

Internet-Based Prevention Efforts

Internet-based prevention efforts, although increasing, seem to still be in an early stage. Research has found that the provision of HIV prevention information that includes information about how to reduce risk sexual behaviors may be acceptable and efficacious when used with men who have sex with men.

There are numerous advantages to using the Internet for HIV prevention efforts. The provision of the information can be accomplished inexpensively in comparison with other approaches. Once loaded onto a Web site, the information can be accessed in private by a large number of people, reducing the possibility that individuals will avoid the topics covered due to embarrassment or fear of discovery by others. The information provided can included graphics, illustrations, photographs, animations, and other visual effects that may help the viewers to understand the material that is presented.

A study conducted by Hooper and colleagues found that there are only minor demographic differences in the acceptability of prevention messages across groups of MSM, suggesting that HIV prevention interventions designed for the Internet can be used with MSM who are demographically diverse. In that study, the researchers found that the HIV prevention topics that were of greater interest to the respondents included men's physical health, developing a long term plan to reduce HIV risk, negotiating safer sex online, and how to date men offline. Images of men who were fully nude and images of men engaging in a variety of sexual behaviors were acceptable to the majority of respondents.

These findings suggest that mental health providers who provide services to MSM and who maintain Web sites may wish to include information designed to reduce HIV risk, or links to credible Web sites that provide this information. Unfortunately, research has not focused on the use of the Internet for HIV prevention among self-identifying heterosexual men and women so that the effectiveness and acceptability of Web-based HIV prevention information for these groups is less clear.

Related Topics: Clinical trials, Coping, Physician-patient relations, Prevention strategies, Risk behaviors

Suggested Readings

Benotsch, E. G., Kalichman, S., & Cage, M. (2002). Men who have met sex partners via the internet: Prevalence, predictors, and implications for HIV prevention. *Archives of Sexual Behavior, 31*(2), 177–183.

Bowen, A. M., Horvath, K., & Williams, M. L. (2007). A randomized controlled trial of internet-delivered HIV prevention targeting rural MSM. *Health Education Research, 22*(1), 120–127.

Carballo-Diéguez, A., Miner, M., Dolezal, C., Rosser, B. R. S., & Jacoby, S. (2006). Sexual negotiation, HIV-status disclosure, and sexual risk behavior among Latino men who use the internet to seek sex with other men. *Archives of Sexual Behavior, 35*, 473–481.

Garofalo, R., Herrick, A., Mustanski, B. S., & Donenberg, G. R. (2007). Tip of the iceberg: Young men who have sex with men, the Internet, and HIV risk. *American Journal of Public Health, 97* (6), 1113–1117.

Gillett, J. (2003). Media activism and internet use by people with HIV/AIDS. *Sociology of Health & Illness, 25*(6), 608–624.

Hogan, T. P., & Palmer, C. L. (2005). Information preferences and practices among people living with HIV/AIDS: Results from a nationwide survey. *Journal of the Medical Library Association, 93*(4), 431–439.

Hooper, S., Rosser, B. R. S., Horvath, K., Oakes, M. J., Danilenko, G., & The Men's INTernet Sex II (MINTS-II) Team. (2008). An online needs assessment of a virtual community: What men who use the internet to seek sex with men want in internet-based HIV prevention. *AIDS Behavior, 12*, 867–875.

Kalichman, S. C., Cain, D., Cherry, C., Pope, H., Eaton, L., & Kalichman, M. O. (2005). Internet use among people living with HIV/AIDS: Coping and health-related correlates. *AIDS Patient Care and STDs, 19*(7), 439–448.

Kalichman, S. C., Cherry, C., Cain, D., Weinhardt, L. S., Benotsch, E., Pope, H., & Kalichman, M. (2006). Health information on the internet and people living with HIV/AIDS: Information evaluation and coping styles. *Health Psychology, 25*(2), 205–210.

Islam

Lucia Volk

Islam emerged in the same region as Judaism and Christianity, and its practitioners consider their holy book, the Qur'an, to be the last revelation of the same God. Prophet Mohammed, who lived as a successful merchant in seventh century Mecca, received the word of God through archangel Gabriel over the span of 20 years. He memorized each line, and later repeated the text to his followers who wrote it down. From its early days, Islam placed high regard on memorization and public recitation of the holy text. Additionally, believers perform five daily prayers, a month of fasting each year, and a pilgrimage to Mecca during a believer's lifetime, which makes Islam a very embodied and praxis-oriented religion. Islam's central text, the Qur'an, is accompanied by two other pieces of scriptures that guide believers: the Hadith and the Shari'a. What the prophet said and did in his life was compiled in Hadith literature, as guidance for believers. The Shari'a is a body of legal texts that evolved over centuries of Islamic jurisprudence, based mainly on the Qur'an and the Hadith.

Like its predecessors Judaism and Christianity, Islam has branched out into various denominations, which together count between 1.2 and 1.5 billion followers worldwide. The differences among Muslims are theological, cultural, political and historical. Some of the most iconic wars of Islamic history are wars between Muslim communities, for instance, the battle of Karbala in 680 C.E. between the leaders of what would become known as Sunni and Shiite communities. The Sunni community became the dominant Muslim group—although divided into several schools of legal interpretation and practice—and Shiites, divided among themselves as well, remain the minority group to this day. Additionally, both Sunni and Shiite communities have been influenced by Sufi thought, an esoteric and, at times, ascetic and monastic form of Islam. Sufis often were outspoken critics of Muslim rulers given to worldly vices rather than the pursuit of justice and well-

L. Volk (✉)
Middle East and Islamic Studies, San Francisco State University, San Francisco, CA, USA
e-mail: lvolk@sfsu.edu

S. Loue (ed.), *Mental Health Practitioner's Guide to HIV/AIDS*,
DOI 10.1007/978-1-4614-5283-6_54, © Springer Science+Business Media New York 2013

being of the community. They rejected traditional Muslim authority and orthodox interpretations of scriptures, and invited individuals to find God within.

Most Muslims today live in South Asia and Southeast Asia; however, Islam's two holiest sites—Mecca and Medina—where Prophet Mohammed lived and preached are in the Arab world. Sizable Muslim immigrant communities exist in the West, including wealthy computer engineers, doctors, and businessmen and semi-illiterate war refugees. As varied as their educational and socio-economic profile is their view of health and health care. Different verses in the Qur'an instruct believers to lead a balanced life and to abstain from intoxicating and polluting substances. The Qur'an also focuses on cleanliness and general hygiene throughout the day via prayer rituals. In Islam, spiritual and physical health are closely linked, although the degree to which individual Muslims follow "the rules" varies.

Sexuality is sanctioned, and even actively encouraged, within the marriage context. However, pre- or extramarital sex, whether with a consenting partner or a paid sex worker, as well as same-sex relationships, carry significant stigma, and may be punishable by Shari'a law. Conservative patriarchal norms in societies that offer little privacy to individuals further discourage sexual freedoms. This has some Muslim theologians proclaim that in a perfect Islamic society, there are no sexually transmitted diseases, and that HIV/AIDS is the disease of others, in particular of immoral Westerners. According to a WHO scientist in 2006, "information about HIV prevalence and trends in the region is insufficient, underreporting is likely, and it is not possible to obtain exact statistics or to ascertain the specific determinant of levels and trends of HIV." In other words, the current spread of HIV/AIDS among Muslim populations is educated guesswork. The available epidemiological evidence suggests that many of the early HIV/AIDS cases reported in the Muslim world were indeed "imported" by migrant workers returning from abroad, or by foreigner workers or visitors (which led, in some Muslim countries, to stringent, discriminating medical exams for foreign workers).

Of course, the reality now is different, and current infection trends show that internal transmission rates, especially in the context of male same-sex partners (MSM), injecting drug use (IDU), and female sex work (FSW), are on the rise. Across the region, condom use remains very low. Consequently, over the past decade theologians across the Muslim world have been debating to what degree the central ethical mandate in Islam "to avoid harm" supersedes the practice of condemning what are considered immoral acts. In other words, politicians, doctors, and clergy in Muslim countries are now discussing different forms of sexuality, condom use, and (mandatory) HIV testing as a way "to avoid harm" in their community.

Currently, HIV/AIDS infections rates in the Muslim world are lower than the global average. Reasons for this kind of data are, possibly, the combination of conservative sexual norms, fewer risk behaviors due to lower alcohol and drug consumption, and near universal male circumcision. However, in urban settings, pre-marital sexuality is on the rise, as is the average age of people at marriage (which fewer young people can afford). Moreover, the recent popularity of contract marriages for an agreed upon time (for the purpose of sex), poses new challenges in a community that already allows a husband up to four wives, if he can treat them equally. In other words, heterosexual sex is breaking out of its normative frame in the Muslim world, as extramarital sex, injection drug use, and same-sex practices continue to exist, stigmatized, at the margins. Encouragingly, more work is being done to educate the general public in Muslim countries about the global trends of HIV/AIDS. It is becoming clear that no community, Muslim or otherwise, can safely consider itself immune from the disease.

Related Topics: Coping, Faith community, Prevention strategies, Religion and spirituality

Suggested Readings

Abu-Raddad, L. J., et al. (2010). Epidemiology of HIV infection in the Middle East and North Africa. *AIDS, 24*(suppl 2), S5–S23.

Armstrong, K. (2007). *Muhammad: A prophet for our time*. New York: Harper.

Esack, F., & Chiddy, S. (Eds.). (2009). *Islam and AIDS: Between scorn, pity, and justice*. Oxford: Oneworld.

Esposito, J. L. (2002). *What everyone needs to know about Islam*. New York: Oxford University Press.

Gray, P. (2004). HIV and Islam: Is HIV prevalence lower among Muslims? *Social Science and Medicine, 58*(9), 1751–1756.

Obermeyer, C. M. (2006). HIV in the Middle East. *BMJ, 333*, 851–854.

Labor Migration

Daniel J. O'Shea

Labor migration is the movement of people both within and across national borders for employment. This is a growing and increasingly important aspect of global, regional, and national economies. Recent estimates indicate as many as 86 million international labor migrants living outside their nation of origin. Migrant employment, however, has become extremely fragile in the context of the current global economic downturn, with migrant workers of all nationalities laid off in construction, manufacturing, agriculture, hotel, catering, and healthcare sectors. This can be a particularly severe blow to their families who may be dependent on money sent home. Already facing particular risks and vulnerabilities to HIV as a result of their migrant status, as work opportunities are reduced, migrant workers are even more likely to seek unsafe, informal work that increases that risk.

The HIV epidemic in many parts of the world is being driven by both rural-to-urban labor migration and by circular labor migration. An example of the former is China's so-called floating population of close to 150 million people. Among these rural-to-urban migrants, frequent substance use, intoxication and elevated rates of sexually transmitted infections are reported. Circular labor migration contributing to two-way HIV transmission has been cited in numerous instances in sub-Saharan Africa, between the USA and Mexico and throughout Latin America, and across the India–Nepal border, sometimes operating in tandem with sexual and/or drug-using networks. High HIV prevalence, including both male migrants and non-migrating female partners, aligns closely with the destination and recruitment points for migrant workers.

Migration and immigration, while not HIV risk factors themselves, may create circumstances that increase susceptibility to infection. United Nations Programme on HIV/AIDS (UNAIDS) data on HIV transmission and risks indicate that migrant and mobile populations, including labor migrants, are at greater risk for HIV infection than the local general populations. UNAIDS attributes this to issues and

D.J. O'Shea (✉)
Public Health Service, County of San Diego, San Diego, CA, USA
e-mail: Dan.OShea@sdcounty.ca.gov

S. Loue (ed.), *Mental Health Practitioner's Guide to HIV/AIDS*, 283
DOI 10.1007/978-1-4614-5283-6_55, © Springer Science+Business Media New York 2013

challenges ranging from financial and environmental conditions to cultural and language barriers, stigma, discrimination and exploitation. Migrant workers often experience isolation and stress as a result of being separated from their spouses, families and communities, food insecurity, harsh working situations, substandard living conditions, and sometimes sexual violence. These factors can lead to risky behaviors, such as unsafe commercial sex or casual sex and/or drug use, compounded by lack of access to appropriate HIV prevention information and basic health services, and fear of being stigmatized for seeking such services. Spouses or partners of migrant workers, left at home with many of the same challenges that caused the husband's migration, may also be forced to exchange sex for food, shelter, protection, or money. In addition, the spouse/partner is also at risk if his or her spouse/partner returns with HIV.

Internationally agreed upon standards for HIV testing with informed consent, confidentiality, counseling and referral to services are not routinely applied for international migrants. Those who acquire HIV in transit or destination countries, or who are already living with HIV, frequently do not have or are denied adequate access to culturally and linguistically appropriate HIV healthcare services, or may delay seeking treatment. Migrants receiving treatment in the destination country may have that treatment regimen disrupted by deportation.

After 22 years, on November 2, 2009, the US Department of Health and Human Services (HHS) finally removed HIV from the list of "communicable diseases of public health significance" that keep non-citizens from entering the USA, effective January 4, 2010. However, over 60 countries still restrict people living with HIV from entering or remaining in their country for any purpose, and international labor migrants may be refused entry or face expulsion if found to be HIV positive.

The United Nations General Assembly adopted declarations in 2001 and 2006 which called for national, regional and international strategies to facilitate access for migrant and mobile workers to HIV/AIDS prevention programs, to fully realize human rights, including access to healthcare, as fundamental to the global HIV response, and to address HIV among international labor migrants as critical to achieving universally agreed upon Millennium Development Goal of halting and reversing the spread of HIV by 2015. International labor migrants, whatever their HIV status or legal status, need access to culturally and linguistically appropriate HIV services, including healthcare, in origin, transit and destination countries at all stages of the migration process, and upon return and reintegration into the countries of origin.

Governments, employers, workers and community organizations and others working with international labor migrants and people living with HIV in origin, transit and destination countries all have an important part to play in addressing HIV among migrant workers. This requires actions directed not only toward the provision of HIV services, but also toward the underlying causes of HIV risk behaviors, including poverty, gender inequality and human rights abuses among both legal and illegal migrant workers.

Mental health care providers who have clients engaged in migrant labor such as agricultural work or factory work should be aware of the increased risks for HIV that have been found to be associated with migrant status as a result of decreased access to health care; long-term or intermittent separation from family, which may lead to increased substance use and/or participation in unprotected sexual relations with multiple partners; and/or poverty, which may encourage participation in sex work in exchange for money, food, or shelter (survival sex work). In situations in which the client's HIV risk appears to be elevated, it is important that mental health care providers review strategies with their clients for HIV risk reduction and provide them with information relating to resources for HIV prevention, testing and treatment.

Related Topics: Access to care, Human rights, Immigration, Stigma and stigmatization

Suggested Readings

Beyrer, C. (2007). HIV epidemiology update and transmission factors: Risks and risk contexts–16th International AIDS Conference epidemiology plenary. *Clinical Infectious Diseases, 44*(7), 981–987.

McKinnon, F., & Kemp, E. (2006). Immigration and HIV. *AIDS Community Research Initiative of America (ACRIA) Update, 15*(4), 15–17.

Suggested Resources

Joint United Nations Programme on HIV/AIDS (UNAIDS) and World Health Organization (WHO) (2009): *AIDS Epidemic Update 2009*. Geneva (November 2010). Retrieved January 30, 2012 from http://www.unaids.org/en/KnowledgeCentre/HIVData/EpiUpdate/EpiUpdArchive/2009/default.asp

Lingga, G. (2009). The impact of financial crisis on labour migration and HIV: The 9th International Congress on AIDS in Asia and the Pacific (ICAAP). *International Labour Organization, Jakarta (August 14, 2009)*. Retrieved January 30, 2012 from http://www.ilo.org/asia/info/public/features/WCMS_112572/lang–en/index.htm

United Nations Programme on HIV/AIDS (UNAIDS) (2008). HIV and international labour migration: Policy Brief, UNAIDS, International Labour Organization, International Organization for Migration. *Geneva (UN AIDS Policy Brief August 2008)*. Retrieved January 30, 2012 from http://data.unaids.org/pub/Manual/2008/jc1513a_policybrief_en.pdf

United Nations Programme on HIV/AIDS (UNAIDS) (2008). New UNAIDS policy on HIV and international labour migration. Geneva (July 16, 2008). Retrieved January 30, 2012 from http://www.unaids.org/en/Resources/PressCentre/Featurestories/2008/July/20080716NewUNAIDSpolicyHIVandintlabourmig/

Latinos

Sana Loue

Incidence and Prevalence Rates of HIV/AIDS

Hispanic/Latino communities in the USA have been disproportionately impacted by HIV/AIDS. Although Latinos accounted for 14% of the population, including Puerto Rico, in 2006 Latinos accounted for 18% of all new HIV diagnoses reported in the 33 areas with long-term confidential name-based HIV reporting. More recently, in 2009, Latinos accounted for 19% of all new HIV diagnoses reported in the 40 states and 5 US dependent areas with long-term confidential name-based HIV reporting. By the end of 2008, approximately 11,438 Latinos in the USA and Puerto Rico had died of AIDS. In 2007, HIV/AIDS became the fourth leading cause of death in the USA for Hispanics ages 35–44 and the sixth leading cause of death among those ages 45–54.

Recent reports indicate that the HIV prevalence rate for Hispanics is 585.3 persons per 100,000 population, 2.6 times the rate for whites. Among Hispanic women, the prevalence rate is 263.0 per 100,000, more than four times the rate for non-Hispanic white women.

It has been estimated that 1 out of every 106 Latina women will become infected with HIV. The rate of new infections among Latina women, 11.8 per 100,000, is also more than four times the rate of new infections among non-Latino white women, which is 2.6 per 100,000. The AIDS diagnosis rate among Latinas is 7.9 per 100,000, compared with 1.5 per 100,000 for non-Hispanic White women; the rate among Latinas is approximately five times the rate of AIDS diagnosis among White women. As of 2006, Latinas accounted for 16% of all AIDS cases diagnosed since the beginning of the epidemic.

S. Loue (✉)
Department of Epidemiology and Biostatistics, Case Western Reserve University, Cleveland, OH, USA
e-mail: Sana.Loue@case.edu

S. Loue (ed.), *Mental Health Practitioner's Guide to HIV/AIDS*, 287
DOI 10.1007/978-1-4614-5283-6_56, © Springer Science+Business Media New York 2013

Approximately 1 out of every 36 Latino men will become infected with HIV. Latino men accounted for 79% of all new infections among Latinos in 2009. Latino men are infected at 2.5 times the rate as non-Hispanic White men. The incidence and prevalence of HIV among Latino gay and bisexual men are high. Latino men who have sex with men accounted for 81% of all new HIV infections among Latino men in 2009. One study of gay and bisexual men in 5 cities found that 17% of Latino gay and bisexual men were HIV-infected and knowledge about HIV prevention and transmission was low.

Of the 114,019 Latino men who have been reported to have AIDS from the beginning of the epidemic in 1981 through December 2000, 42% contracted the infection through unprotected sex with men, 35% through injection drug use, 6% as the result of unprotected heterosexual intercourse, and 7% were engaged in both injection drug use and unprotected sexual intercourse with men. In Puerto Rico, unlike the US mainland, injection drug use accounted for a greater proportion of AIDS cases than did unprotected sex with men.

AIDS diagnosis rates among Latinos are highest in the northeastern part of the USA. Approximately 88% of all AIDS cases have occurred in 10 states, with the majority occurring in New York, California, Puerto Rico, and Texas. Approximately 37% of the individuals with AIDS diagnoses were born in the mainland USA, with an additional 18% born in Mexico and 14% born in Puerto Rico. The geographic differences in prevalence are believed to result from the greater prevalence of injection drug use in the northeastern part of the USA and the possible reluctance of non-US citizens, such as individuals who were born in Mexico and reside in the southwestern states of the USA, to present for care due to provisions in the immigration law that may affect their legal status in the USA.

Risk Factors for HIV Transmission

The Centers for Disease Control and Prevention have identified various factors that affect the risk of transmission and/or prevention efforts. These include infection with other sexually transmitted diseases, which facilitates the transmission of HIV; avoidance of HIV testing due to embarrassment and stigma; socioeconomic factors such as poverty, migration, lack of adequate health insurance coverage, limited access to health care, and language barriers; fear of disclosure of HIV test results; the use of alcohol and drugs, including injection drug use; and, for women especially, a lack of awareness of their partner's sexual- and drug-related HIV risk behaviors that may put the woman at risk. Traditional gender roles may also affect HIV risk. One study conducted by Noland with heterosexual Puerto Rican men and women in Puerto Rico reported negative effects of *machismo* on sexual communication, the use of risk reduction practices in sexual relationships, and the practice of sexual monogamy.

Poverty, which has been found to be associated with HIV, is particularly problematic. Poverty affects HIV risk and progression to AIDS both directly and indirectly. In 2010, approximately 15.1% of all Americans lived in poverty, but 26.6% of Hispanics/Latinos were poor. Approximately one-quarter of all Latinos with HIV/AIDS have been found to lack any health insurance coverage, compared to 17% of non-Hispanic Whites with HIV/AIDS. Almost 40% of Latinos who present for HIV testing obtain the test late in their illness and are diagnosed with AIDS within 1 year of their HIV test, suggesting that they may have delayed diagnosis and treatment of HIV due to lack of available funds and health care insurance. Additionally, individuals may engage in survival sex, trading sexual relations to obtain safety, shelter, and/or food that would otherwise not be available or accessible to them.

Prevention efforts must consider the diversity that exists across Latino communities; interlinking issues of fatalism, religion, gender role, and denial; lack of knowledge about HIV; and the stigma associated with same-sex sexual relations, drug use, and HIV. Various subgroups, such as migrant farmworkers, homeless individuals, and severely mentally ill individuals encounter additional difficulties accessing services due to transiency and/or impaired cognition.

Suggested Readings

Loue, S. (2011). *"My nerves are bad": Puerto Rican women managing mental illness and HIV risk*. Nashville, TN: Vanderbilt University Press.

Noland, C. M. (2006). Listen to the sound of silence: Gender roles and communication about sex in Puerto Rico. *Sex Roles, 55*, 283–294.

Suggested Resources

Academy for Educational Development Center for Community-Based Health Strategies, Centers for Disease Control and Prevention, National Alliance of State & Territorial AIDS Directors, National Association of People With AIDS, National Minority AIDS Council, & U.S.-Mexico Border Health Association. (2002). *The state of Latinos in HIV prevention community planning*. Retrieved December 23, 2011 from http://www.cdcnpin.org/Reports2/SLCP.pdf

Anderson, R.N., & Smith, B.L. (2005). Deaths: Leading causes for 2002. National Vital Statistics Report, 53, 17: 51 Table 2. Retrieved from http://www.cdc.gov/nchs/data/nvsr/nvsr53/nvsr53_17.pdf

Centers for Disease Control and Prevention. (2011). *HIV among Latinos*, November. Retrieved December 23, 2011 from http://www.cdc.gov/hiv/latinos/index.htm

Centers for Disease Control and Prevention. (2009). HIV prevalence estimates—United States, 2006. *Journal of the American Medical Association, 301(1)*, 27–29.

Centers for Disease Control and Prevention. (2006). *HIV/AIDS among Hispanics*, June.

Centers for Disease Control and Prevention. (2008). *HIV/AIDS among Hispanics*, April. Retrieved August 13, 2008 from http://www.cdc.gov/hiv/hispanics/resources/ factsheets/hispanic.htm

Kaiser Family Foundation. (2011). *Fact sheet: Latinos and HIV/AIDS*. Retrieved December 23, 2011 from http://www.kff.org/hivaids/upload/6007-09.pdf

Lesbians

Elena Cristina Chinole Cazacu

A lesbian, according to most dictionaries, is a woman who is sexually attracted to other women or a "female homosexual." The term is derived from the name of the island of Lesbos where, in ancient Greece, a school for young women was organized by poetess Sappho who mostly wrote poetry about love between women. However, there is no set definition of what a "lesbian" is, since definitions of what it means to be a "lesbian" can differ across cultural, racial, and ethnic groups. Some women who identify themselves as lesbians may also engage in sexual activity with men and others may be having sex with women, without considering themselves lesbians.

Medical professionals often fail to recognize such distinctions and usually use the term WSW: women having sex with women. However, this term defines the women who have, or have had, sex with women who may or may not self-identify as lesbian. In various cultures, women who have sex with women (WSW) often engage in heterosexual relations, especially young ones, or as a result of social pressure, in order to avoid stigma or to have children.

HIIV Risk

Lesbians and WSWs are often overlooked by many health care providers as a risk group for HIV. They are hardly targeted or included in HIV prevention or service programs, due to a widespread perception that they are a "low risk" population when compared to male/male or male/female sexual contact. Such generalization is harmful since lesbians and WSWs are not a homogenous population, having diverse sexual practices and different risk behaviors. For example, some WSWs and lesbians are at a heightened risk of getting HIV, as well as other STDs, as they may be

E.C. Chinole Cazacu (✉)
Center for Ethics and Public Policies, Bucharest & Iasi, Romania
e-mail: cchinole@yahoo.com

S. Loue (ed.), *Mental Health Practitioner's Guide to HIV/AIDS*,
DOI 10.1007/978-1-4614-5283-6_57,

injection drug users, sex workers, prisoners, or have unprotected sex with men who have sex with men (MSM), or with men who inject drugs. Homophobia, sexism, and racism that LGBT communities face in health care access exacerbate these risks.

Available statistics make the point that women from certain ethnic minorities are especially affected by HIV infection and AIDS as the rates of HIV diagnosis are significantly higher for African American and Hispanic women than for Non-Hispanic White, Asian and Pacific Islander, or American Indian and Alaska Native women. Also, rates for Black women are higher than the rates for all men, except Black men.

According to the Centers for Disease Control and Prevention (CDC), there are as yet no confirmed cases of female-to-female transmission of HIV in the USA. Existing research shows that the risk of contracting HIV is directly related to a woman's experiences and behavior. Female-to-female HIV transmission from the use of sex toys without protection has been documented. The *National AIDS Manual* (NAM) points out that oral sex, sharing sex toys, and fisting are high risk behaviors for HIV; women who have sex with other women need to be aware of that. Lesbians and WSW, like bisexuals or heterosexuals, may be at high risk of getting HIV if they have unprotected sex with men of unknown health status, have multiple sexual partners, inject drugs, use sex toys without condoms, or engage in any sexual activity that includes exchanging fluids known to transmit HIV, such as menstrual blood or vaginal secretions.

Surveillance of infection among women having sex with women has not been adequate. The reality of the epidemic and actual number of cases, as well as modes of HIV transmission in the lesbian/WSW community will become more visible as data collection improves.

Multiple studies have indicated that many women who have sex with women believe that they are at little to no risk for HIV infection, and that only a few lesbians/WSWs practice safe sex. Sex between women should not be ignored as a possible means of HIV infection, since the virus may be transmitted through body fluids such as blood, menstrual blood, breast milk, and vaginal secretions. Sexual practices such as genital to genital rubbing, oral stimulation of genital and anal areas, and the use of fingers and sex toys usually pose a risk of HIV transmission, unless forms of protection such as condoms, dental dams, or female condoms are used. Sexual education is needed not only for HIV prevention but also because there are many other sexually transmitted diseases which are communicable between women, such as chlamydia, genital herpes, human papillomavirus (HPV), genital warts, trichomoniasis, and syphilis.

Access to Care

Lesbians, as well as other sexual minorities, face specific obstacles in getting adequate health care and often avoid routine health check-ups. Sometimes women are embarrassed or afraid to reveal their sexuality or sexual history to the health professionals. Lack of medical insurance may be another obstacle, since lesbians/WSWs often do not have the same health insurance benefits as married couples. Stigma and fear of discrimination and disclosure are also important barriers in seeking HIV testing, counseling, care, and treatment for lesbians/WSW.

There is a need for more education, not only for WSW/lesbians about HIV prevention, but also for medical practitioners, as many lack knowledge or training about specific health issues that lesbians and WSW face, thus failing to give tailored advice on SDTs prevention. Health practitioners should bear in mind the limitation of judging risk of HIV exposure solely on somebody's (apparent) sexual orientation. Often, sexual orientation is not being asked about for female patients, when taking personal health histories, and therefore important information about experiences, practices and behaviors that may risky for HIV infection is missing. Prevention and policy interventions have to incorporate culture and gender relevant materials, according to the needs of lesbian and WSW community. Otherwise women who partner with women will continue to fall through the cracks of the surveillance and medical systems.

Related Topics: Bisexuals and bisexuality, Sex toys, Sexual orientation, Women

Suggested Readings

Diaz, T., Vlahov, D., Greenberg, B., Cuevas, Y., & Gartein, R. (2001). Sexual orientation and HIV infection prevalence among young Latino injection drug users in Harlem. *Journal of Women's Health & Gender-Based Medicine, 10*(4), 371–380.

Dworkin, S. L. (2005). Who is epidemiologically fathomable in the HIV/AIDS epidemic? Gender, sexuality, and intersectionality in public health. *Culture, Health and Sexuality, 7*(6), 615–623.

Friedman, S. R., Ompad, D. C., Maslow, C., Young, R., Case, P., Hudson, S. M., et al. (2003). HIV prevalence, risk behaviors, and high-risk sexual and injection networks among young women injectors who have sex with women. *American Journal of Public Health, 93*(6), 1–8.

Suggested Resources

The American Heritage Medical Dictionary. (2007). New York: Houghton Mifflin Company

Centers for Disease Control and Prevention. (2008). *HIV/AIDS fact sheet: HIV/AIDS among women, August 2008*. Retrieved February 2012 from http://www.cdc.gov/hiv/topics/women/resources/factsheets/pdf/women.pdf

Centers for Disease Control and Prevention. (2006). *HIV/AIDS fact sheet: HIV/AIDS among women who have sex with women.* Retrieved March 23, 2012, from http://www.cdc.gov/hiv/topics/women/resources/factsheets/pdf/wsw.pdf.

Centers for Disease Control and Prevention. (2008). *HIV/AIDS Facts, August 2008*. Retrieved February 2012 from http://www.cdc.gov/hiv/resources/factsheets/index.htm

HIV risk for lesbians, bisexuals & other women who have sex with women, June 2009. Retrieved March 9, 2012 from http://www.gmhc.org/files/editor/file/GMHC_lap_whitepaper_0609.pdf

The Lesbian handbook, Retrieved January 18, 2012, from http://lesbianhandbook.net/definitions.html

Media

Mihaela-Catalina Vicol

Mass media plays an important role in portraying HIV and AIDS and also in educating people about the disease. Unfortunately, media's impact on people brought sometimes fear, even panic, stigmatization and discrimination attitudes.

During the 1980s, the representations of HIV/AIDS in the media related with gay men, drug addicts and even African origin, so that such associations determined attitudes of stigmatization, of labeling people, of promoting racism. Some of the studies relating to the representation of HIV/AIDS in the media report the use of metaphors that had a negative impact rather than a positive one. It had been spectacular to talk and write about AIDS in terms of "Sex is danger," "AIDS as crime," "AIDS is a moral reformer" on the front page. Unfortunately, media induced panic by sensationalizing HIV and some authors even conceptualized this into "media panic," similar to the concept of the British sociologist Stanley Cohen "moral panic," when talking about media's exaggerations far beyond the boundaries of the reality. Most of the representations of HIV and AIDS in the media during the 1980s framed the disease as a result of deviant behavior restricted to gays, naming it "gay plague," a metaphor that suggested gays are the people to blame. This is why the social construction of this representation fostered stigmatization and rejection of the gay communities. Many authors suggest that the image of HIV/AIDS in the media in the early period had been a disease of deviance.

Another important aspect of the representation of HIV in the media was that it made a social division between people as "innocents" and "guilty villains," simplifying incorrectly the spread of the disease. Subsequently, the association of HIV with deviance and with homosexuality and the division of people into "innocents" and "givers" or "transmitter," created a simplified world that was composed of the general population and the dangerous, infectious, homosexual population.

M.-C. Vicol (✉)
Department of Bioethics, University of Medicine and Pharmacy "Gr. T. Popa", Iasi, Romania
e-mail: mihavicol@yahoo.com

S. Loue (ed.), *Mental Health Practitioner's Guide to HIV/AIDS*,
DOI 10.1007/978-1-4614-5283-6_58, © Springer Science+Business Media New York 2013

In this context, people that were found to be HIV positive were not only responsible for contracting the disease but were also a dangerous threat to the "general population." To warn the population about the danger, mainly sexual and drug-using partners, some politicians even suggested that the individuals who were HIV-positive should be given two tattoos, one on the forearm and one on the buttocks.

Other press articles created reactions of racism against Africans and West Indians, by writing sensational news about the origin of HIV. The social attitudes resulting from this sensationalism were race and gender inequities, marginalization, and sometimes even hate.

During the late 1980s, media has modified its representation of the disease, showing that it is also heterosexually transmitted. People's reactions towards gays remained in the sphere of "homophobia," as some authors call it, sympathizing more with people with medically acquired disease, than with gay men carrying HIV.

From 1990, in the attempt to emphasize individuals' responsibility, the representation of HIV has fortunately changed, from a disease of deviance to a disease that may affect everyone. Still, in some countries, the sensationalistic approach of the news related to the disease continues and the result has been the social construction of a deadly disease that made more and more victims and could spread to the entire population.

After this period, the sensationalism weakened in relationship to HIV/AIDS, letting in its place educational articles and campaigns that would provide people with accurate medical and scientific information. The press even became involved in campaigns against racism and homophobia showing that HIV can affect every individual regardless of his or her race, origin, or sexual orientation.

Related Topics: AIDS activism, Internet

Suggested Readings

Alcorn, K. (1988). Illness, metaphor and AIDS. In P. Aggleton & H. Homans (Eds.), *Social aspects of AIDS* (pp. 63–74). Lewes: Falmer Press.

Cohen, S. (1972). *Folk devils and moral panics*. London: MacGibbon and Kee.

Cullen T. (2003). HIV/AIDS: 20 years of press coverage. *Australian Studies in Journalism, 12*.

Gilman, S. (1988). *Disease and representations: Images of illness from madness to AIDS*. New York: Cornell University Press.

Shevory T. (2004). *Notorious H.I.V: The media spectacle of Nushawn Williams*. Minneapolis, MN: University of Minnesota Press.

Suggested Resources

Howe, A. (1998). *Sexed crime in the news*. Australia: The Federation Press.

Medicaid

Robert W. Stephens

Medicaid is the US health program for certain people and families with low incomes and resources. Medicaid is a means-tested program that is jointly funded by state and federal governments and managed by the states. People eligible for Medicaid are US citizens or legal permanent residents, including low-income adults, their children, and people with certain disabilities. As explained further below, poverty alone does not necessarily qualify someone for Medicaid. Medicaid is the largest source of funding for medical and health-related services for people with limited income in the USA.

Medicaid was created by the Social Security Amendments of 1965 which added Title XIX to the Social Security Act. Each state administers its own Medicaid program while the federal Centers for Medicare and Medicaid Services (CMS) monitors the state-run programs and establishes requirements for service delivery, quality, funding, and eligibility standards.

States may bundle together the administration of Medicaid with other programs such as the Children's Health Insurance Program (CHIP), so the same organization that handles Medicaid in a state may also manage the additional programs. Separate programs may also exist in some localities that are funded by the states or their political subdivisions to provide health coverage for indigents and minors. State participation in Medicaid is voluntary; however, all states have participated since 1982. In some states Medicaid is subcontracted to private health insurance companies, while other states pay providers (i.e., doctors, clinics and hospitals) directly.

During the 1990s, many states received waivers from the federal government to create Medicaid managed care programs. Under managed care, Medicaid recipients are enrolled in a private health plan, which receives a fixed monthly premium from the state. The health plan is then responsible for providing for all or most of the

R.W. Stephens (✉)
Rynearson, Suess, Schnurbusch & Champion, L.L.C., St. Louis, MO, USA
e-mail: rstephens@rssclaw.com

S. Loue (ed.), *Mental Health Practitioner's Guide to HIV/AIDS*,
DOI 10.1007/978-1-4614-5283-6_59, © Springer Science+Business Media New York 2013

recipient's healthcare needs. Today, all but a few states use managed care to provide coverage to a significant proportion of Medicaid enrollees.

Unlike Medicare, Medicaid is a program that is not solely funded at the federal level. States provide up to half of the funding for the Medicaid program. In some states, counties also contribute funds. Unlike the Medicare entitlement program, Medicaid is a means-tested, needs-based social welfare or social protection program rather than a social insurance program. Eligibility is determined largely by income. The main criterion for Medicaid eligibility is limited income and financial resources, a criterion which plays no role in determining Medicare coverage. Medicaid covers a wider range of health care services than Medicare. Some people are eligible for both Medicaid and Medicare and are considered to have dual eligibility.

While Congress and the Centers for Medicare and Medicaid Services (CMS) set out the general rules under which Medicaid operates, each state runs its own program. Under certain circumstances, an applicant may be denied coverage. As a result, the eligibility rules differ significantly from state to state, although all states must follow the same basic framework.

Having limited assets is one of the primary requirements for Medicaid eligibility, but poverty alone does not qualify a person to receive Medicaid benefits unless they also fall into one of the defined eligibility categories. According to the CMS Web site, "Medicaid does not provide medical assistance for all poor persons. Even under the broadest provisions of the Federal statute (except for emergency services for certain persons), the Medicaid program does not provide health care services, even for very poor persons, unless they are in one of the designated eligibility groups."

There are a number of Medicaid eligibility categories; within each category there are requirements other than income that must be met. These other requirements include, but are not limited to, assets, age, pregnancy, disability, blindness, income and resources, and one's status as a US citizen or a lawfully admitted immigrant. In order to receive Medicare coverage an individual must produce documents to prove that he or she is a US citizen or resident alien. An exception is made for Emergency Medicaid where payments are allowed for the pregnant and disabled regardless of immigration status. Special rules exist for those living in a nursing home and disabled children living at home.

A child may be covered under Medicaid if she or he is a US citizen or a permanent resident. A child may be eligible for Medicaid regardless of the eligibility status of his or her parents or guardians. Thus, a child can be covered by Medicaid based on his or her individual status even if his or her parents are not eligible. Medicaid does not pay benefits to individuals directly; Medicaid sends benefit payments to health care providers. In some states Medicaid beneficiaries are required to pay a small fee (co-payment) for medical services.

Both the federal government and state governments have made changes to the eligibility requirements and restrictions over the years. The Deficit Reduction Act of 2005 (DRA) significantly changed the rules governing the treatment of asset transfers and homes of nursing home residents. The DRA created a 5-year "look-back period." That means that any transfers without fair market value, gifts of any kind, made by the Medicaid applicant during the preceding 5 years can be penalized, dollar for dollar. Gifts of any size during the 5 years preceding a Medicaid application are totaled and penalized dollar for dollar.

Medicaid planners typically advise retirees and other people facing high nursing home costs to adopt strategies that will protect their financial assets in the event of nursing home admission. State Medicaid programs do not consider the value of one's home in calculating eligibility; therefore, it is often recommended that retirees pursue home ownership. Legal asset protection can be done at any point since it is not a transfer without fair market value and is not governed by the 5-year look-back period.

On November 25, 2008, a new federal rule was passed that allows states to charge premiums and higher co-payments to Medicaid participants. This rule will enable states to take in greater revenues, limiting financial losses associated with the program. Estimates figure that states will save $1.1 billion while the federal government will save nearly $1.4 billion. However, this means that the burden of financial responsibility will be placed on 13 million Medicaid recipients who will face a $1.3 billion increase in co-payments over 5 years.

Medicaid provided the largest portion of federal money spent on health care for people living with HIV/AIDS until the implementation of Medicare Part D when the prescription drug costs for those eligible for both Medicare and Medicaid shifted to Medicare. Unless low income people who are HIV positive meet some other eligibility category, they must progress to AIDS before they can qualify under the "disabled" category to receive Medicaid assistance. More than half of people living with AIDS in the US are estimated to receive Medicaid payments. Two other programs that provide financial assistance to people living with HIV/AIDS are the Social Security Disability Insurance (SSDI) and the Supplemental Security Income. Once someone is approved as a beneficiary in the Supplemental Security Income program they may automatically be eligible for Medicaid coverage (depending on the laws of the state they reside in).

Also included in the Social Security program under Medicaid are dental services. These dental services are an optional service for adults above the age of 21; however, this service is a requirement for those eligible for Medicaid and below the age of 21.

Related Topics: Access to care, Medicare

Suggested Resources

The Henry J. Kaiser Family Foundation. Medicaid and HIV/AIDS. Retrieved January 30, 2012 from http://www.kff.org/hivaids/upload/7172_04.pdf

Medicaid—Wikipedia, the free encyclopedia: Retrieved January 30, 2012 from: http://en.wikipedia.org/wiki/Medicaid..

Medicaid & CHIP Program Information by Population. Medicaid.gov: Retrieved January 30, 2012 from http://www.medicaid.gov/Medicaid-CHIP-Program-Information/By-Population/By-Population.html.

Medicaid Eligibility: Overview. Centers for Medicare and Medicaid Services (CMS). Retrieved January 30, 2012 from http://www.cms.gov/MedicaidEligibility/.

Medical Marijuana

Brandy L. Johnson

Marijuana refers to a preparation of the flowering plant from a genus called *Cannabis*. Cannabis, which includes several different species, has harvested and utilized throughout history for fiber, oil, seeds, medicine, and recreational drugs. *Cannabis Sativa*, for example, is one species of cannabis and is utilized, among other things, for medical purposes.

There are more than 60 cannabinoids, or chemical compounds that are psychoactive substances, found in cannabis. When utilized for medicinal purposes, delta-9-tetrahydrocannabinol (THC), delta-8-tetrahydrocannabinol, cannabidiol (CBD), cannabinol (CBN), β-caryophyllene, and cannabigerol (CBG) are some of the more important cannabinoids. THC is the primary compound responsible for cannabis' psychoactive effect. The highest amount of THC can be found in the flowers of the plant, with a lesser amount found in the stems, seeds, and leaves.

Cannabis has been used for medicinal purposes since ancient times. The Chinese Emperor, Chen Nung is thought to have discovered the healing properties of cannabis around the twenty-eighth century B.C. Cannabis was also used, among other places, in ancient India, Persia, Egypt, Greece, the Middle East, and South East Asia.

In the early nineteenth century, William O'Shaughnessy, a British doctor, introduced cannabis to Western Medicine. He used cannabis for the treatment of rheumatism, convulsions, and muscle spasms from tetanus and rabies. By 1854, cannabis was recognized in the US Dispensary for the treatment of neurologia, gout, tetanus, hydrophobia, cholera, convulsions, spasticity, hysteria, depression, insanity, uterine hemorrhage, and contractions during childbirth delivery. During the mid- to late 1800s and early 1900s, cannabis was also used to treat symptoms of dysmenorrhea (painful menstruation), insomnia, gonorrhea, stomach pain, loss of appetite, migraines, withdrawal, excessive coughing, and the plague and typhoid fever.

B.L. Johnson (✉)
Rynearson, Suess, Schnurbusch & Champion, L.L.C, St. Louis, MO, USA
e-mail: bjohnson@rssclaw.com

S. Loue (ed.), *Mental Health Practitioner's Guide to HIV/AIDS*,
DOI 10.1007/978-1-4614-5283-6_60,

In the USA, cannabis preparations were widely available until the Marihuana Tax Act of 1937. The tax of $1.00 per ounce when used for medicinal purposes had a prohibitory effect. The *National Formulary and Pharmacopoeia* then removed cannabis in 1942. Subsequent legislation, such as the Narcotics Control Act and the Controlled Substances Act, further penalized the use of cannabis. Cannabis, or marijuana, remained completely banned until 1996, when California passed legislation permitting the use of proscribed medical marijuana. Since 1996, 15 other states have followed California's lead and legalized marijuana for medicinal purposes. The federal government, however, has not legalized the use of medical marijuana. Therefore, both medical marijuana distributors and its users could face federal charges if caught with the drug.

The US history with medical marijuana is not unique. Cannabis was outlawed in many counties after the 1971 Convention on Psychotropic Substances instituted by the United Nations. Nonetheless, countries such as the UK and Canada now recognize the therapeutic use of medical marijuana. As in the USA, before the use of medical marijuana is permitted, specific conditions must be met. The conditions vary from jurisdiction to jurisdiction, but usually include the involvement of a physician.

Medical marijuana has been found to help with symptom management for diseases including, but not limited to, cancer, multiple sclerosis, HIV/AIDS, spinal cord injuries, glaucoma, amyotrophic lateral sclerosis (also known as ALS or Lou Gehrig's disease), and Parkinson disease. Medical marijuana has been reported as helping individuals with nausea, vomiting, appetite stimulation, pain reduction, spasticity control, improved sleep, bladder spasms, inflammation, and mood disturbances. It should be noted further studies are needed to determine all of medical marijuana's therapeutic uses, benefits, and effectiveness.

With regard to HIV/AIDS, medical marijuana may help with nausea, anorexia, cachexia, the reduction of pain associated with peripheral neuropathy, and distal sensory predominant polyneuropathy. As it has been estimated that 30% or more individuals with HIV will experience neuropathic pain, the ability to successfully use medical marijuana instead of, or in conjunction with, other pain management measures could significantly improve the quality of life for many.

In the early nineteenth century, the ability to deliver opiates by injection was one of the reasons marijuana began to fall out of favor. Ironically, opiate dependence is now one of the concerns that are helping medical marijuana regain support and legitimization. Marijuana has been found to be far less addictive than opiates. According to a 2009 CBS News report, 14–23% of prescription drug abusers either cannot stop using the medication or experience withdrawal when they want to stop. Only 9% of marijuana users, on the other hand, develop problems. The same news report indicated that medication that had been approved by the US Food and Drug Administration (FDA) was suspected as the primary cause of 10,008 deaths and a secondary cause in another 1,679 deaths. Conversely, there were no deaths in which marijuana was the primary suspect and it was a suspected secondary cause in 279 deaths. As the number of individuals dependent on prescription drugs is now greater than the number of those who are dependent on marijuana, marijuana is becoming seen, more and more, as the lesser threat for some conditions.

The criminalization of cannabis/marijuana in the USA and abroad has limited the extent to which testing and studies have been conducted. This is starting to change. The exploration and recognition of the benefits of medical marijuana could potentially help to improve the lives of millions of people, including those with HIV/AIDS, who are suffering from painful, debilitating, and/or chronic conditions. As further study is conducted, it is also possible that scientists will develop delivery systems that are more expedient, effective, longer lasting, and without side-effects.

Related Topics: Substance use

Suggested Reading

Aggarwal, S., Carter, G., Sullivan, M., ZumBrunnen, C., Morrill, R., & Maye, J. (2009). Medicinal use of cannabis in the United States: Historical perspectives, current trends, and future directions. *Journal of Opiate Management, 5*(3), 153–168. Available at http://www.letfreedomgrow.com/cmu/JOM_5-3-03-Carter.pdf

Ben Amar, M. (2006). Cannabinoids in medicine: A review of their therapeutic potential. *Journal of Ethnopharmacology, 105,* 1–25. Available at http://www.doctordeluca.com/Library/WOD/WPS3MedMj/CannabinoidsMedMetaAnalysis06.pdf

Clark, E. (2011). *Cannabis sativa for health and hemp (Public Health in the 21st Century).* Hauppauge, NY: Nova Science Pub, Inc.

Ellis, R., Toperoff, W., Viada, F., van den Brande, G., Gonzales, J., Gouaux, B., Bentley, H., & Atkinson, J. (2008). Smoked medicinal cannibis for neuropathic pain in HIV: A randomized, crossover clinical trial. *Neuropsychopharmacology*, *34*(3), 672–680. Available at http://www.ncbi.nlm.nih.gov/pmc/articles/PMC3066045/

Green, A. & De-Vries, K. (2010). Cannabis use in palliative care – An examination of the evidence and implications for nurses. *Journal of Clinical Nursing*, *19,* 2454–2462. Available at http://www.advancedholistichealth.org/PDF_Files/Palliative%20care.pdf

Mack, A., & Joy, J. (2000). *Marijuana as medicine? the science beyond the controversy.* Washington, D.C.: The National Academic Press.

Mikuriya, T. (1969). Marijuana in medicine. *California Medicine, 110*, 34–40.

Russo, E. (2002). *Cannabis therapeutics in HIV/Aids,* 1st ed. New York: Routledge.

Medicare

Robert W. Stephens

Medicare is a social insurance program administered by the US government (CMS), providing health insurance coverage to people who are aged 65 and over; to those who are under 65 and are permanently physically disabled or who have a congenital physical disability; or to those who meet other special criteria. The Medicare program also funds residency training programs for the vast majority of physicians in the USA. The Medicare program was established under The Social Security Act of 1965, which was signed into law by President Lyndon B. Johnson on July 30, 1965, as amendments to existing Social Security legislation.

The Centers for Medicare and Medicaid Services (CMS), a component of the Department of Health and Human Services (HHS), administers Medicare and Medicaid. The Social Security Administration is responsible for determining Medicare eligibility and processing premium payments for the Medicare program. Since the beginning of the Medicare program, CMS has contracted with private companies to operate as intermediaries between the government and medical providers. These contractors are commonly already in the insurance or health care area. Contracted processes include claims and payment processing, call center services, clinician enrollment, and fraud investigation.

Medicare is financed by payroll taxes imposed by the Federal Insurance Contributions Act (FICA) and the Self-Employment Contributions Act of 1954. Until December 31, 1993, the law provided a maximum amount of compensation on which the Medicare tax could be imposed each year. Beginning January 1, 1994, the compensation limit was removed. Beginning in 2013, the 2.9% hospital insurance tax will continue to apply to the first US$200,000 of income for individuals or $250,000 for couples filing jointly and will rise to 3.8% on income in excess of those amounts.

In general, all persons 65 years of age or older who have been legal residents of the USA for at least 5 years are eligible for Medicare. People with disabilities under

R.W. Stephens (✉)
Rynearson, Suess, Schnurbusch & Champion, L.L.C., St. Louis, MO, USA
e-mail: rstephens@rssclaw.com

S. Loue (ed.), *Mental Health Practitioner's Guide to HIV/AIDS*,
DOI 10.1007/978-1-4614-5283-6_61,

65 may also be eligible if they receive Social Security Disability Insurance (SSDI) benefits. Specific medical conditions may also help people become eligible to enroll in Medicare. Those who are 65 and older must pay a monthly premium to remain enrolled in Medicare if they or their spouse have not paid Medicare taxes over the course of 10 years while working.

People with disabilities who receive SSDI are eligible for Medicare while they continue to receive SSDI payments; they lose eligibility for Medicare based on disability if they stop receiving SSDI. The 24-month exclusion means that people who become disabled must wait 2 years before receiving government medical insurance, unless they have one of the listed diseases or they are eligible for Medicaid.

Many beneficiaries are dual-eligible. This means they qualify for both Medicare and Medicaid. In some states for those making below a certain income, Medicaid will pay the beneficiaries' Part B premium for them (most beneficiaries have worked long enough and have no Part A premium), and also pay for any drugs that are not covered by Part D. In 2008, Medicare provided health care coverage for 45 million Americans. Enrollment is expected to reach 78 million by 2030, when the baby-boom generation is fully enrolled.

Medicare has four parts: Part A is Hospital Insurance. Part B is Medical Insurance. Medicare Part D covers prescription drugs. Medicare Advantage plans, also known as Medicare Part C, are another way for beneficiaries to receive their Part A, B, and D benefits. All Medicare benefits are subject to medical necessity. The original program included Parts A and B. Part D was introduced in January 2006; before that, Parts A and B covered prescription drugs in a few special cases.

Part A covers inpatient hospital stays (at least overnight), including semiprivate room, food, and tests. Part A covers brief stays for convalescence in a skilled nursing facility if certain criteria are met.

Part B medical insurance helps pay for some services and products not covered by Part A, generally on an outpatient basis. Part B is optional and may be deferred if the beneficiary or his/her spouse is still working. There is a lifetime penalty (10% per year) imposed for not enrolling in Part B unless actively working. Part B coverage begins once a patient meets his or her deductible, then typically Medicare covers 80% of approved services, while the remaining 20% is paid by the patient.

Part B coverage includes physician and nursing services, X-rays, laboratory and diagnostic tests, influenza and pneumonia vaccinations, blood transfusions, renal dialysis, outpatient hospital procedures, limited ambulance transportation, immunosuppressive drugs for organ transplant recipients, chemotherapy, hormonal treatments such as Lupron, and other outpatient medical treatments administered in a doctor's office. Medication administration is covered under Part B if it is administered by the physician during an office visit. Part B also helps with durable medical equipment (DME), prosthetic devices, as well as one pair of eyeglasses following cataract surgery, and oxygen for home use is also covered.

Part C, also known as, Medicare Advantage, offers health plans options run by Medicare approved private insurance companies. Medicare plans are a way to get the benefits and services covered under Part A and Part B. Most Medicare

Advantage plans cover Medicare prescription drug coverage (Part D). With Medicare Advantage health plan, Medicare pays the private health plan a fixed amount every month. Members typically also pay a monthly premium in addition to the Medicare Part B premium to cover items not covered by traditional Medicare Parts A and Part B.

Medicare Part D is Medicare Prescription Drug Coverage. This plan helps to cover the cost of prescription drugs. Part D is run by Medicare approved private insurance companies. Anyone with Medicare Part A or Medicare B is eligible for Medicare Part D. Unlike Medicare Part A and B, Part D coverage is not standardized. Plans choose which drugs they wish to cover, at what tier they wish to cover it, and are free to choose not to cover some drugs at all. Beneficiaries who are dual-eligible under both Medicare and Medicaid, should note that Medicaid may pay for drugs not covered by Part D of Medicare.

There are several differences between Medicare and Medicaid. Medicaid is a state governed program while Medicare is a federally governed program. Medicaid is for low income individuals who are pregnant women, children under 19, individuals over 65, individuals who are blind, individuals who are disabled and people who need nursing home care. Applications for Medicaid are processed through the State's Medicaid Agency.

Medicare, on the other hand, is for individuals over 65, individuals of any age who have kidney failure or long term kidney disease, or individuals who are permanently disabled and cannot work. Medicare applications are processed through the Social Security Office. As noted above, some individuals are eligible for both Medicaid and Medicare. For these people, Medicaid is sometimes used to help pay for Medicare premiums.

Related Topics: Access to care, Medicaid

Suggested Resources

Medicare basics—Medicare benefits. Retrieved January 25, 2012 from: http://www.medicare.gov/navigation/medicare-basics/medicare-benefits/medicare-benefits-overview.aspx

What is the difference between Medicare and Medicaid? Retrieved January 25, 2012 from http://questions.medicare.gov/app/answers/detail/a_id/2038.

Mindfulness

Sana Loue

The concept of mindfulness has been subject to various definitions. In general, the term has been used to refer to interventions that focus on maintaining purposeful attention to the present moment, without judgment. It has been described as a way of being, rather than a way of doing. Mindfulness is also characterized by an open, receptive attitude. Additional key elements of mindfulness include an ability to recognize and label one's emotions, the development of more refined self-awareness, and movement towards becoming more responsive and less reactive. Some scholars have distinguished between mindfulness interventions and concentrative meditations, such as Transcendental Meditation. Concentrative meditations are distinguished by their focus on a specific stimulus, such as breathing, and a refocusing on that stimulus when attention drifts from it.

Mindfulness has been integrated with various other modalities in intervention efforts with individuals with mental illness. These mindfulness based interventions include, for example, Mindfulness-Based Stress Reduction (MBSR), Trauma Sensitive MBSR for women with posttraumatic stress disorder, and Mindfulness-Based Cognitive Therapy (MBCT). MBCT has been shown to help reduce the likelihood of depression relapses in individuals with major depression and to reduce the anxiety experienced by individuals with bipolar disorder that is in remission. These interventions may include both formal and informal components. MBSR, for example, includes the formal practices of mindful awareness of the body, such as through yoga exercises, and sitting meditation. Informal components include being conscious of oneself as one goes about one's daily activities of living and maintaining an awareness of the present moment even under trying circumstances, such as pain or grief.

Mindfulness practices have also been utilized with individuals suffering from physical ailments. MBSR has been found to reduce distress and improve well-being

S. Loue (✉)
Department of Epidemiology and Biostatistics, Case Western Reserve University, Cleveland, OH, USA
e-mail: Sana.Loue@case.edu

S. Loue (ed.), *Mental Health Practitioner's Guide to HIV/AIDS*,
DOI 10.1007/978-1-4614-5283-6_62,

in patients with rheumatoid arthritis and to help reduce pain in individuals suffering from chronic pain. MBSR had also been used beneficially among individuals with fibromyalgia.

Mindfulness-based practices have also been used beneficially with HIV-positive individuals. Mindfulness practices have been found to be associated with reductions in impulsivity, use of intoxicants, and sexual and drug-related HIV risks among HIV-positive drug users. The decrease in impulsivity may be the result of a decreased identification with one's thoughts and the associated emotional intensity, due to the practice of detached observation and non-judgment of one's thoughts. Another study of the use of MBSR techniques among HIV-positive men found that the use of these techniques was associated with an increase in positive psychological functioning and a reduction in distress. It has been hypothesized that the use of mindfulness-based techniques may also help to reduce the cognitive dysfunction that is common among HIV-infected persons.

Use of mindfulness-based practices has also been found to be beneficial to mental health providers. One study found that the use of MBSR by mental health care providers is associated with reduced stress, rumination, negative affect and anxiety and increases in positive affect and self-compassion.

Research efforts have attempted to understand the mechanism by which mindfulness practices operate. Studies indicate that mindfulness meditation practices activate the prefrontal cortex and the anterior cingulate cortex and that long-term meditation practice is associated with changes in the areas of the brain associated with attention. Studies have also suggested that mindfulness meditation may improve immune system functioning. As an example, researchers conducting a study that examined the effect of mindfulness meditation on immune functioning among HIV-infected persons concluded that mindfulness training can help to mitigate against a decline in the immune functioning of HIV-infected adults.

Related Topics: Coping, Mental health comorbidity and HIV/AIDS, Religion and spirituality

Suggested Readings

Greeson, J. M. (2009). Mindfulness research update: 2008. *Complementary Health Practice Review, 14*(1), 10–18.

Grossman, P., Niemann, L., Schmidt, S., & Walach, H. (2004). Mindfulness-based stress reduction and health benefits: A meta-analysis. *Journal of Psychosomatic Research, 57*, 35–43.

Kabat-Zinn, J. (1994). *Wherever you go, there you are*. New York: Hyperion.

McCown, D., Reibel, D., & Micozzi, M. S. (Eds.). (2010). *Teaching mindfulness: A practical guide for clinicians and educators*. New York: Springer.

Shapiro, S. L., Brown, K. W., & Biegel, G. M. (2007). Teaching self-care to caregivers: Effects of mindfulness-based stress reduction on the mental health of therapists in training. *Training and Education in Professional Psychology, 1*(2), 105–115.

Monogamy

Beatrice Gabriela Ioan

The term *monogamy* comes from two Greek words; *monos*, which means alone/one and *gamos*, which means union or marriage. Monogamy refers to a situation in which a person has only one sexual partner at a time, whether in an informal or formal relationship within a marriage. The norm promoted by the Judeo-Christian tradition is monogamy within marriage between a man and a woman, while in Islam polygamy is accepted, i.e., marriage of a man with several women at the same time.

Because HIV can be transmitted sexually, it is assumed that monogamous relationships between HIV negative persons will prevent transmission of the infection. This concept emerged in the early epidemic in gay communities, when monogamy was considered to be a more reliable prevention method than the use of condoms. However, monogamy may be falsely perceived as an element of security, because one or both partners may actually not be "safe" due to current or past risk behaviors.

Monogamy is not just the sexual side of relationships, but also involves emotional and interpersonal issues. Research has suggested, for example, that in relations between gay men, *emotional monogamy* may be more important than a commitment to sexual exclusivity. In this situation, the most important element is the emotional integrity of the couple and the sexual relationships outside the couple are allowed only if they do not destroy it. For this reason the partner who has an affair at some point in time may fear its disclosure to the other partner, increasing the likelihood that the faithful partner becomes HIV infected.

A US study involving 6,864 heterosexuals, lesbians, and gay men, identified an increase in monogamy from 1975 until 2000. The study indicates that the prevalence of sexual relationships outside the couple among heterosexual men decreased from 28% in 1975 to 10% in 2000, and among heterosexual women from 23 to 14%. Among gay men, there was a decrease from 83 to 59%, and among lesbians from 28

B.G. Ioan (✉)
Legal Medicine, Medical Deontology and Bioethics Department, University of Medicine and Pharmacy "Gr. T. Popa", Iasi, Romania
e-mail: ioanbml@yahoo.com

S. Loue (ed.), *Mental Health Practitioner's Guide to HIV/AIDS*,
DOI 10.1007/978-1-4614-5283-6_63, © Springer Science+Business Media New York 2013

to 8%. The authors hypothesized that this might be due, at least in part, to an awareness of the danger of HIV and other STDs transmission in extramarital relationships. Also, half of the gay men in the study were involved in civil unions, the rest being involved in committed relationships. Married couples adopt less risky sexual behaviors and have fewer sexual partners than unmarried couples, suggesting that formalization of the relationship could be a protective factor against extramarital affairs.

Mutual influences operating within a couple can increase the incidence of either risky or protective behaviors for HIV transmission. Increased trust and intimacy between the members of a couple can promote risky behaviors; for example, the incidence of sharing injecting equipment is more common in couples. In this context, one of the partners can contract HIV outside of the couple as those who share needles in couples often share them with others outside the couple; thus the other partner may become HIV-infected as well.

The use of condoms during sexual relationships in monogamous couples is rare, often due to a false perception that they are at low risk of HIV transmission. However, gay male couples have been found to use condoms more frequently than do heterosexual couples, probably due to the recognition that monogamy is difficult to maintain, even in a long-term loving relationship. Good information about HIV/AIDS increases awareness of HIV risk and HIV testing. It is important that both members of the couple be informed as information limited to only one of the partners may have insufficient impact on the couple's common behaviors.

There are gender differences in the behaviors and attitudes associated with risk of HIV/AIDS. Thus, men assess their HIV risk as lower than women, although they report adopting more risky sexual behaviors and less HIV testing.

It is estimated that many women face a higher risk of HIV from their primary partners than from more casual ones, because they believe that they are safe within monogamous relationships and are consequently more likely to engage in riskier behaviors within that relationship, such as sexual relations without the protection of a condom. However, it is recognized that the increased rates of HIV infection in heterosexual men and women are largely due to their participation in concurrent relationships, which are more common among men than women. Sexual activity of the partners outside of the couple, without the protection afforded by consistent condom use, leads to a dramatic increase of the risk of introducing HIV in the primary relationship.

Partner violence may also increase individuals' risk of contracting HIV. A study of 1,600 women victims of intimate partner violence in their primary relationships found that the women are more likely to report more than one sexual partner, infection with a sexually transmitted disease, inconsistent use of condoms and acceptance of sexual partners with known HIV risk factors compared to women who have not experienced intimate partner violence in their primary relationships. Violence and fear of violence are important contextual factors in terms of risk of HIV infection as the women may be abused if they try to talk about condom use with their partner, despite knowledge of a partner's sexual relations with other women and/or men. In many traditional relationships, the social and economic power of women is compromised, so that women may yield to their male partner's authority, including sexually. Many of these women are unable to control their involvement in the couple's common behaviors, which increases their risk of contracting HIV.

The development of a firm belief in the partner's fidelity could be an adaptive response when women are unable to negotiate with partners to adopt safer sex behaviors. A study on women participating in a methadone treatment program who were victims of intimate partner violence showed that many of them initially desired a monogamous relationship. However, they gradually abandoned this wish due to the deteriorating quality of their relationship, because they lost their motivation to be vigilant, and because they did not attribute sufficient value to their relationship to try to maintain it after they had been physically abused. For others who experience feelings of powerlessness and hopelessness, monogamy may not have any importance.

Sexual partner concurrency refers to a situation in which an individual has overlapping sexual partners over a period of time. This may take any one or more of several forms: individuals may have long-term concurrent relationships, such as with polygamy; people may be involved in long-term relationships, but have sporadic or isolated sexual relationships with other partners during the course of that long-term relationship; or individuals may have multiple sporadic relationships that overlap. Concurrent sexual partnering represent an additional HIV risk factor, and more so for the multiple partners than for the person who practices this kind of relationship. Concurrency promotes the efficient transmission of infection, because the infectivity is high during the acute phase of HIV infection (during the first months after contracting the infection), after which infectivity is reduced significantly. During the chronic phase, transmission occurs in approximately 1 out of every 1,000 incidents of unprotected sexual intercourse. The risk increases again during the final symptomatic phase, many years after the initial infection.

Serial monogamy refers to the situation in which a person has multiple sexual partners at different points in time; the relations do not overlap and there is only one sexual partner at a time. The risk of HIV transmission in this case is lower than in the case of concurrent sexual partners because a relationship begins only after the previous one ends, with no overlap between them.

Related Topics: Partner violence, Prevention strategies, Risk behaviors

Suggested Readings

De Souza, R. (2010). Women living with HIV: stories of powerlessness and agency. *Women's Studies International Forum, 33*, 244–252.

Gotta, G., Green, R. J., Rothblum, E., Solomon, S., Balsam, K., & Schwartz, P. (2011). Heterosexual, lesbian, and gay male relationships: A comparison of couples in 1975 and 2000. *Family Process, 50*(3), 353–376.

Hearn, K. D., O'Sullivan, L. F., El-Bassel, N., & Gilbert, L. (2005). Intimate partner violence and monogamy among women in methadone treatment. *AIDS and Behavior, 9*(2), 177–186.
Mah, T. L., & Shelton, J. D. (2011). Concurrency revisited: Increasing and compelling epidemiological evidence. *Journal of the International AIDS Society, 14*, 33.
Stein, J. A., Nyamathi, A., Ullman, J. B., & Bentler, P. M. (2007). Impact of marriage on HIV/AIDS risk behaviors among impoverished, at-risk couples: A multilevel latent variable approach. *AIDS and Behavior, 11*(1), 87–97.
Wu, E., El- Bassel, N., Gilbert, L., & Chang, M. (2003). Intimate partner violence and HIV among urban minority women in primary health care settings. *AIDS and Behavior, 7*, 291–301.

Suggested Resources

Fox, A. Monogamy. *The Body. The complete HIV/AIDS resource*. Retrieved February 1, 2012 from http://www.thebody.com/content/art14030.html?ts=pf
http://www.newworldencyclopedia.org/entry/Monogamy. Retrieved February 1, 2012

Orphans

Ezer Kang and Cabrina Kang

In regions disproportionately affected by HIV in Africa, Asia, and South America, the Joint United Nations Programme on HIV/AIDS (UNAIDS) defined "orphans" as children who have lost one or both parents to HIV. Given the discrediting nature of the term "AIDS orphan," and the inaccurate labeling of orphans as necessarily HIV-positive, the description is referenced less in scholarship. In the context of the epidemic, orphans are also referred to as children made vulnerable by AIDS. Although the definition of orphan carries significant programmatic and policy implications, few studies clearly define the term in the context of their work. Moreover, medical and social science research have not reached a consensus on the sociodemographic characteristics that define children orphaned by AIDS. Lack of clarity and consensus on the definition have rendered accurate and detailed epidemiological surveillance and the development of evidenced-based psychosocial interventions challenging at best. Specifically, there is considerable variability in published studies on the age (under 19 or 15 years) and serostatus of a child orphaned by AIDS, definition of caregiver who died (e.g., single or both parents; maternal or paternal), and the child's relationship to the caregiver who died (e.g., biological parents or kinship guardians).

Although reports have provided estimates of paternal, maternal, and double (death of mother and father) orphans in regions of sub-Saharan Africa, it remains unclear how many have been orphaned due to AIDS in each parental death category. Of note, the challenge of identifying children orphaned by AIDS is further complicated by the secrecy and stigma carried by families affected by HIV. The United Nations Children's Fund (UNICEF) for example, provided specific estimates of maternal (28,500,000), paternal (34,800,00), and double (10,300,000)

E. Kang (✉)
Department of Psychology, Wheaton College, Wheaton, IL, USA
e-mail: ezer.kang@wheaton.edu

C. Kang
Wellesley College, Wellesley, MA, USA

S. Loue (ed.), *Mental Health Practitioner's Guide to HIV/AIDS*, DOI 10.1007/978-1-4614-5283-6_64, © Springer Science+Business Media New York 2013

orphans in Sub-Saharan Africa in 2010, and estimated that 15,700,000 children would be orphaned by AIDS without further defining nature parental death.

Some researchers have argued the merits of understanding orphans in African countries as a socially constructed category based on loss and need. This raised nuanced considerations as to whether children were to be considered orphans if they were well cared for by kin and had adjusted in culturally normative ways to parental deaths. Furthermore, would this broaden the definition of orphans to include young adults with fewer social and economic resources who face adjustment challenges? In Malawi, for example, researchers challenged the conventional premise that family and social infrastructure were in complete disarray as a result of parental death. They argued that children orphaned by AIDS underwent a process of social reconfiguration that could be normative when faced with familial disruption. As such, categorizing them as orphans carried unnecessary stigma that further perpetuated perceptions of them as passive victims.

In the USA, children orphaned by AIDS gained national attention with the emerging "boarder babies" crisis in New York City, particularly in Harlem where HIV-exposed and infected infants and children were left to board at hospitals because of parental abandonment, postpartum complications, and an inadequate foster care referral system. Between 1983 and 1989, 3–5% of pregnant women at Harlem Hospital were infected with HIV. Many of the newborns of these women were abandoned by their mothers and were referred to as boarder babies because they were cared for in hospitals until they were eventually placed with foster families. During this period of the crack cocaine epidemic, nearly 10% of babies born in Harlem went directly to foster care, primarily due to maternal drug-related problems, and these babies were eight times more likely to be HIV exposed than those babies discharged to their mothers.

The challenge of consistently defining children orphaned by AIDS across disciplines has resulted in equivocal findings on the extent of their vulnerabilities. Studies that examined the physical and emotional-behavioral effects of orphan-hood have been hampered by sampling, methodological, and construct operationalization inconsistencies, rendering comparison of findings across studies unfeasible. Moreover, systematic reviews of studies that generally showed adverse developmental outcomes among variously defined orphans did not adequately consider potential confounding affects of baseline family functioning, support networks, or poverty. As such, the implications drawn from studies indicating the detrimental effects of orphan-hood (e.g., poor emotional and behavior functioning, academic achievement decline, poor reproductive health, high-risk sexual behavior) should be interpreted with caution, as the causal relationship between paternal/ maternal or parental death due to AIDS per se and reported adverse outcomes remains unclear. Other factors that predate a child's orphan-hood such as the developmental stage of the child, guardian-child relationships, child HIV serostatus, family wealth, extended family network, communal HIV stigma, and gender inequalities are important to consider when explicating the degree of vulnerability of orphans. It is noteworthy that several studies did not report negative outcomes, highlighting the importance of identifying individual and familial/ communal strengths and resources that contribute to a child's resiliency.

Studies in sub-Saharan Africa have consistently noted the general benefits of preserving family caretaking roles and challenging the long-term merits of institutional care. Concerns have included sustainability of institutional care, adaptive reintegration into society where HIV stigma persists, inadequate monitoring and accountability, and cost effectiveness of supporting residential facilities compared to community- or family based care. Recent studies in economically disadvantaged rural regions of Asia and Africa have found that double orphans residing in government supported community-based small group homes, managed by houseparents for a small number of children orphaned by AIDS, generally reported higher levels of mental health, physical, and educational functioning compared to orphans under kinship or institutional care (e.g., orphanage). The advantages of community group homes lie in a child's proximity to family settings, and living in a family oriented household. Moreover, economic assistance mitigates the stressors of meeting basic daily needs. Pervasive poverty in these regions coupled with community members and families emerging to collectively care for children orphaned by HIV have led to external funding and capacity building efforts to help ensure community ownership and sustainability of responses.

Related Topics: Caregiving and caregivers, Children, Stigma and stigmatization, United Nations

Suggested Readings

Chirwa, W. C. (2002). Social exclusion and inclusion: Challenges to orphan care in Malawi. *Nordic Journal of African Studies, 11*(1), 93–113.

Chuong, C. & Operario, D. (2012). Challenging household dynamics: Impact of orphanhood, parental absence, and children's living arrangements on education in South Africa. *Global Public Health, 7*(1), 42–57.

Hong, Y., Li, X., Fanf, X., Zhao, G., Zhao, J., Zhao, Q., et al. (2010). Care arrangements of AIDS orphans and their relationship with children's psychosocial well-being in rural China. *Health Policy and Planning, 26*, 115–123.

Nicholas, S. W., & Abrams, E. J. (2002). Boarder babies with AIDS in Harlem: Lessons in applied public health. *American Journal of Public Health, 92*, 163–165.

Richter, L. M., Sherr, L., Adato, M., Chandan, U., Desmond, C., Drimeie, S., et al. (2009). Strengthening families to support children affected by HIV and AIDS. *AIDS Care, 21*(S1), 3–12.

Sherr, L., Mueller, J., & Varrall, R. (2009). Evidence-based gender findings for children affected by HIV and AIDS – a systematic overview. *AIDS Care, 21*(S1), 83–97.

Sherr, L., Varrall, R., Mueller, J., & Workgroup, J. L. I. C. A. (2008). A systematic review on the meaning of the concept 'AIDS Orphan': Confusion over definitions and implications for care. *AIDS Care, 20*(5), 527–539.

Suggested Resources

UNICEF (2006). Africa's orphaned and vulnerable generations: Children affected by AIDS. Retrieved 12/13/11 from http://www.unicef.org/publications/files/Africas_Orphaned_and_-Vulnerable_Generations_Children_Affected_by_AIDS.pdf

Partner Notification

Abishek Jain

Partner notification is the process of informing an HIV-positive individual's sexual and/or needle-sharing partners of possible HIV exposure. In a review of nine studies, approximately 20% of HIV-positive individuals' tested partners were found to be newly diagnosed with HIV infection. With an estimated two-thirds of HIV infections transmitted by individuals unaware of being HIV-positive, partner notification can help reduce the spread of HIV by promoting testing, awareness, and prevention among high-risk populations.

Partner notification can be performed by (1) *provider referral* (public health professional or medical care provider informs partners), (2) *patient referral* (infected individual informs his or her partners), (3) *dual referral* (both provider and patient inform the partners), or (4) *contract referral* (patient agrees to notify his or her partners by a predetermined date, with the understanding that a third party will notify the partners if the patient does not do so).

In one study of a high-risk population, 65% were unaware of partner notification. In various studies, having a long-term relationship with a sex partner, talking to health department staff about partner notification, and having a sense of moral obligation can increase a patient's likelihood of notifying partners. Fear of verbal and physical attacks, concerns about confidentiality, and unawareness of partner notification services can decrease a patient's likelihood of notifying partners.

An analysis comparing provider, patient, and dual referrals found that provider referral is the most cost-effective. In comparing provider and patient referrals, provider referral resulted in 1.5–6.5 times more partners being notified, and more partners presenting for medical evaluation. However, in a study of Massachusetts men who have sex with men, most preferred to be notified directly by their partner. E-card notification, such as through Internet Sexuality Information Services (ISIS), is an option for anonymous patient referral.

A. Jain (✉)
Cleveland, OH, USA
e-mail: beesh.jain.md@gmail.com

S. Loue (ed.), *Mental Health Practitioner's Guide to HIV/AIDS*,
DOI 10.1007/978-1-4614-5283-6_65, © Springer Science+Business Media New York 2013

Partner Counseling and Referral Services (PCRS), or simply "partner services," are available to assist with partner notification. These services can link infected partners with additional resources, such as mental health care, housing assistance, and legal counsel. They can also help prioritize notifying certain groups, such as recently exposed partners who may be candidates for post-exposure prophylaxis, partners at increased risk for transmission to others, or pregnant partners.

Guidelines of the Centers for Disease Control and Prevention (CDC) encourage partner services to be confidential, collegial, and sensitive to potential consequences of notification, including violence. Partner services are highly under-used, despite potential benefits and strong CDC recommendations. Some federally sponsored HIV-prevention programs require states to have partner services.

Partner notification laws differ state-by-state and can be complex. Many states *permit* practitioners to warn at-risk partners; some states *require* practitioners to warn at-risk partners. Furthermore, certain states permit disclosure to spouses or sexual partners, but not necessarily to needle-sharing partners. Physicians and laboratories in all states are legally required to report the names of all persons newly diagnosed with AIDS to their local or state health departments. Learning the specific state law is necessary, and legal consultation is highly recommended, before a health practitioner assumes having a duty or privilege to warn.

Many advocacy groups have opposed mandatory HIV partner notification, arguing that it can compromise confidentiality, cause individuals to avoid HIV testing, and result in further suffering. Regardless of specific partner notification laws, a reasonable approach for practitioners can include educating HIV-positive individuals about potential criminal prosecution under willful exposure statutes, present in at least 34 states, and about avoiding risky behaviors that expose others.

Related Topics: Contact tracing, Disclosure, Disclosure laws, HIV testing

Suggested Reading

Centers for Disease Control and Prevention. (2008). Recommendations for partner services programs for HIV Infection, syphilis, gonorrhea, and chlamydial infection. *Morbidity and Mortality Weekly Report, 57*(RR09), 1–63.

Lin, L., & Liang, B.A. (2005). HIV and health law: Striking the balance between legal Mandates and medical ethics. *American Medical Association Journal of Ethics, 7*(10). Retrieved November 23, 2011 from http://virtualmentor.ama-assn.org/2005/10/toc-0510.html

Mathews, C., Coetzee, N., Zwarenstein, M., Lombard, C., Guttmacher, S., Oxman, A.D., & Schmid, G. (2009). Strategies for partner notification for sexually transmitted diseases (Review). *The Cochrane Collaboration*, 1.

Mimiaga, M. J., Tetu, A. M., Gortmaker, S., Koenen, K. C., Fair, A. D., Novak, D. S., Vanderwarker, R., Bertrand, T., Adelson, S., & Mayer, K. H. (2009). Partner notification after STD and HIV exposures and infections: Knowledge, attitudes, and experiences of Massachusetts men who have sex with men. *Public Health Reports, 124*, 111–119.

Suggested Resources

Guide to Community Preventive Services. (2010, Nov. 28). *Interventions to identify HIV-positive people through partner counseling and referral services*. Retrieved April 11, 2012 from www.thecommunityguide.org/hiv/partnercounseling.html.

Partner Violence

Susan Hatters Friedman

HIV and intimate partner violence (IPV) are interrelated public health issues. IPV is a term encompassing physical violence, sexual violence, emotional abuse and threats of violence, perpetrated by an intimate partner or date. In the US, between 9 and 30% of women are victims of physical IPV in their lifetime, and 8% are victims of sexual IPV. Eight percent of men report IPV victimization. Some studies suggest that men and women are equally likely to be victims but that women are more seriously injured.

IPV may occur at home, in the street, or in the workplace. Violence occurs for various reasons such as power, control, anger, revenge and self-defense. Common characteristics of perpetrators of IPV include those with a history of violence, substance abuse, physical victimization in their own childhood, fears of abandonment, moodiness, insecurity, jealousy, temper problems, low self-esteem and externalizing blame. Those who are young, less educated, low income, urban dwellers, with a history of being abused, substance abuse, mental illness, and current pregnancy are at higher risk of IPV victimization.

Researchers have explored the intersection of IPV and HIV from various angles. Yet, many questions remain. Rates of IPV among HIV positive individuals have been explored, as have transmission of HIV risk, and HIV testing behaviors among IPV victims. Various cultures and subcultures have varying results. Among HIV-positive patients at an urban clinic, 73% reported lifetime IPV victimization and 20% reported current IPV, most commonly physical IPV. Rates were highest among men who have sex with men (MSM) and Blacks. Over one-quarter believed that the violence was related to the HIV positivity. A Nigerian study of pregnant HIV-positive women found a 6% prevalence of physical IPV and 28% prevalence of psychological IPV. Risk factors included IPV before diagnosis, having an HIV-positive child, having more than one child and lower partner education.

S.H. Friedman (✉)
Department of Psychiatry, School of Medicine, Case Western Reserve University, Cleveland, OH, USA
e-mail: Susan.Hatters-Friedman@UHhospitals.org

S. Loue (ed.), *Mental Health Practitioner's Guide to HIV/AIDS*,
DOI 10.1007/978-1-4614-5283-6_66,

Mediators of HIV transmission in IPV may include: use of sexual force, refusal of condom use, fear of violence, lack of disclosure in a relationship with power imbalance and comorbidity of substance abuse. In a US sample, women victimized by IPV in the past 3 months had more episodes of unprotected sex than non-victims. Among poor Chilean women, those who had experienced IPV in the past 6 months had a higher risk of HIV than non-victims. An Indian study found that women who suffered sexual violence in marriage were more likely to be HIV positive than those who did not. HIV positive men appear to experience more severe and frequent IPV than their HIV negative counterparts.

Those who abuse their partners may engage in other risky sexual behaviors. Men who have perpetrated IPV are more likely to have HIV. Among men with multiple concurrent female partners in South Africa, 41% had perpetrated IPV. IPV perpetration was associated with: less condom use, STD symptoms, transactional sex, alcohol abuse, belief in partner's unfaithfulness and more than five partners. Among US urban men attending health clinics, one-third reported perpetrating physical or sexual IPV in their lifetime, which was associated with HIV risk behaviors and HIV diagnosis. Among HIV-positive persons in a US sample, who were in a relationship, 27% reported IPV—approximately half of which was mutual abuse. More than two-fifths of HIV-positive injection drug using men reported physical or sexual IPV against their female partner and this was correlated with unprotected sex. Among heterosexual Black men in urban clinics who had more than one partner in the past year, 21% reported IPV perpetration in their current relationship, which was correlated with HIV diagnosis, transactional sex and unprotected anal sex.

Overall, IPV victimization increases vulnerability to STDs and decreases safer sex practices. IPV victimization appears to be both a risk factor for HIV infection and a consequence of HIV infection. (IPV has a similar relationship to substance abuse.) However, some studies have not found a consistent association, particularly in lower income countries. Among US women in relationships, IPV was associated with HIV infection when controlling for socioeconomic status (SES) and risky sexual behaviors. Similarly a Rwandan study found a correlation between IPV and HIV in women with no or few sexual risk factors.

The American Medical Association recommends routine screening for IPV. Screening should take place in emergency rooms, dental offices, and community health centers. Victims may not report abuse because they are embarrassed, consider it private, have low self-esteem, have a secret relationship, or fear additional violence. Asking about victimization and perpetration can occur in various ways. The clinician may wish to discuss decision making in the relationship to approach the topic, or gender equity, or proceed with direct inquiry. Formal screening may be used (e.g., Sharon and colleagues' HITS scale—which inquires about hurting, insulting, threatening, and screaming). Support and validation of the patient are important, as is documentation of injuries and reports.

Screening for IPV is particularly important among both those at risk for HIV and persons with HIV. Screening may take place in the STD testing center (where both problems may be addressed simultaneously), through social services and other medical locations. Screening should occur in a culturally appropriate manner with attention to how the person defines his or her own experience. Practitioners may routinely ask about IPV during HIV screening because many may seek testing but not other medical care. Violence and gender inequality may be discussed. Condom use discussions should be empowered. Similarly, women who screen positive for IPV may be offered HIV prevention information. Even when screening HIV-positive persons for IPV was required by New York law it was sporadic and not standardized.

IPV leads to both physical and psychological symptoms. IPV may have negative effects on medication adherence. Mental health concerns include depression and anxiety, post-traumatic stress disorder, suicidal thoughts, low self-esteem and substance abuse. Victims may blame themselves, lose self-esteem, and feel unsafe in their own homes. Clinicians should provide information about shelters, domestic violence services, legal help (for protection orders) and crisis management services, such as by providing local phone numbers. Victims should not make the decision to leave a violent relationship lightly, because separation and restraining orders increase the risk of serious violence in some relationships. Also, even when reported, offenders may not be arrested, and protection orders are often violated. The clinician may work with the patient on issues of self-esteem, emotional isolation and trust. Treatment programs also exist for batterers, often accessed through the courts or anger management.

Related Topics: Adherence, Housing and homelessness, Mental health comorbidity and HIV/AIDS, Women

Suggested Readings

El-Bassel, N., Gilbert, L., Witte, S., Wu, E., & Chang, M. (2011). Intimate partner violence and HIV among drug-involved women: Contexts linking these two epidemics. *Substance Use Misuse, 46*(2–3), 295–306.

Friedman, S. H., Stankowski, J. E., & Loue, S. (2008). Intimate partner violence and the clinician. In R. Simon & K. Tardiff (Eds.), *Textbook of violence assessment and management* (pp. 483–500). Arlington: The American Psychiatric Press.

Loue, S. (2001). *Intimate partner violence: Societal, medical legal and individual responses*. New York: Plenum.

Physician–Patient Relationship

Simona Irina Damian

Ever since the emergence of the AIDS pandemic, it became obvious that HIV was much more than just a disease. Unlike any other condition, HIV not only affects the lives of those infected, but it also impacts the lives of virtually everyone around, clearly becoming one of the most significant public health issues. Beyond an accurate diagnosis and appropriate prescription, the physician must work to create a health-sensitive interpersonal relationship with the patient. A cooperative doctor–patient relationship has inherent therapeutic value. The physician's major role is to educate and encourage the patient to take responsibility for his health. It is the patient, not the doctor, who ultimately creates or accomplishes healing. The physician must strive to inspire hope as well as understanding.

Apart from the treatment itself, the physician contributes to the efficacy of the healing process, primarily by conveying a sense of empowerment to the person seeking the healing, managing related issues as well, such as treating psychiatric co-morbidities, preserving the patient's hope and motivation, and giving him an adequate amount of information regarding the disease and its possible developments. Areas of best practice that enhance access to health care include doctors' interactional styles, ways of providing treatment options and treatment information, and ways of addressing the specific needs and life circumstances of patients tackling a cureless disease.

The care of people with HIV and AIDS is a life-changing challenge due to its multidisciplinary nature, its medical complexity, physical manifestations, the need for infection control procedures and the associated stigma. Despite gains in knowledge, several problems have affected the provision of proper care. The most commonly reported barriers that prevent physicians from managing the care of HIV-infected patients include fear of contagion, fear of losing patients, unwillingness to care, inadequate knowledge/training about treating HIV patients, homophobia, burnout, and religious attitudes. Financial risk, the lack of insurance, a lack of

S.I. Damian (✉)
University of Medicine and Pharmacy Gr. T. Popa, Iasi, Romania
e-mail: si_damian@yahoo.com

S. Loue (ed.), *Mental Health Practitioner's Guide to HIV/AIDS*,
DOI 10.1007/978-1-4614-5283-6_67,

support staff, the structure of general practice, a lack of speciality backup support for patients in whom complications develop, or the lack of community social services or resources have also posed impediments to treatment and care by doctors. Professional staff and health care students have frequently reported fear of occupational exposure, which is further fueled by the potential discrimination against health professionals who do become infected. However, the U.S. Centers for Disease Control and Prevention have assessed the risk of HIV infection and AIDS among physicians after a single accidental exposure to HIV at work to be 0.5% or less. This figure is lower than the published risk of contracting most other infectious diseases after a single exposure, e.g., the risk for hepatitis B is 10–20%. The stigma of caring for and treating patients with HIV and AIDS could pose a significant barrier as well.

From classic paternalism to enhanced autonomy and team care, the physician–patient relationship has evolved tremendously. Health care is being revolutionarily transformed by improvements in e-health and by the empowered, computer-literate public. As part of this era of enhanced patient role in decision making, people are prone to become partners in their own health and to seize the opportunity of the online feedback, health portals, and physician web pages; this type of health care consumer is certainly redefining the physician–patient relationship. Web interaction, through social networking with other persons with the same condition, may further promote patients' active role in developing a greater sense of responsibility, accountability, and self-efficacy associated with higher confidence in the patients' perceived ability to manage the disease and more willingness to ask doctors pertinent questions. Undoubtedly such changes can generate positive results as: improved clinical decision-making, increased efficiency, and strengthened communication between physicians and patients..

Related Topics: Adherence, Informed consent

Suggested Readings

Bradford, J., Coleman, S., & Cunningham, W. (2007). HIV system navigation: An emerging model to improve HIV care access. *AIDS Patient Care and STDs, 21*(Suppl. 1), S49–S58.

Baer, H. (2008). Comparison of treatment of HIV patients in naturopathic and biomedical settings. *Journal of Evidence-Based Complementary and Alternative Medicine, 13*(3), 182–197.

Friedland, G. H. (1995). A journey through the epidemic. *Bulletin of the New York Academy of Medicine, 72*(1), 178–186.

Lo, B., & Parham, L. (2010). The impact of web 2.0 on the doctor-patient relationship. *Journal of Law, Medicine & Ethics, 38*(1), 17–26.

Naidoo, P. (2006). Barriers to HIV care and treatment by doctors: A review of the literature. *South Africa Family Practice, 48*(2), 55. Retrieved April 1, 2012 from http://www.safpj.co.za/index.php/safpj/article/viewFile/513/467.

Szasz, T. (1956). A contribution to the philosophy of medicine: The basic models of the doctor-patient relationship. *Archives of Internal Medicine, 97*(5), 585–592.

Wald, H. S., Dube, C. E., & Anthony, D. C. (2007). Untangling the web—The impact of internet use on health care and the physician-patient relationship. *Patient Education and Counseling, 68*(3), 218–224.

Suggested Resources

American Academy of HIV Medicine. (2009, January 20). *Connecting HIV infected patients to care: A review of best practices*. Retrieved April 2, 2012 from http://www.aahivm.org/upload_module/upload/provider%20resources/aahivmlinkagetocarereportonbestpractices.pdf.
American Public Health Association. (2004, June). *Adherence to HIV treatment regimens: Recommendations for best practices*. Retrieved April 2, 2012 from http://www.apha.org/NR/rdonlyres/A030DDB1-02C8-4D80-923B-7EF6608D62F1/0/BestPracticesnew.pdf.
Maldonado, J., Gore-Felton, C., Durán, R., Diamond, S., Koopman, C., & Spiegel, D. (1996). *Supportive-expressive group therapy for people with HIV infection: A primer*. Stanford, CA Retrieved April 12, 2012 from http://stresshealthcenter.stanford.edu/research/documents/GroupLeaderPrimerforHIVGroupTherapyStudy.pdf

Prevention Strategies

Sana Loue

Prevention programs frequently emphasize one or more of the following behavioral modifications, depending upon the individuals who are the focus of the program and the context in which the program is situated: abstinence, condom use, reduction in number of partners/monogamy, and the use of clean injection paraphernalia. Additionally, the development and/or dissemination of prevention strategies are often premised on one or more theories of behavior change, such as the theory of reasoned action, diffusion theory, the health belief model, and others. This entry addresses various behavior modifications that are often utilized as the basis of HIV prevention efforts.

Abstinence

Abstinence has been promoted as a strategy to prevent HIV transmission. While it is true that sexual transmission of HIV cannot occur in the absence sexual relations, research suggests that abstinence may not be an effective prevention approach. Research has found that reliance on an abstinence-only approach is correlated with increased teenage pregnancy and birth rates, suggesting that it would be similarly ineffective as a HIV prevention strategy. In contrast, abstinence-plus programs, which include a focus on abstinence as one component of a program that also includes safer sex messages, appear to lead to reduced HIV risk.

S. Loue (✉)
Department of Epidemiology and Biostatistics, Case Western Reserve University, Cleveland, OH, USA
e-mail: Sana.Loue@case.edu

S. Loue (ed.), *Mental Health Practitioner's Guide to HIV/AIDS*,
DOI 10.1007/978-1-4614-5283-6_68, © Springer Science+Business Media New York 2013

Antiretroviral Regimens and Prevention of Mother-to-Child Transmission

It has been estimated that more than one-half million infants worldwide become HIV-infected as the result of mother-to-child transmission. Transmission can occur during pregnancy, during labor and delivery, or following birth through the mother's breast milk. It has been estimated that, in the absence of breastfeeding, approximately 30% of infant HIV infections occur in utero and an additional 70% occur during the process of labor and delivery. Research suggests that as much as 40% of infant infections may be attributable to breastfeeding, with the vast majority of the infections occurring during the first few months of the infant's life. Increased viral load appears to be associated with an increased risk of maternal transmission of the virus during breastfeeding.

Results from clinical trials indicate that the incidence of perinatal transmission can be drastically reduced through the use of a short course of zidovudine (AZT) treatment of the mother and the child. Some studies have demonstrated a 50% reduction in HIV transmission among mothers who did not breastfeed and who were administered AZT twice a day beginning at 36 weeks of pregnancy and every 3 h during labor. One clinical trial, known as the PACT 076 trial, found that mother-to-infant transmission was reduced by 68% in women who received AZT during 14–34 weeks of pregnancy and intravenously during labor, and whose infants received AZT during the first 6 weeks of life.

Condom Use

Condoms have been consistently recommended as a mechanism for HIV risk reduction and prevention for individuals regardless of their biological sex or sexual orientation. Clinical trials indicate that condoms are very effective in preventing HIV transmission between individuals engaged in opposite-sex (heterosexual) sexual relations. One study found that among individuals who always use condoms, the incidence of HIV is 0.9 per 10 person-years, while among those who never use condoms, the incidence of HIV transmission is 6.8 per 100 person-years. In general, the condom has been found to be approximately 87% effective in preventing HIV transmission among heterosexuals. Various factors have been found to be associated with increased condom use, including knowledge of HIV, perceived susceptibility to HIV , later age at initiating sexual relations, a belief that one's peers and friends utilize condoms, previous condom use, carrying a condom, communication with one's sexual partner about condom use, and more positive attitudes towards condom use. Individuals with higher educational levels and socioeconomic status have also been found to be more likely to use condoms.

There are, however, significant barriers to women's use of prevention strategies with their male sexual partners. These include unequal power in the relationship and the threat of or use of partner violence; the cultural context of the relationships, which may discourage women from engaging in communication about sexuality with their sexual partners; and a cultural emphasis on the role of motherhood, which precludes the use of condoms. Although prevention programs that stress self-management skills and sexual communication skills can reduce these barriers to some extent, they emphasize factors at the level of the individual and fail to address the social and cultural influences that make consistent condom use difficult.

HIV Testing and Counseling

The Centers for Disease Control and Prevention has recommended that HIV testing be made a routine part of medical care for individuals in high HIV-prevalence clinical settings, those with high risk behaviors in low HIV-prevalence clinical settings, and those in clinical settings characterized by high HIV risk, such as clinics that provide diagnosis and treatment of sexually transmitted infections. Testing can be accomplished with a blood test at a clinic, a public health facility, or with a home testing kit. HIV counseling provides the individual with not only the results of his or her HIV test, but also information relating to the meaning of the test result and strategies to prevent transmission. If the individual is HIV-infected, HIV counseling can also provide him or her with referrals for care and services.

Monogamy/Reduction in Number of Sexual Partners

Monogamy can work as a HIV prevention strategy if both partners involved in the sexual relationship, whether same-sex or opposite-sex, define their sexual relationship as exclusive. However, research findings indicate that although women in heterosexual relationships may be engaging in unprotected sexual relations with only one partner, they may be at risk of HIV transmission due to their sexual partner's risk behaviors such as unprotected sexual relations with others or the sharing of injection paraphernalia with others. Risk for either partner may be increased, even if they are monogamous within their relationship, if they have engaged in unprotected sexual relations with others prior to the current relationship and do not know their HIV serostatus. Similar issues exist within same-sex relationships in that an individual who is monogamous within that relationship may be at increased risk depending upon his or her sexual partner's risk behaviors and his or her own prior sexual relationships.

Research has also found that HIV risk increases with an increased number of sexual partners. These sexual relationships may occur sequentially or concurrently. An increased rate of change of sexual partners is likely to increase an individual's risk of HIV infection, as well as the risk for other sexually transmitted infections.

Syringe Exchange

Syringe exchange is a public health approach to reduce the health risks associated with injection drug use, including HIV transmission. Research conducted in various countries has consistently demonstrated that individuals' use of syringe exchange programs lowers their risk of contracting HIV infection. Syringe exchange programs typically offer a wide range of services in addition to syringe exchange and sterilizing equipment such as alcohol and cotton swabs. These include information about HIV//AIDS and strategies for preventing its transmission; HIV testing and counseling; the provision of condoms; referrals to substance abuse treatment, medical and social services; screening for diseases such as tuberculosis (TB) and hepatitis C and B; and the provision of primary health care services.

Implications for Mental Health Care Providers

Although many mental health care providers believe that their clients are not sexually active, particularly those with severe mental illness such as schizophrenia and major depression, research findings indicate that individuals with mental illness may actually be at elevated risk for HIV transmission. It is critical, therefore, that mental health care providers discuss with their clients their sexual relationships, the measures that the clients are utilizing to prevent HIV and other sexually transmitted infections, and additional measures that can be used to prevent infection. This review of prevention strategies should include the need to use condoms and to reduce the number of sexual partners, whether they are concurrent or sequential. Clients who share injection paraphernalia can be referred to syringe exchange programs if one exists in the geographic area and/or to recovery services. Clients who appear to be engaging in high risk behaviors, or who have partners who are engaging in high risk behaviors, should be referred for HIV testing and counseling. Clients who are pregnant or who are contemplating pregnancy should be provided with referrals for HIV testing and counseling and, if they are found to be HIV seropositive, with referrals to physicians or clinic who are able to advise the mother about the risks of perinatal transmission and the availability of preventive treatment regimens. Engaging clients in a discussion of their sexual- and drug-related risk behaviors will likely be easier if the mental health care provider is comfortable discussing issues related to sexuality and sexual behavior.

Related Topics: Case management, Contact tracing, Harm reduction, HIV counseling, HIV testing, Partner notification, Quarantine and isolation, Risk behaviors, Syringe exchange

Suggested Readings

Amaro, H. (1995). Love, sex, and power: Considering women's realities in HIV prevention. *American Psychologist, 50*(6), 437–447.

Davis, K. R., & Weller, S. C. (1999). The effectiveness of condoms in reducing heterosexual transmission of HIV. *Family Planning Perspectives, 31*(6), 272–279.

De Cock, K. M., Fowler, M. G., Mercier, E., de Vincenzi, I., Saba, J., Hoff, E., et al. (2000). Prevention of mother-to-child HIV transmission in resource-poor countries: Translating research into policy and practice. *Journal of the American Medical Association, 283*(9), 1175–1182.

Sheeran, P., Abraham, C., & Orbell, S. (1999). Psychosocial correlates of heterosexual condom use: A meta-analysis. *Psychological Bulletin, 125*(1), 90–132.

Shelton, J. D., Halperin, D. T., Nantulya, V., Potts, M., Gayle, H. D., & Holmes, K. K. (2004). Partner reduction is crucial for balanced "ABC" approach to HIV prevention. *British Medical Journal, 328*, 891–894.

Stanger-Hall, K.F., & Hall, D.W. (2011). Abstinence-only education and teen pregnancy rates: Why we need comprehensive sex education in the U.S. *PLoS One, 6*(10), e24658. Retrieved April 20, 2012 from http://www,plosone.org.

Underhill, K., Operario, D., & Montgomery, P. (2007). Systematic review of abstinence-plus HIV prevention programs in high-income countries. *PLoS Medicine, 4*(9), e275, Retrieved April 20, 2012 from http://www.plosmedicine.org

Protease Inhibitors

Todd Wagner

Antiretroviral drugs are classified by the viral life cycle they inhibit and, in some cases, by their chemical structure. There are currently five classes of antiretroviral drugs: nucleoside reverse transcriptase inhibitors (NRTI), non-nucleoside reverse transcriptase inhibitors (NNRTI), protease inhibitors (PI), integrase inhibitors, and entry inhibitors. Although grouped in classes, these medications have unique side effect profiles, drug–drug interactions, and potency. All currently recommended treatment regiments consist of a backbone of two NRTIs and a third antiretroviral drug, typically a NNRTI, a ritonavir-boosted protease inhibitor, or an integrase inhibitor. It is important for care providers of HIV-infected patients with psychiatric or substance abuse disorders to recognize the potential interactions between psychotropic and antiretroviral medications, especially with respect to protease inhibitors.

All protease inhibitors are metabolized by the cytochrome P450 (CYP) system and possess enzyme-inhibiting or enzyme-inducing properties. Cytochrome P450 enzymes are responsible for drug metabolism and bioactivation of various substrates, including many psychotropic medications. Drugs that interact with the CYP system usually do so in one of three ways—by acting as a substrate, through inhibition, or through induction. A drug can at the same time be a substrate for and induce or inhibit one or more CYP enzymes. Enzyme inhibition usually involves competition with another drug for the enzyme binding site. Enzyme induction occurs when a drug stimulates the synthesis of more enzyme protein, enhancing the enzyme's metabolizing capacity. Individuals may also exhibit genetic polymorphisms which result in varying levels of activity for specific enzymes, and therefore altered levels of drug metabolism.

Inhibition of CYP metabolic pathways by ritonavir, a protease inhibitor, forms the basis for its use with other "boosted" protease inhibitors. Ritonavir is a potent inhibitor of CYP3A4, the enzyme primarily involved in the metabolism of most

T. Wagner (✉)
University Hospitals Case Medical Center, Cleveland, OH, USA
e-mail: todd.wagner@case.edu

S. Loue (ed.), *Mental Health Practitioner's Guide to HIV/AIDS*,
DOI 10.1007/978-1-4614-5283-6_69, © Springer Science+Business Media New York 2013

protease inhibitors. Ritonavir's inhibition of the CYP3A4 enzyme reduces the metabolism of a concomitantly administered protease inhibitor, resulting in increased bioavailability and penetration of the boosted-protease inhibitor, despite reduced doses and less frequent administration. Although the drug interaction involving ritonavir has proven beneficial in antiretroviral therapy regiments with respect to boosted-protease inhibitors, other potential CYP interactions may lead to toxicity or failure.

Numerous medications used to treat individuals with psychiatric and substance abuse disorders interact with the CYP system and are at risk for drug interaction. Although the clinical significance of such interactions is not always known, additional monitoring and consideration of dose adjustments are warranted. For example, selective serotonin reuptake inhibitors all have the potential to interact with protease inhibitors given they are all metabolized by CYP enzymes. Serotonin syndrome is a potential risk when selective serotonin reuptake inhibitors are combined with a potent CYP inhibitor, such as ritonavir. Tricyclic antidepressants are also metabolized by CYP enzymes. Close observations for signs and symptoms of tricyclic toxicity is necessary when combining tricyclic antidepressants with CYP inhibitors.

Given the prevalence of psychiatric and substance abuse disorders among HIV-infected individuals, addressing their mental health is critical to maintaining quality of life, antiretroviral therapy adherence, and limiting HIV disease progression. The potential interaction of psychotropic medications with antiretroviral drugs, such as protease inhibitors, should not prohibit their use, rather should demand careful consideration and close monitoring for potential interactions.

Related Topics: Adherence, Antiretroviral therapy

Suggested Readings

Johns, M., & Tracy, T. (1998). Cytochrome P450: New nomenclature and clinical implications. *American Family Physician, 57*(1), 107–116.

Nijhawan, A., Kim, S., & Rich, J. D. (2008). Management of HIV infection in patients with substance abuse problems. *Current Infectious Disease Reports, 10*(5), 432–438.

Thompson, A., Silverman, B., Dzeng, L., & Treisman, G. (2006). Psychotropic medications and HIV. *Clinical Infectious Diseases, 42*, 1305–1310.

Quarantine and Isolation

Nicholas K. Schiltz

Introduction

The act of removing sick individuals away from the rest of society dates back to ancient times. Quarantines have been imposed throughout history to protect a society from infected foreigners or sailors or in response to outbreaks of diseases like yellow fever, cholera, and tuberculosis. The words "quarantine" and "isolation" are often used interchangeably, though they are in fact different. *Quarantine* confines people who have been exposed to a communicable disease for the disease's presumed incubation period. *Isolation* is the practice of isolating an individual known to be contagious, commonly in a health facility, for the duration of the illness.

Isolation of HIV-infected persons was discussed as a potential approach to controlling the disease as AIDS was emerging in the 1980s. Opposition from advocacy groups, health practitioners, and researchers, as well as public apprehension toward mandatory isolation, curtailed any efforts to quarantine the HIV/AIDS population in most of the world. One notable exception was Cuba, which implemented mandatory HIV testing and required infected individuals to live in sanatoriums, although these policies have since been lifted. Two states in the USA currently isolate HIV-positive inmates from the general prison population. Many social, legal, ethical, and epidemiological issues arise out of the practice of quarantine, including the relationship between individual civil rights and population health.

N.K. Schiltz (✉)
Department of Epidemiology and Biostatistics, School of Medicine, Case Western Reserve University, Cleveland, OH, USA
e-mail: nks8@case.edu

S. Loue (ed.), *Mental Health Practitioner's Guide to HIV/AIDS*,
DOI 10.1007/978-1-4614-5283-6_70,

Epidemiology

The majority of HIV transmissions occur through sexual contact with an infected person. Other forms of transmission include contact with infected blood or mother-to-child transmission. HIV is not airborne and casual contact with infected persons is not a risk factor. HIV/AIDS is pandemic; an estimated 33 million people worldwide are currently infected. The incidence of new cases is 2.6 million per year, and mortality is estimated at 1.8 million deaths annually.

The purpose of quarantine is to stop the spread of infectious disease in the general population. Because most infectious diseases transfer by human to human contact, isolating infected individuals from society until they are no longer contagious can prevent the further spread of disease. The following conditions should be present for quarantine or isolation to be effective and practical: the duration of the incubation period must be relatively short, the number of persons infected should be low, infected individuals should be easily identifiable, and the attack rate of disease (i.e., how contagious it is through casual contact) should be high. None of these conditions are true for HIV/AIDS. Therefore, quarantine and isolation of the HIV/AIDS population is not an effective or practical strategy to control the spread of disease.

Legal Issues

The International Health Regulations is binding international law authored by the World Health Organization that deals with global health risks. This document reaffirms the State's right to implement procedures such as quarantine and isolation to prevent the spread of communicable diseases.

The US government has the legal right to enforce quarantine and isolation. These laws address diseases that are communicated through casual contact, such as through airborne transmission, and therefore HIV has never been included among the diseases listed for quarantine. Any attempt to quarantine HIV patients would be arguably unconstitutional unless the state can show it meets the specific goal of public health protection.

Thirty-four states in the USA and multiple countries have laws against the criminal transmission of HIV, whereby a known infected individual has unprotected sex with others to purposefully spread the virus. Several states also have laws that require HIV-positive individuals to notify their sexual partners or face criminal prosecution or civil lawsuits. In rare cases, states have detained HIV-positive individuals that were believed to be a risk to others, but usually only for a brief period.

Social Issues

Quarantine and isolation of HIV-positive individuals has been denounced as unnecessary and stigmatizing by UNAIDS and the World Health Organization (WHO). If the disease in question is associated with a particular race or ethnic group this can lead to stigmatization of that group. At the beginning of the outbreak, HIV/AIDS was associated with gay men and intravenous drug users—two groups of people already marginalized by society.

Surveys of public attitudes toward AIDS in the USA have shown that a majority of Americans do not think that persons with AIDS should be isolated from society. While 34% said they should be isolated in 1991, just 12% thought the same in 1999, indicating public support for isolation of persons with AIDS is minimal. However, the same survey found that stigmatization exists in other areas, and that as many as 50% believed casual social contact (e.g., sharing a glass, sneezing, coughing) increased the risk of transmission.

Ethical Issues

The ethical issues around quarantine generally revolve around the trade-off between individual autonomy and the greater public welfare. Liberalism tends to place great emphasis on individual autonomy and civil rights, and therefore measures such as mandatory testing and quarantine are usually not implemented in Western liberal democracies. Communist, autocratic, and tribal societies may place more value on the community, and countries with these forms of government are often more likely to implement compulsory measures for the good of the public.

The U.N. Declaration of Human Rights tends to favor individual autonomy and civil rights. Quarantine and isolation are often done in violation of international documents such as the U.N. Declaration of Human Rights. Quarantine involves a sacrifice of certain rights in that a person is held in detention, despite the fact they have done nothing criminal.

HIV-positive persons who behave recklessly by having unprotected sex or sharing needles do put others in society in danger of infection. There will be people who will contract the HIV virus who otherwise may not have if known-infected individuals were isolated from society. Cuba, which does require isolation for a brief period, has the lowest prevalence of HIV in the Caribbean. Proponents of isolation will argue that it is more unethical to expose the general public to the risk of future transmission than to protect the rights of those already infected.

The general consensus among health organizations and health professionals is against the quarantine of persons with HIV/AIDS on grounds that it is impractical, ineffective, and unethical.

HIV/AIDS Quarantine in Cuba

In the 1980s, Cuba diverged from the rest of the world by requiring HIV-positive persons to live in sanatoria that were isolated from the general population permanently. In addition, the centralized government of Cuba implemented compulsory testing of HIV. An estimated 12 million tests were performed on the population of 11 million citizens prior to 1994. In 1994 these laws were relaxed to require quarantine of infected individuals for an 8-week education program. After the 8 weeks persons are free to leave, but many stay for free care. Supporters have pointed out that, based on statistics, Cuba's HIV/AIDS program is one of the best in the world. Cuba has a very low incidence rate of HIV, compared to other low-income countries and has a mortality rate 35 times lower than the USA. Critics contend that this program violated basic human rights and trampled on individual autonomy. Others have insisted that Cuba's low incidence rates can be attributed to other factors such as isolation from most of the developed world and their universal health care system.

Isolation in Prison Populations

At one time 47 out of 51 state and federal prison systems in the USA had laws segregating HIV-positive prisoners from the rest of the population. Today, two states still have laws that require isolation of HIV-positive patients: South Carolina and Alabama. Federal courts have upheld a state's right to segregate prisoners based on HIV status. Poor health facilities, lack of condoms, and shared needles may contribute to higher risk of transmission among the prison population. The WHO guidelines declare that isolation among prisoners is not useful and should only be done in case-specific situations deemed necessary by medical personal.

Conclusion

Due to the nature of the disease and how the HIV retrovirus is transmitted, the quarantine or isolation of persons with HIV/AIDS is not recognized as a viable strategy by most of the public health community. The ethical, legal, and social ramifications of quarantine are high relative to the net public health benefits. Efforts to control the disease through behavioral change are preferred through mechanisms such as education, health promotion campaigns, or programs that make condoms more readily available.

Related Topics: HIV testing, Human rights, Legal issues for HIV-infected clients, Prevention strategies, Stigma and stigmatization

Suggested Readings

Anderson, T. (2009). HIV/AIDS in Cuba: A rights-based analysis. *Health and Human Rights, 11* (1), 93–104.

Fee, E., & Parry, M. (2008). Jonathan Mann, HIV/AIDS, and human rights. *Journal of Public Health Policy, 29*(1), 54–71. doi:10.1057/palgrave.jphp. 3200160.

Hansen, H., & Groce, N. E. (2001). From quarantine to condoms: Shifting policies and problems of HIV control in Cuba. *Medical Anthropology, 19*(3), 259–292. doi:10.1080/01459740.2001.9966178.

Harrington, J. A. (2002). The instrumental uses of autonomy: A review of AIDS law and policy in Europe. *Social Science & Medicine (1982), 55*(8), 1425–1434.

Herek, G. M., Capitanio, J. P., & Widaman, K. F. (2002). HIV-related stigma and knowledge in the United States: Prevalence and trends, 1991–1999. *American Journal of Public Health, 92*(3), 371–377.

Musto, D. F. (1986). Quarantine and the problem of AIDS. *The Milbank Quarterly, 64*(Suppl. 1), 97–117.

Webber, D. W. (1997). *AIDS and the law* (3rd ed.). New York: John Wiley & Sons, Inc.

Relativism

Nicole M. Deming

Relativism is a philosophical theory that states that there are no absolute truths, only subjective truths based on an individual, group or custom. To determine what is right or wrong, a relativist would look to the social norms of the society that raises the question. This theory is based on the observation that beliefs vary and that these beliefs are based upon an individual's upbringing, education, and community. Initially, relativism is a very attractive theory because we observe that our patients have different values. These values are tied to family, religion and the patient's experiences. We are taught to respect different views, and be sensitive to how our behavior will be interpreted by different cultures. However, there are many problems with relativism as a moral theory and most ethicists do not considered it a strong theory. If we accept relativism, we could say nothing against the practices of Nazi scientists in concentration camps, infanticide, or slavery because these practices were accepted in pastsocieties. Our current society believes these practices are wrong, but we cannot say we are more ethical, just different.

The study of ethics and moral philosophy is often separated into two categories: (1) Nonnormative and (2) Normative. Nonnormative ethics is concerned with descriptive ethics and metaethics (defining terms or theories of reasoning). Nonnormative ethics are often useful when describing a culture or code of ethics. Nonnormative ethics explains the ethics that exist but does not make a value judgment about the ethics being practiced. In contrast, normative ethics deals with claims of right and wrong. When we are dealing with a patient and working in the clinical context, we may observe the ethics of a particular patient (nonnormative), but we are ultimately looking for how to act ethically in a given situation (normative).

The benefits of considering relativism include the recognition that we are influenced and situated in a particular time and place. Relativism calls into question the justification of our moral beliefs and what, if anything, is different from the

N.M. Deming (✉)
Department of Bioethics, Case Western Reserve University, Cleveland, OH, USA
e-mail: Nicole.Deming@case.edu

S. Loue (ed.), *Mental Health Practitioner's Guide to HIV/AIDS*, DOI 10.1007/978-1-4614-5283-6_71, © Springer Science+Business Media New York 2013

concepts we use to justify our ethical framework. How can I claim that my beliefs are better or more ethical than my patients? On the other side, we must recognize that we do not live in a world where we accept all actions as ethical. When values conflict or oppose each other, we generally try to find the action that is more ethical.

It is important that mental health care providers be cognizant of this distinction between normative and nonnormative ethics. Although an understanding of a patient's values and the context in which those values were developed are critical in both forming and maintaining a therapeutic alliance, a patient's values and behaviors may not be congruent with his or her health, the health or safety of others, or the law. As an example, providers may understand why an HIV-positive patient with severe anxiety does not disclose his HIV seropositivity to sexual partners and chooses to engage in unprotected sexual relations. However, this conduct places his own health and that of others at risk and, depending upon the particular state, may be in violation of state law.

Related Topics: Cultural sensitivity, Declaration of Helsinki, Universalism

Suggested Readings

Barnes, B., & Bloor, D. (1982). Relativism, rationalism and the sociology of knowledge. In M. Hollis & S. Lukes (Eds.), *Rationality and relativism* (pp. 21–47). Oxford, UK: Basil Blackwell.

Sulmasy, D., & Sugarman, J. (Eds.), (2001). The many methods of medical ethics (or thirteen ways of looking at a blackbird). In *Methods in medical ethics* (pp. 3–18). Washington, D.C.: Georgetown University Press.

Wood, A. (2002). Chapter 5: Relativism. In *Unsettling obligations: Essays on reason, reality, and the ethics of belief.* Stanford, CA: Center for the Study of Language and Information, Publishers.

Suggested Resources

Santa Clara University Markkula Center for Applied Ethics. Retrieved February 29, 2012 from http://www.scu.edu/ethics/practicing/decision/ethicalrelativism.html

Stanford encyclopedia of philosophy. Retrieved February 29, 2012 from http://plato.stanford.edu/entries/relativism/

Religion and Spirituality

Sana Loue

Religion and spirituality have been found to be important resources for individuals living and coping with HIV/AIDS. These coping methods include spiritual transformation, a belief in a higher power and/or miracles, prayer, and collaboration between the individual and God or a higher power. Studies have found that individuals' reliance on such methods is associated with greater levels of optimism, hope, self-esteem, social support, and helping others; less emotional distress; lower cortisol levels, which indicate lower stress levels; and longer survival. Individuals may also derive a sense of purpose and of peace from their religious or spiritual beliefs. Increased frequency of church attendance has been found to be associated with keeping current with medical appointments. Among injection drug users, more church attendance has been found to be associated with HIV testing, HIV-positive status, and receiving medical care for HIV, suggesting that the church may be both an important source of support and friendship for injection drug users.

However, researchers have also found that some religious/spiritual beliefs may have negative effects. A stronger belief that HIV is a sin has been found to be associated with not being in medical care, and a belief that HIV is a punishment from God has been linked to longer delay between the time of HIV diagnosis and the initiation of treatment for HIV. HIV-positive individuals who are experiencing religious struggles may suffer ill effects such as increased depression, alienation, shame, and/or guilt. This may be due to the stigma associated with HIV in some religious groups or with risk behaviors that led to the HIV infection, such as injection drug use and same-sex sexual relations.

Religious or spiritual beliefs may also be critical to HIV prevention among individuals who are HIV-negative. Individuals who ascribe to particular religious tenets, such as abstinence from intoxicants, may refrain from using alcohol and illicit substances, which may directly or indirectly increase the risk of HIV

S. Loue (✉)
Department of Epidemiology and Biostatistics, Case Western Reserve University, Cleveland, OH, USA
e-mail: Sana.Loue@case.edu

S. Loue (ed.), *Mental Health Practitioner's Guide to HIV/AIDS*,
DOI 10.1007/978-1-4614-5283-6_72,

transmission. Similarly, those who adhere to religious beliefs that permit sexual intercourse only within the context of marriage may be less likely to engage in sexual relations with multiple partners, thereby decreasing the risk of HIV transmission associated with their own behaviors.

These research findings suggest that it is important that mental health care providers understand their clients' religious/spiritual beliefs, regardless of the client's HIV serostatus. The provider may wish to reinforce client beliefs that help the HIV-negative client to reduce his or her HIV risk or encourage the HIV-positive client to adhere to treatment and provide adequate self care. In contrast, beliefs that appear to exacerbate a client's mental health symptoms, such as depressive symptoms associated with guilt or shame, or erect a barrier to the client's presentation for adequate treatment, should be addressed. It will be important for mental health care providers to help clients counter negative internalized messages that stem from religious beliefs of sin and punishment.

Related Topics: Coping, Faith community, Social support

Suggested Readings

Latkin, C. A., Tobin, K. E., & Gilbert, S. H. (2002). Sun or support: The role of religious behaviors and HIV-related health care among drug users in Baltimore, Maryland. *AIDS and Behavior, 6* (4), 321–329.

Loue, S., & Sajatovic, M. (2006). Spirituality, coping, and HIV risk and prevention in a sample of severely mentally ill Puerto Rican women. *Journal of Urban Health, 83*(6), 1168–1182.

Pargament, K. I., McCarthy, S., Shah, P., Ano, G., Tarakeshwar, N., Wachholtz, A., et al. (2004). Religion and HIV: A review of the literature and clinical implications. *Southern Medical Journal, 97*(12), 1201–1209.

Parsons, S. K., Cruise, P. L., Davenport, W. M., & Jones, V. (2006). Religious beliefs, practices and treatment adherence among individuals with HIV in the southern United States. *AIDS Patient Care, 20*(2), 97–111.

Reproduction

Bryan R. Taylor and Susan Hatters-Friedman

Since many women with HIV are either diagnosed during pregnancy or desire to become pregnant, healthcare providers, including mental health care providers, should have a basic understanding regarding HIV and reproduction. The progression of HIV disease does not appear to be influenced by pregnancy. Advancements in drug therapy, access to healthcare, and increased information regarding HIV's lifecycle, transmission, and pathology affect the way we treat individuals who are pregnant or planning for pregnancy.

Epidemiology

In the USA, the number of women infected with HIV/AIDS has rapidly increased. According to 2007 Centers for Disease Control and Prevention (CDC) data, women accounted for 27% of newly acquired HIV/AIDS cases. Eighty percent of new cases in women are contracted through heterosexual intercourse, and 20% from infected needles and other methods of infection including vertical transmission from mother to infant. The majority of women are diagnosed between the ages of 25–44 years, suggesting that many women contract the virus during their reproductive years.

Vertical transmission rates from mother to infant in the absence of treatment are estimated to be as high as 25–30%. Prior to the development of antiretroviral medications, approximately 2,000 babies were born infected with HIV each year in the USA. Currently only 300 infants in the USA are infected with HIV per year despite the increasing prevalence of HIV. In the USA, the mother-to-infant risk of

B.R. Taylor (✉)
Cleveland, OH, USA
e-mail: brytay22@gmail.com

S. Hatters-Friedman
Department of Psychiatry, School of Medicine, Case Western Reserve University, Cleveland, OH, USA

S. Loue (ed.), *Mental Health Practitioner's Guide to HIV/AIDS*,
DOI 10.1007/978-1-4614-5283-6_73,

transmission has decreased to less than 2% due to implementation of HIV antiretroviral medication, testing availability, counseling, and delivery by cesarean section prior to onset of delivery.

Pregnancy Planning

Individuals with HIV of reproductive age who are interested in pregnancy should be encouraged to plan pregnancy to reduce the risk of transmission. Depending on which partner is infected, different strategies help decrease the risk of transmission in disconcordant couples. Studies have shown that women with HIV are less fertile. Women's viral load should be stable and maximally suppressed prior to conception. On average, conception occurs after 6 months with two acts of intercourse per ovulatory cycle. Therefore, based on what is known about decreased fertility, couples must weigh the risk of transmission even with an undetectable viral load. Females with HIV should consider alternative reproductive techniques in order to prevent transmission.

If the male partner is infected, adoption and sperm donation should be considered due to risk of infection. Assisted reproduction techniques may be considered with an infected male if the couple will not consider adoption or sperm donation. Despite antiretroviral therapy, viral load is typically greater in seminal fluid than in plasma. Therefore, blood viral load levels are not fully representative of transmission risk. Undetectable seminal viral load levels are considered for insemination. However, when seminal viral load levels are elevated despite antiretroviral therapy, semen washing may decrease HIV RNA and DNA to undetectable levels and may be used for intrauterine insemination or in-vitro fertilization. When both partners are infected, it is important to determine HIV serology to ensure partners do not co-infect with different strains of the HIV virus.

It is important to conduct a discussion about planning pregnancy and risks with individuals diagnosed with HIV. Because half of all pregnancies are unintended in the USA, the CDC and the American Congress of Obstetrics and Gynecology (ACOG) recommend preconception counseling to all women of childbearing age as a component of routine primary care. Since HIV-infected women who refuse contraceptive use are more likely to become pregnant, open communication between provider and patient about mother-to-infant transmission of HIV is essential to reduce likelihood of infant infection. Current and future pregnant HIV-positive women will need special consideration to determine optimal antiretroviral therapy in order to minimize the risk of teratogenic effects of some medications. The discussion should also stress the importance of compliance with medication regimens, cessation of smoking, and updating immunizations.

Screening

Screening for HIV is recommended by the CDC for all pregnant women as part of routine prenatal tests. Testing should be done early in pregnancy in order to start appropriate antiretroviral therapy, and strategically plan to decrease risk of transmission to the fetus. A woman's reasons for declining testing should be discussed and she should be encouraged to be screened. Furthermore, a second HIV test during the third trimester should be considered if the woman is at high risk or shows signs of acute infection. Despite current recommendations, 30% of pregnant women are not tested for HIV as part of the prenatal workup. Furthermore, 15–20% of women in the general population do not receive any form of prenatal care.

When HIV status is unknown during labor, rapid testing should be considered. Antiretroviral therapy should be initiated without waiting for confirmatory testing if a rapid test is positive. If postpartum HIV status is unknown, it is recommended that both mother and infant be tested. Newborn antiretroviral therapy is most effective within the first 12 h after birth.

Antiretroviral Medications

Increased risk of perinatal transmission of HIV is related to viral load. Antiretroviral therapy (ART) should be considered by all pregnant women to decrease the risk of transmission, as it has been shown to decrease risk to below 2%. Combination ART is recommended for all cases of HIV and should include Zidovudine—which is the only antiretroviral to demonstrate a decrease in perinatal transmission—both intrapartum and antepartum. The choice of therapy should take into account ART response history, resistance to medications, fetal gestational age, potential toxicity to fetus, drug interaction, pill burden, and lifestyle.

Once therapy has been initiated, it should not be discontinued due to possible increase in viral resistance (unless the regime is not tolerated or resistance occurs). CD4 count, viral load, transaminases, lactate levels, and hemoglobin should all be monitored for adverse effects of therapy, to ensure adequate suppression of viral load, to decrease the chance of transmission, and to monitor for resistance.

The goal of the various medications that are prescribed for the treatment of HIV infection—nucleotide analogue reverse transcriptase inhibitors (NRTIs), non-nucleoside reverse transcriptase inhibitors (NNRTIs) and protease inhibitors (PIs)—is to decrease the maternal viral load. Additionally, these drugs can cross the placenta and potentially provide fetal prophylaxis as well. The Antiretroviral Pregnancy Registry has not reported any congenital malformations with exposure to antiretrovirals even in the first trimester, with the exception of enfavirenz. However, combination therapy has been associated with preeclampsia (when a pregnant woman develops high blood pressure and protein in the urine after the 20th week of pregnancy).

NRTIs in general are well tolerated and cross the placenta. Adversely, these drugs may cause mitochondrial dysfunction (inability of mitochondrial structures to carry out their designated functions within a cell, namely energy production in the form of ATP) leading to cardiomyopathy (deterioration of the function of the heart muscle), neuropathy (damage to a nerve which results in loss of movement, sensation or function), lactic acidosis (a condition defined by low pH in the blood and body tissues accompanied by buildup of lactate which is produced when oxygen levels in the body decrease), and liver dysfunction. These effects usually subside once the medication has been discontinued. Didanosine/stavudine combination should only be used in the case of resistance or toxicity to other NRTIs, due to possible hepatic (liver) failure from mitochondrial toxicity (a condition that occurs when the body's mitochondria become damaged or significantly decreased in number) and lactic acidosis.

Less information about the effects of NNRTIs in pregnancy is known. Nevirapine and enfavirenz cross the placenta. Neural tube defects have been reported after exposure to enfavirenz in the first trimester. Rash is the most common side effect seen with nevirapine. However, fatal hepatotoxicity appears to be increased in pregnancy; therefore, nevirapine should be avoided unless no other option is available or it was already part of therapy when pregnancy was diagnosed.

In contrast, protease inhibitors (PIs) do not easily cross the placenta and have not been noted to have teratogenic effects (abnormal embryonic development) in animals. Though studies show contrasting results, there may be an elevated risk of prematurity and low birth weights among infants exposed to combination therapy with PIs. Glucose intolerance has been associated with the use of PIs and should be closely monitored throughout pregnancy.

Treatment Recommendations

HIV-infected pregnant women currently receiving therapy generally should continue the regime as long as it is tolerated. Stopping therapy could lead to increased viral load –consequently leading to disease progression and decreased immunity as well as an increased risk of transmission to the fetus. Drug resistance testing should be utilized if viral load is detectable on current therapy. Virally suppressed patients already on nevirapine should continue treatment as long as they are tolerating the regimen. Efavirenz-containing therapy should be avoided where possible during the first trimester. Due to the long half-life of efavirenz and nevirapine, they must be stopped with a nucleoside backbone for 3–5 days to provide coverage during the process and reduce resistance evolution.

In HIV-infected pregnant women who are not currently receiving ART medications but have previously received ART, obtaining a detailed history of the prior treatment regimen and resistance is imperative. Before initiating therapy, resistance testing must be performed. A combination ART regimen is recommended and chosen based on resistance testing and prior history of viral suppression. Once therapy has been initiated, virologic response should be followed and provide guidance for future therapy.

Antiretroviral naïve HIV-infected pregnant women who meet the standard criteria for ART therapy (as outlined by adult ART guidelines) should receive combination therapy as recommended for non-pregnant adults, taking into account what is known about risks of teratogenicity and adverse effects. Treatment should be initiated immediately for women who require therapy for their own health. For women who do not require urgent therapy for their own health, initiation of three-drug combination therapy aimed at reducing perinatal transmission is recommended after completion of resistance testing.

For HIV-infected laboring women with no antepartum treatment, intravenous (IV) lidovudine should be immediately initiated. Zidovudine administration to the infant for 6 weeks following delivery is recommended. For infants of HIV-infected women who present following delivery, the same 6-week Zidovudine course is recommended. Furthermore, because of the risk of transmission, breastfeeding should be avoided in HIV-infected women if replacement feeding is a possibility.

Elective C-Section

Cesarean (C-section) delivery before the onset of labor eliminates viral exposure from blood and vaginal secretions during delivery and may avoid microtransfusion (when maternal blood passes across the placenta due to force of contractions) that occurs with contractions. Cesarean delivery is recommended for all HIV-infected women who have a viral load titer greater then 1000 copies/mL at 36 weeks gestation, in order to decrease transmission risk. Prophylactic antibiotics should be administered prior to cesarean section given the increased risk of morbidity and mortality associated with infection and decrease immune function.

Scheduled cesarean section should be discussed as early as possible in pregnancy to allow the HIV-infected woman to have adequate time to consider and plan for the procedure. The mother must decide if the benefits to her and her baby outweigh the risks involved.

Conclusion

Despite current efforts to halt the spread of HIV infection, women are now considered to have a rapidly increasing prevalence rate. Prenatal screening has been shown to play an important role in the diagnosis of HIV in women, and should be a part of routine prenatal testing. Both ACOG and CDC recommend that all HIV-infected women receive counseling regarding pregnancy immediately after a diagnosis has been made. Couples that desire to conceive should seek out assistance in a way that reduces the risk of transmission to the uninfected partner, and the fetus. It is recommended that HIV-infected women initiate treatment immediately in order to reduce the risk of mother-to-infant transmission. Zidovudine is the only antiretroviral proven to decrease the risk of transmission to the fetus, and therefore plays an important role in the treatment of both the mother and infant. Elective C-section should be discussed in the early stages of pregnancy, and is recommended for all HIV-infected women with viral loads greater then 1,000 copies/mL at 36 weeks gestation.

Related Topics: Antiretroviral therapy, Children, Protease inhibitors, Women

Suggested Readings

Centers for Disease Control and Prevention (CDC). (2006). Revised recommendations for HIV testing of adults, adolescents, and pregnant women in health-care settings. *Morbidity and Mortality Weekly Report, 55*(14), 1–17. Retrieved August 10, 2011 from http://www.cdc.gov/mmwr/preview/mmwrhtml/rr5514a1. htm?s_cid=.

Jamieson, D., Read, J., Kourtis, A., Durant, T., Lampe, M., & Dominguez, K. (2007). Cesarean delivery for HIV-infected women: recommendations and controversies. *American Journal of Obstetrics and Gynecology, 97*(3), S96–S100.

Rahangdale, L., & Cohan, D. (2008). Rapid human immunodeficiency virus testing on labor and delivery. *Obstetrics & Gynecology, 112*(1), 159–163.

Watts, H. (2002). Management of human immunodeficiency virus infection in pregnancy. *New England Journal of Medicine, 346*, 1879–1891.

Suggested Resources

http://aidsinfo.nih.gov/ContentFiles/Perinatal_FS_en.pdf
http://www.americanpregnancy.org/pregnancycomplications/hivaids.html
http://www.avert.org/pregnancy.htm
http://www.womenshealth.gov/hiv-aids/living-with-hiv-aids/pregnancy-and-hiv.cfm
http://whqlibdoc.who.int/publications/2008/9789241596596_eng.pdf

Risk Behaviors

Sana Loue

HIV can be transmitted through four mechanisms: unprotected intercourse with an HIV-infected sexual partner; the use of HIV-contaminated injection and other medical paraphernalia; mother-to-child transmission during pregnancy, labor and delivery, or through breastfeeding; and through contaminated blood. Sexual intercourse includes vaginal, anal, and oral intercourse. Transmission through injection drug use with contaminated injection equipment can occur due to the use of contaminated needles, syringes, cookers, and/or cotton. Although the HIV virus is present in tears and saliva, it cannot be transmitted through contact with these fluids. However, it can be transmitted through semen, vaginal and cervical secretions, blood and blood products, tissue and organs from HIV-infected donors, and breast milk.

Although HIV can be transmitted through any of these four mechanisms, the likelihood of transmission varies across these mechanisms. As an example, the risk of HIV transmission from an insertive HIV-infected partner to an uninfected receptive partner during an unprotected act of anal intercourse is approximately 1 in 50 compared to a risk of 1 in 1,000 or 2,000 that is associated with unprotected vaginal intercourse. However, the risk of transmission is increased in the presence of various other factors, such as infection with a sexually transmitted disease.

Research has found that individuals are less likely to practice safer sex behaviors with partners with whom they have been involved for an extended period of time compared to more casual partners. As a result, even though an individual may be in a monogamous relationship, he or she may be exposed to a risk of HIV transmission from his or her partner if the serostatus of that partner is unknown. Additionally, many individuals may have serially monogamous relationships, whereby they engage in a sequence of sexually exclusive relationships. Others may be realistically monogamous, meaning that they have serially monogamous relationships that

S. Loue (✉)
Department of Epidemiology and Biostatistics, Case Western Reserve University, Cleveland, OH, USA
e-mail: Sana.Loue@case.edu

S. Loue (ed.), *Mental Health Practitioner's Guide to HIV/AIDS*,
DOI 10.1007/978-1-4614-5283-6_74, © Springer Science+Business Media New York 2013

are interspersed with shorter, more casual sexual relationships. In either case, individuals may be engaging in sexual relations with individuals who do not know their HIV serostatus.

Some sexual practices may also be associated with increased HIV risk. These include felching (ejaculating into a partner's rectum and then using one's mouth to pull semen from the partner's rectum), fisting (inserting one's fist or hand into the partner's rectum), group sex, and snowballing (exchanging semen between mouths). Fisting, for example, can result in tears of the rectal tissue, which may increase the risk of HIV transmission through anal intercourse. Some domination–-submission practices may also increase the risk of HIV transmission if a partner is HIV-infected or his or her HIV serostatus is unknown. As an example, the use of a whip for play with sequential partners could potentially increase the risk of HIV transmission to subsequent partners if the whip draws blood from an HIV-infected individual and is not cleaned before it is used on the next person.

Injection drug use with shared paraphernalia also increases the likelihood of HIV transmission due to the transfer of the virus through the sharing of injection equipment such as needles, syringes, or cotton. This may occur because the initial user of the syringe may draw blood into the syringe prior to injecting in order to verify that the needle is actually inside the vein. After injecting, he or she may refill the syringe with blood from the vein in order to wash out any drug that remains in the syringe. In either case, the sharing of the uncleaned syringe with a subsequent user may result in HIV transmission if the initial user was HIV-positive because only a small amount of HIV-infected blood is required to transmit the virus. Injection drug use may involve the use of heroin, cocaine, and/or methamphetamine.

Non-injection drug use has also been implicated as a risk factor for HIV transmission. Due to the effect of the particular substance ingested, such as alcohol, individuals may experience impaired judgment, reducing their ability to evaluate situations for risk. Other substances, such as methamphetamine, may increase libido and sexual confidence, leading to sexual relations with multiple persons over a prolonged period of time.

Other behaviors may also lead to an increase in the risk of HIV transmission. As an example, individuals may engage in amateur tattooing or body piercing, using shared tattooing implements such as needles, knives, and blades. This shared usage may inadvertently result in contact with the blood of a HIV-infected individual, who may or may not be aware of his or her positive serostatus. At least one study has found that the prevalence of tattooing and body piercing is higher among individuals who inject drugs and that the practice of cleaning shared tattooing equipment is much less common than the practice of cleaning shared injection equipment. These research findings suggest that the risk of HIV transmission associated with the sharing of paraphernalia for tattooing and body piercing may be relatively high. Similar issues relate to the shared use of sex toys. Because sex toys may come into contact with body fluids that can serve as a mechanism for HIV transmission, such as vaginal fluid or blood, the sharing of sex toys also presents a risk of HIV transmission.

In some cultures, individuals may self-inject with vitamins or antibiotics or inject their children with vitamins as a preventive strategy for health maintenance. This practice is culturally acceptable in many places, particularly in those countries in which antibiotics, injectable vitamins, and needles and syringes are available over-the-counter without a prescription. The use of the same needle and syringe for multiple family members may increase HIV risk if individuals are HIV-seropositive or are unaware of their HIV serostatus. Individuals providing these injections in their home environments often do not perceive themselves to be at risk of disease transmission because the practice is not equated with illicit drug usage. And, because prevention programs targeting injection drug users rarely make mention of these practices as a possible vehicle for transmission, individuals do not have the information necessary to safeguard against HIV transmission.

Mental health care providers may wish to provide their clients with basic information relating to HIV risk behaviors, particularly those clients who they know are sexually active with multiple partners or who are engaging in drug use. These discussions of HIV risk can be accompanied by frank discussions of prevention strategies that can be utilized by clients to reduce their risk of contracting HIV or, if they are HIV seropositive, of transmitting the infection to others. Individuals engaging in risk behaviors should also be provided with information about available HIV testing and counseling should they wish to follow up with this.

Related Topics: Denialism, HIV counseling, HIV testing, Prevention strategies, Risk groups, Sex toys, Sexually transmitted infections, Substance use, Survival sex

Suggested Readings

Grov, C., Parsons, J. T., & Bimbi, D. S. (2010). Sexual compulsivity and sexual risk in gay and bisexual men. *Archives of Sexual Behavior, 39*(4), 940–949.

Loue, S., Loarca, L. E., Ramirez, E. R., & Ferman, J. (2002). Penile marbles and potential risk of HIV transmission. *Journal of Immigrant Health, 4*, 117–118.

Loue, S., & Oppenheim, S. (1994). Immigration and HIV: A pilot study. *AIDS Education and Prevention, 6*(1), 74–80.

Makkai, T., & McAllister, I. (2001). Prevalence of tattooing and body piercing in the Australian community. *Communicable Disease Intelligence, 25*, 67–72.

Misovish, S. J., Fisher, J. D., & Fisher, W. A. (1997). Close relationships and elevated HIV risk behavior: Evidence and possible underlying psychological processes. *Review of General Psychology, 1*(1), 77–107.

Risk Groups

Beatrice Gabriela Ioan

At the beginning of the HIV/AIDS epidemic, the US Centers for Disease Control and Prevention (CDC) identified a number of groups at risk for HIV infection based on the characteristics of the persons known to be affected by this then-mysterious and unknown disease. It later became clear that behavior, rather than presumed commonality of characteristics, was responsible for disease transmission. Accordingly, it is important that mental health care providers counsel their clients regarding behaviors that may increase their risk of becoming infected and the behavioral strategies that they can use to reduce their risk of infection. This is particularly important because clients may be misinformed and believe that because they do not self-identify as a member of one of these initially named risk groups, they are not at risk of the disease.

The first risk group, identified in June 1981, was that of gay men, among whom the first cases of AIDS were recorded. In 1982, this infection was given names suggestive for the group: "gay related immune deficiency (GRID)," "gay cancer," "community- acquired immune dysfunction," or "gay compromise syndrome." The second risk group, identified in 1982, was that of injecting drug users (IDUs), followed shortly by heterosexual hemophiliacs who had received blood transfusions and then by Haitians. In this way, AIDS became known as the disease of the "4-H club" (homosexuals, heroin users, hemophiliacs, and Haitians), even if there were cases that did not fit into any of these risk groups. The inclusion of Haitians in risk groups for HIV infection provoked heated reactions from American Haitians, who accused the CDC of stigmatization and racism, Indeed, that assessment was not based on valid data that could support the categorization of a whole people as a group at risk for a disease. Similar objections were raised to the classification of all homosexuals as a risk group.

B.G. Ioan (✉)
Legal Medicine, Medical Deontology and Bioethics Department, University of Medicine and Pharmacy "Gr. T. Popa", Iasi, Romania
e-mail: ioanbml@yahoo.com

S. Loue (ed.), *Mental Health Practitioner's Guide to HIV/AIDS*,

DOI 10.1007/978-1-4614-5283-6_75, © Springer Science+Business Media New York 2013

Society has often distinguished between individuals who acquired the virus through blood transfusions (e.g., people with hemophilia) or by perinatal transmission, calling them "innocent victims," and those who became infected due to behaviors not accepted by the larger society, such as homosexuals, IDUs, commercial sex workers, and people belonging to certain ethnic groups. Some voices even claimed that persons who had contracted the infection through their behavior had been punished by God for their behavior.

The AIDS epidemic was from the beginning a disease that caused social stigma and discrimination because, on the one hand, it came to be associated with traditionally stigmatized groups such as homosexuals and heroin users. On the other hand, it was in part due to the limited data available regarding the mechanisms of HIV transmission. It is estimated stigma and ostracism of persons belonging to certain groups have been the primary environmental factors that have facilitated HIV transmission. The social stigmatization of gay men, for example, favored the transmission of HIV by creating an environment that promotes short-term relationships, often with anonymous partners, instead of supporting and promoting stable and long-term relations, as is the case for heterosexual couples. The stigmatization of African Americans gradually led to the creation of a counterculture, characterized by increased illegal substance use, self-neglect, low self-esteem, poverty, increased unemployment, and poor access to health care. These conditions have favored short-term relationships, serial monogamy, the initiation of sexual relationships at a very young age, and risk taking behaviors such as unsafe illicit drug injection and unsafe sexual intercourse.

The identification of risk groups for HIV infection had a double negative effect. First, those who were members of the enumerated risk groups were socially stigmatized and ostracized. Second, those who did not belong to the risk groups felt protected from the infection and did not consider necessary preventive measures, which favored the expansion of the epidemic. For example, the identification of IDUs as a risk group has created the misconception that injecting substances other than illicit drugs would not involve the risk of HIV transmission and that non-injecting drug users are protected from infection because they are not injecting. In fact, many people contracted the virus through iatrogenic injection during the administration of medically prescribed treatment or dental treatment. Also, non-injecting drug users, in turn, can acquire the infection by adopting sexual risk behaviors facilitated by the effects of the drugs.

Individuals are at increased risk of HIV transmission not by belonging to one of these groups, but because of the adoption of certain risky behaviors. For example, injecting drug users are at increased risk of HIV infection due to both the sharing of non-sterile injection equipment and to participation in unsafe sex while under the influence of drugs. The introduction of needle exchange programs that promote a safer injection style by providing sterile injecting equipment in exchange for the used one have led to lower rates of HIV transmission, even if not accompanied with reduced drug use. Key behaviors that promote HIV transmission among men having sex with men (MSM) are practicing unprotected sex and acceptance of multiple sexual partners and drug and alcohol abuse.

Risk behaviors for HIV transmission can be identified, however. Modes of transmission and risk behaviors for HIV vary, depending on many factors, causing a different prevalence of infection in different parts of the world and in different periods of time. For example, blood transfusions are still an important route of HIV transmission in sub-Saharan African countries. In India, HIV prevalence increased among women, who are primarily infected through unprotected sexual intercourse with their husbands who engage in unprotected extramarital sex or unsafe drug injection.

Therefore, in terms of HIV prevention it is more useful to look at the risk behaviors for HIV transmission. The reasons and causes for which people voluntarily or involuntarily adopt risk behaviors are different. Women have an increased risk of HIV infection worldwide; they represent about 50% of all people affected by HIV/AIDS, with the highest prevalence in Sub-Saharan African countries. The increased risk of HIV infection among women is due to several factors, such as low decision making power in their sexual relationships due to intimate partner violence and social and economic inequities. They are most often infected in monogamous heterosexual relationships, often because of partners' infidelity or drug injecting behavior. Vaginal lesions produced during forced sex increase the chance of HIV transmission, especially in young women. Women are also more susceptible biologically to HIV infection; HIV transmission from men to women is two times more frequent than transmission from women to men.

Currently, commercial sex workers are at high risk for HIV transmission. This is frequently due to physical violence, unsafe sex practices often motivated by the impossibility of requiring the use of condoms, and increased consumption of illicit drugs and alcohol. Detention environments facilitate the adoption of HIV risk behaviors such as the practice of tattooing, the injection of drugs with shared non-sterile paraphernalia, and voluntary or forced unprotected sexual intercourse.

Social and economic conditions existing in different countries have frequently led to increased emigration. This in turn favors the transmission of HIV due to the isolation of families; the practice of unprotected sex with multiple partners, often with commercial sex workers; and the increased consumption of illegal drugs and alcohol. At their return, migrants can unknowingly transmit the virus to their stable sexual partners, thereby increasing transmission of HIV infection in areas with little or no previous prevalence.

Armed conflict facilitates HIV transmission through the poor living conditions and trauma suffered by victims, such as rape, physical violence, and a lack of prevention and treatment for HIV. Victims may later engage in risk behaviors themselves, such as unprotected sexual relations and unsafe drug use, due to the physical and psychological trauma experienced. This is particularly true if the victims of these crimes are stigmatized and ostracized by their families and communities.

HIV transmission may also occur as a result of reduced access to programs for the prevention and treatment of HIV infection and the low level of knowledge about HIV infection that may result. Reduced access to prevention and treatment of HIV infection programs can be due to either stigma and social exclusion, as in the case of

MSM, IDUs, and commercial sex workers or because of the fear of possible legal consequences, as in the case of illegal migrants and refugees or IDUs and MSM in countries where the law criminalizes these practices. In addition, the limited resources of the medical systems, as is the case in many of the origin countries of migrants, refugees, and internally displaced persons favor HIV transmission.

Related Topics: Risk behaviors, Sex work and sex workers, Stigma and stigmatization, Substance use

Suggested Readings

Altman, L.K. (1983, July 31). Debate grows on U.S. listing Haitians in AIDS category. *New York Times.*

De Souza, R. (2010). Women living with HIV: Stories of powerlessness and agency. *Women's Studies International Forum., 33*, 244–252.

Novick, A. (1997). Stigma and AIDS: Three layers of damage. *Journal of the Gay and Lesbian Medical Association, 1*(1), 53–60.

Suggested Resources

http://globalhealth.org/hiv_aids/risk_groups/. Last accessed December 28, 2011

The history of HIV and AIDS in America. Retrieved from December 28, 2011 www.avert.org/aids-history-america.htm.

Ryan White Care Act

Sana Loue

The Ryan White CARE Act, formally known as the Ryan White Comprehensive AIDS Resources Emergency Act, was first passed by the US Congress in 1990 to provide funding for the provision of HIV/AIDS-related services. The legislation was named after Ryan White, a child with hemophilia who was diagnosed with AIDS at the age of 13. White and his mother fought for the right to attend school. Congress has reauthorized the legislation four times since its initial passage, in 1996, 2000, 2006, and 2009. The legislation is now known as the Ryan White HIV/AIDS Program.

The legislation currently consists of eight parts. Part A provides funding to Eligible Metropolitan Areas and Transitional Grant Areas that have been the most severely impacted by HIV/AIDS. An area must have reported at least 2,000 AIDS cases within the previous 5 years and have a population of at least 50,000 to be considered an EMA. EMAs currently include Houston, New York, Philadelphia, San Francisco, and others. Areas designated as TGAs must have reported between 1,000 and 1,999 new AIDS cases during the preceding 5 years and have a population of at least 50,000. Current TGAs include Austin, Las Vegas, Oakland, Seattle, and others. Funding is allocated for the care of individuals living with HIV. Core services that can be covered by Part A funding include outpatient and ambulatory medical care, AIDS drug assistance, AIDS pharmaceutical assistance, medical nutrition therapy, home health care, medical case management, mental health services, substance abuse outpatient care, hospice services, early intervention services, oral health services, and health insurance premium and cost sharing assistance for those with low incomes. All support services must be linked to medical outcomes.

Part B funding is available to all 50 states, the District of Columbia, Puerto Rico, Guam, the US Virgin Islands, and 5 US Pacific Territories. Emerging Communities that have reported a cumulative number of AIDS cases between 500 and 999 during

S. Loue (✉)
Department of Epidemiology and Biostatistics, Case Western Reserve University, Cleveland, OH, USA
e-mail: Sana.Loue@case.edu

S. Loue (ed.), *Mental Health Practitioner's Guide to HIV/AIDS*, 363
DOI 10.1007/978-1-4614-5283-6_76, © Springer Science+Business Media New York 2013

the preceding 5 years are eligible for Part B funds. These funds are distributed based on a formula and cover core medical and support services, such as oral health care, early intervention services, medical nutrition therapy, medical case management, treatment adherence services, and others. Funding may also be available for linguistic services and medical transportation. Respite care is available for caregivers under some circumstances.

Service providers are able to receive grants directly under Part C of the program for early intervention services, planning grants, and capacity development grants. Organizations can receive funding for early intervention services if they fall within a list of eligible organizations. Examples of such organizations include rural health clinics and nonprofit private entities that provide comprehensive primary care to individuals that are at risk of HIV/AIDS, among others. Costs under early intervention services must be allocated into the following categories: early intervention services, core medical services, support services, quality management, and administrative costs. Early intervention services are associated with the direct provision of medical services and include services such as lab and x-ray services and medical and dental equipment and supplies. Core medical services include early intervention services as well as HIV counseling, home health care, hospice care, and several other types of services. Organizations can use quality improvement funding for such things as involving consumers as a means of improving services and staff training and technical assistance. Support services include patient transportation to medical appointments, respite care, and patient education materials.

Family centered care can be funded under Part D, which specifically addresses services needed by women, children, and their families. Funding is limited to nonprofit, governmental, faith-based, and community-based organizations meeting specified criteria. These funds support service delivery, clinical quality management, and administrative expenses.

Part F funding refers to *Special Projects of National Significance*. Funding priorities as of the time of this writing include initiatives focused on hepatitis C treatment, capacity building to develop electronic client information systems, increasing access to and retention in HIV care of HIV-infected women of color, the development of innovations in oral health care, the evaluation of existing electronic network systems for persons living with HIV/AIDS in underserved communities, and enhancing linkages to care for those in jail settings. Part F provides funding for reimbursement to eligible service providers of dental care and for a community-based dental partnership program that seeks to increase the access of individuals living with HIV/AIDS to dental care.

Related Topics: Access to care, Case management, Medicaid, Medicare

Suggested Resources

United States Department of Health and Human Services, Health Resources and Services Administration. (n.d.). *About the Ryan White HIV/AIDS program*. Retrieved April 24, 2012 from http://hab.hrsa.gov/abouthab/aboutprogram.html.

Sex Toys

Elena Cristina Chinole Cazacu

The use of objects to generate or enhance sexual arousal can be traced from ancient times. The oldest artifacts that seemed to be used for stimulating sexual pleasure are approximately 2,000–4,000 years old and originated from China. Most of the sex toys sold nowadays are made in China, as well. Ancient sex toys were made of jade, stone or bones; modern ones are made of rubber, glass, plastics, steel, and they are available in many shapes or geometries, colors, and designs. The progress of technology has also brought progress in powering sex toys—many have batteries, like vibrators or dildos—while others, more advanced ones, may be operated and controlled using a remote control. Many are still powered by simple hand power and their use is limited only by each individual's imagination.

Some sex toys resemble human genitalia; others are simply devices in the shapes or forms that allow them to be either inserted into body orifices or attached to various body parts. Depending on the way they are used, there are several categories of sex toys, such as inserting toys, such dildoes and vibrators that may be used for vaginal or anal stimulation; male-oriented toys, which may mimic vaginas, or various contraptions that prolongue male erection; nipple toys; fetish toys; or erotic furniture. Many household objects or appliances, as well as fruits and vegetables, may be used as well as sex toys.

In spite of a long time history of sex toy usage, there is limited scholarly research on the use, manufacturing process, and commercialization of sex toys. In some countries sex toys are sold like any other merchandise; in others, sex toys may be bought only from the Internet. There are still some federal regulations in place in the USA that prohibit the sale of sex toys by mainstream retailers. Mores and opinions are changing, mainly due to the rise of the Internet and e-commerce, which are expanding the cultural visibility and availability of sex toys for the general public. This phenomenon is also enhanced by the change in consumer culture. It has been noted that women are becoming important customers for sex toys and are

E.C. Chinole Cazacu (✉)
Center for Ethics and Public Policies, Bucharest, Iasi, Romania
e-mail: cchinole@yahoo.com

S. Loue (ed.), *Mental Health Practitioner's Guide to HIV/AIDS*,
DOI 10.1007/978-1-4614-5283-6_77,

demanding not only quality products but also sexual information. Regardless of what the general public may think about the morality/necessity of using sex toys, their use entails several health concerns. Some are related to the materials they are made of, and the lack of health and safety regulations imposed upon manufacturers/ merchants by relevant bodies, such as the Food and Drug Administration (FDA) in the USA. Unfortunately, nowadays the sex toy industry is flooded with inexpensive, harmful products that are often mass produced by manufacturers that disregard the various dangerous health effects they pose to their users. The vast majority of sex toys available on the market are made from cheap materials containing toxic ingredients, such as products containing phthalates, which are not only harmful for human health but also for the environment. Chemical substances found in sex toys may include solvents and other rubber chemicals or plasticizers, as well as other components that have been proven to cause harmful neurotoxic and/or reproductive effects.

Another health concern, even more pressing, is related to the use of sex toys and STD and HIV transmission. Research shows that sex toys are used as tools to enhance pleasure, and, if used properly, they may help reduce sexually transmitted infections. Some basic rules apply to reduce the risk of transmitting or contracting HIV or other STDs when using sex toys. The safest sex method is to use condoms each time for vaginal, anal and oral sex when sharing sex toys. This can help prevent the transmission of HIV and reduce the risk of many STDs. Safer sex involves preventing one person's body fluids get into someone else's body. Sharing uncleaned sex toys bring a high risk of HIV and other STDs transmission as they come into contact with infected body fluids (such as semen or blood) which can be introduced into someone else's body, even without direct sexual intercourse. Also, because sex toys are used during foreplay or after other sexual activities, they may cause inflammation or injury to the vaginal tissue or anal lining, like other forms of play, such as fingering or fisting. This is why sharing unprotected sex toys may result in the transmission of sexually transmitted infections and blood-borne infections. At least one case of HIV infection was reported as the result of swapping sex toys between one woman who had sex with a HIV-infected woman. Rough sex play, including the use of sex toys that cause abrasions or bleeding of the skin or mucous membranes, may be another aggravating risk factor for HIV transmission. Therefore, safe sexual practices are always necessary also when sharing sexual toys.

There is no risk of HIV transmission when sharing sex toys if they are covered with new condoms each time they are used for a new partner. Having a separate collection of sex toys for each partner should also be considered as an option for risk reduction. Another measure to prevent HIV infection or STD transmission is to ensure that, if not using condoms, sex toys are thoroughly cleaned or disinfected between use with different partners. Cleaning sex toys before and after each use would not only decrease the risk of infection but may also significantly prolong the toys' usefulness. Depending on the materials they are made of, and the instructions placed on or inside their packaging, they may be washed with soap, detergent, or bleach; the use of specific disinfectants is also recommended. It is important also that sex toys not only be cleaned thoroughly, but also be dried after each use. Regular checks on the integrity of the sex toys is necessary; they should be replaced if scratched or broken, as cracks may hide harmful bacteria and viruses.

Related topics: Prevention strategies, Risk behaviors

Suggested Readings

Satinsky, S., Rosenberger, J. G., Schick, V., Novak, D. S., & Reece, M. (2011). USA study of sex toy use by HIV-positive men who have sex with other men: Implications for sexual health. *International Journal of STD & AIDS, 22*(8), 442–448.

Weitzer, R. (Ed.). (2000). *Sex for sale: Prostitution, pornography, and the sex industry*. New York: Routledge.

Suggested Resources

Danish Technological Institute. (2006). *Survey of chemical substances in consumer products, no. 77: Survey and health assessment of chemicals substances in sex toys*. Retrieved March 7, 2012 from http://www2.mst.dk/udgiv/publications/2006/87-7052-227-8/html/helepubl_eng.htm.

HIV and gay men—safe sex. Retrieved March 7, 2012 from http://www.betterhealth.vic.gov.au/bhcv2/bhcarticles.nsf/pages/HIV_and_gay_men_safe_sex

Reducing the sexual health risks from using sex toys. Retrieved March 7, 2012 from http://www.hiv-wakeup.org.uk/know-your-risk/do-you-know-your-risk/safer-sex-toys/

Sex toys. Retrieved March 7, 2012 from http://www.aidsmap.com/Sex-toys/page/1323537/

Sexual risk factors. Retrieved September 29, 2011 from http://aids.gov/hiv-aids-basics/prevention/reduce-your-risk/sexual-risk-factors/#risky.

Sex Work and Sex Workers

Vanessa A. Forro

The emergence of HIV/AIDS in the Western world has revived the association of sex workers with sexually transmitted diseases and HIV/AIDS. The issues underlying sex work are diverse and require consideration of the linkages between policy, behavior, attitude and contextual factors involved in transactional sex and HIV transmission. Many sex workers rights groups and human rights groups contend that it is not sex work per se that makes sex workers vulnerable to HIV/AIDS, but rather the policies associated with sex work. The double stigma against sex workers infected with HIV is often used to justify abuse and repression in many countries.

Sex work is broadly defined as the exchange of money or goods for sexual services, either on a regular basis or occasionally, involving male, female, and transgender individuals; coercion or voluntary decision may be involved. For some, it may be the only income-generating option, or it may be a formal or informal temporary activity. Individuals who have exchanged sex for food, shelter, or protection (also known as "survival sex") would not consider themselves to be a formal sex worker.

The World Health Organization (WHO) has identified sex workers as one of four key populations globally for HIV/AIDS health initiatives. A core issue for WHO with regard to sex work is the vulnerability and lack of rights and the causal role they play in HIV transmission worldwide. Sex workers often lack the personal or social status to negotiate safe sexual practices. HIV prevalence among poorer sex workers is higher mostly due to the inability to negotiate condom use. HIV prevalence among sex workers in the West tends to be relatively low and fairly stable, with injection drug use as a major risk factor. Sex workers who also inject are at a greater vulnerability because of their work and the illegality of their drug use, which opens them up to exploitation and abuse, including sexual violence and harm as well as incapacity to negotiate condom use.

V.A. Forro (✉)
Neurological Outcomes Center, Case Western Reserve University, Cleveland, OH, USA
e-mail: Vanessa.Forro@case.edu

S. Loue (ed.), *Mental Health Practitioner's Guide to HIV/AIDS*,
DOI 10.1007/978-1-4614-5283-6_78, © Springer Science+Business Media New York 2013

A high HIV prevalence among female sex workers has been reported in a number of Southeast Asian countries where rates range from 3 to 6%, and in China where female sex workers and their clients make up approximately 20% of all HIV cases. In Latin America and the Caribbean, HIV rates among female sex workers are reported to range from 16 to 27%. In Russia and the former Czech Republic, HIV prevalence is highest (33%) among female sex workers under the age of 19. Reports have shown the highest rates of HIV among female sex workers in Ethiopia (73%), Zambia (68%), Ghana and South Africa (50%). Rates of HIV infection among sex workers in India appear to be stable, with most HIV infections occurring among unprotected heterosexual contact. In Mumbai and Pune, where rates of HIV infection among sex workers have been found to be 54 and 49% respectively, the likelihood of transmitting HIV to clients can be high. Other factors related to the transmission of HIV among female sex workers include lack of information about HIV/AIDS, early entry into the sex work industry, and migration patterns.

The United Nations (UN) authored a guidance note on HIV and sex work which was adamantly opposed by many sex workers rights groups. The note recommends a reduction of demand for sex work as a strategy to reduce HIV transmission among sex workers and their clients. Activists argue that this does not address the need to improve the occupational and health conditions of sex work or the empowerment of sex workers, which is important in fighting HIV in this population. In addition, the UN Guidance Note is at odds with international guidelines on HIV/AIDS and human rights, which state that sex work should be decriminalized and then legally regulated to improve the safety and health of both sex workers and clients.

Many programs worldwide have been developed to provide comprehensive HIV prevention and treatment programs for sex workers. Of these, the major focus combines sexually transmitted disease treatment, condom promotion and provision, and prevention education interventions through peer outreach. In Thailand, the "100% Condom Use" policy was initially very successful. Implemented in the early 1990s, it sought to enforce consistent condom use in all commercial sex establishments. Data from the program evaluation of this policy showed a steady and rapid decline in STDs and increase in condom use among brothel-based sex workers and their clients. In addition, studies found a tenfold reduction in STD incidence and HIV prevalence among young Thai men during the period from 1991 to 1993. Similarly, in Santo Domingo, Dominican Republic, low HIV prevalence has been attributed in part to safe sex behaviors resulting from the city's 100% condom use program. The achievements of the Sonagachi Project in Kolkata, India have served as a model elsewhere. The Durbar Mahila Samanwaya Committee (DMSC) runs the project, which organizes over 65,000 sex workers and their children. Other programs have focused on the provision of alternative employment for sex workers.

A number of studies on transgendered female-to-male sex workers (TFSW) in the USA indicate a high incidence of mental illness, lack of social support, and physical assault with HIV risk behavior. Depression and suicide ideation is common among TFSW which has been shown to lead to risky behaviors, such as unprotected sex, sex in exchange for drugs, food, or shelter. Due to the criminality of sex work in the USA, it is often difficult to reach the most vulnerable groups (i.e., street-based sex workers) and self-initiated prevention needs are not met largely as a result of stigma and fear of being reported to the police. Several US cities, including Denver, Colorado have first-time offender diversion programs that target street-based sex workers going through the criminal justice system. All of the sex workers who are offered diversion in lieu of criminal charges must be subject to an HIV test. If they test HIV positive, and were knowingly engaging in sex work, then they face up to 2 years in prison. The customers, or “johns,” who are commonly not arrested during prostitution stings, are not required to take an HIV test.

In 2004, the US President’s Emergency Plan for AIDS Relief (PEPFAR) was implemented despite huge criticism by the HIV/AIDS and sex worker communities. The initiative includes an anti-prostitution clause forbidding grant recipients from providing any kind of HIV/AIDS prevention services unless they specifically state that they are against prostitution. As a result of this pledge there has been a decline of services for sex workers; drop-in centers have closed; sex workers have reduced access to places where they can bathe, rest, or receive safe-sex materials; and reports of sex workers being denied health care in clinics has increased. In some organizations, peer education programs about safer sex techniques have ended and campaigns to raise awareness about violence against sex workers have been eliminated. Some organizations have chosen not to work with sex workers altogether for fear of losing important USAID funding. However, the Brazilian government refused $40 million (USD) in 2005 due to the imposition of the “prostitution clause,” arguing that the policy undermines the country’s efforts to fight HIV/AIDS. The consensus among a number of organizations has been to modify the terminology used to describe programs in order to offer services to sex workers without compromising US funding.

Future global health initiatives to reduce and address HIV/AIDS prevalence among sex worker populations must include fighting social stigma, decriminalization of sex work, and empowerment initiatives. Policy should be formed around reducing HIV infection rates and providing sex workers the resources to protect themselves. Mental health providers who have clients engaged in sex work will want to be aware of community resources that can assist their clients in accessing needed resources such as HIV testing and counseling.

Related Topics: Human trafficking, Prevention strategies, Stigma and stigmatization

Suggested Readings

Ditmore, M., & Allman, D. (2010). Implications of PEPFAR’s anti-prostitution pledge for HIV prevention among organizations working with sex workers. *HIV/AIDS Policy & Law Review, 15*(1), 63–64.

Nemoto, T., Bödeker, B., & Iwamoto, M. (2011). Social support, exposure to violence and transphobia, and correlates of depression among male-to-female transgender women with a history of sex work. *American Journal of Public Health, 101*(10), 1980–1988.
Scambler, G., & Paoli, F. (2008). Health work, female sex workers and HIV/AIDS: Global and local dimensions of stigma and deviance as barriers to effective interventions. *Social Science & Medicine, 66*(8), 1848–1862.
Seshu, M., Hunter, A., Hunter, E., Strack, F., Mollet, S., Morgan Thomas, R., Overs, C., Ditmore, M., & Allman, D. (2008). U.N. guidance note on HIV and sex work "reworked" by activists. *HIV/AIDS Policy & Law Review, 13*(2–3), 95–97.

Suggested Resources

Fisher, L. (3 March 2011). *Fact sheet memorandum: SB 11–085 prostitution offender program.* Sen. Shaffer & Rep. McCann. Office of Sen Mike Johnston. Colorado General Assembly. Available at http://www.mikejohnston.org/images/stories/110313_FactSheet_11-085_v2.pdf.
UNAIDS guidance note on HIV and sex work. March 2009. Available from http://www.unaids.org/en/media/unaids/contentassets/dataimport/pub/basedocument/2009/jc1696_guidance_note_hiv_and_sexwork_en.pdf
United Nations Population Fund (UNFPA). UNAIDS Inter-Agency Task Team on Gender and HIV/AIDS. HIV/AIDS, Gender, and Sex Work. Available from http://www.unfpa.org/hiv/docs/factsheet_genderwork.pdf

Sexual Orientation

Beatrice Gabriela Ioan

Introduction

Human sexuality is characterized by the sense that a person assigns to his/her sexuality. To avoid confusion in characterizing a person's sexuality, a specific terminology is necessary to describe its different aspects: sexual acts (hetero- or homosexual, that is, with a partner of the opposite or same sex, respectively), sexual orientation (androphilic, gyneophilic, bisexual) and gender identity. Sexual identity has, in turn, several levels: biological (male, female, intersexual), social (man, woman), or sexual orientation (heterosexual, homosexual, bisexual). These categories can interact with each other, resulting in complex categories, such as gay-man, male-to-female transsexual, and non-gay homosexual. Sexual orientation refers to sexual attraction, sexual fantasies, and sexual behavior of an individual.

The choice of sexual partner may be motivated, however, by factors other than sexual desire or sexual orientation, such as power (power differences between partners, as happens in prisons or during the war), economic relations, and the availability of alternative partners. Depending on the cultural context, homosexuality may be considered essential for boys to reach physical maturity; the homosexual act may be motivated by a desire to transmit or receive what are thought to be the healing powers of semen, by the fear that a heterosexual act could be harmful to a man due to woman's polluting features, or by the relative unavailability of female sexual partners.

A partner's sex is not always essential to characterize the sexual act and one's sexual orientation. Many Native Americans communities recognize *berdache* or *halfman-halfwoman* or *two-spirit people*. These people, although showing male morphological traits, assumed many of the characteristics and roles associated with

B.G. Ioan (✉)
Legal Medicine, Medical Deontology and Bioethics Department, University of Medicine and Pharmacy "Gr. T. Popa", Iasi, Romania
e-mail: ioanbml@yahoo.com

S. Loue (ed.), *Mental Health Practitioner's Guide to HIV/AIDS*,
DOI 10.1007/978-1-4614-5283-6_79, © Springer Science+Business Media New York 2013

the status of women. Homosexual behavior was only a secondary aspect of their status. Men who had sex with *berdache* were not labeled differently from men who had sex only with women. Currently, these people identify themselves as *gay*.

In India, *hijras* are people with religious duties who are physically males, but they are impotent and have no sexual desire towards women, either because of a congenital defect of their sexual organs or due to intentional emasculation. Because they are impotent, they are not considered men; because they cannot carry a pregnancy, they are not considered women. *Hijras* adopt female clothing and roles but also have some of the social behaviors that are characteristic of men. Although *hijras* have sex only with men, they are not considered and do not consider themselves homosexuals. Due to these qualities, *hijras* are considered by the members of the community *neither man nor woman and woman and man*.

In the late 1800s, in Western countries, only vaginal intercourse between a man and a woman was considered normal sexual activity. Other types of sexual acts were believed to be abnormal or perverse, including homosexuality, which was defined as a sexual act between persons of the same sex.

The term *homosexuality* was introduced in 1869 by Karl Maria Kertbeny, who believed that homosexuality is innate and therefore unchangeable. Kertbeny was one of the first promoters of homosexuals' rights, arguing that the State should not interfere in its citizens' lives and privacy. In 1899, Magnus Hirschfeld introduced the concept of *the third sex*, which included a wide range of expressions of sexuality, which could not be labeled as feminine or masculine; these expressions did not necessarily refer to sexual intercourse. Ulrichs used, in turn, the notion of *the third sex* to describe individuals who have a masculine body but are female both in spirit and sexual activity.

In the twentieth century, homosexuality was until relatively recently considered to be a pathological condition. This belief provided the impetus for research designed to identify its cause. Homosexuality had long been used as a diagnostic label for a mental disorder. It was not until 1973 that homosexuality was removed from the *Diagnostic and Statistical Manual of Psychiatric Disorders*. The diagnosis of *gender identity disorder* has been retained in the most current edition of the manual to characterize those persons who are experiencing clinically significant distress or impairment in an important area of functioning due to their sexual orientation. The *Manual* no longer contains any reference to homosexuality as a mental disorder per se.

During the period from 1960 to approximately 1970, homosexual men and women (who gradually adopted the label *gay* and *lesbian,* respectively) set up political organizations to fight against the laws, practices and social beliefs which were stigmatizing and discriminatory. They argued that homosexuality is not a pathological condition or a perverse feature, but a difference in sexual orientation, which should be accepted and tolerated in an open and free society.

Homosexuality refers to the erotic desire or interest of a person directed to members of their own sex or gender, without having, usually, the desire to belong to the opposite sex. This latter feature essentially differentiates homosexuals from transsexuals, who identify themselves as members of the opposite sex and exhibit the desire to belong to the opposite sex. Thus, even if they have sex with people with the same body morphology, transsexuals do not necessarily consider themselves as homosexual and may even be offended by the assignment of this term to them.

The terms *homosexual* or *heterosexual* can be problematic when it comes to transgenic or intersexual persons. In these cases is necessary to explain in what sense we refer to homosexuality: biological, gender role or sexual identity. For this reason the terms *androphilic*, *gyneophilic*, *bisexual* are considered most suitable to describe a person's sexual orientation.

In 1986, Money introduced the concept of *lovemap*, which includes one's conceptualization of an idealized lover, and idealized or real erotic and sexual activity. Subsequently, he introduced two additional concepts: *gender map* and *sexual orientation map*. Homosexuality, according to these concepts, is the gender transposition of the ideal lover in the *lovemap*, accompanied by a wide variety of ideal erotic and sexual activity, either imaginary or real. This approach may explain the large interindividual variation of sexuality that exists in the human species.

An important and necessary distinction is made between *homosexuality*, which involves erotic desire, and *homosexual behavior*, which refers only to sexual intercourse between a person and someone of the same body morphology, without the need for erotic desire to be directed to the partner and without the two partners necessarily considering themselves to be homosexuals. Terms such as *transgendered*, *gay*, *lesbian*, *bisexual* refer primarily to a person identifying him- or herself with a certain group and only secondarily to his or her sexual behavior.

Sexual Orientation and HIV

At the beginning of the HIV epidemic, the sexual orientation of those infected was considered a significant epidemiological factor. Homosexuals were considered a risk group for HIV infection, among other categories of individuals: Haitians, intravenous drug users, and commercial sex workers. In the public's perception, HIV infection was related to socially marginalized identities and communities.

In 1983, during a meeting of the National Association of People with AIDS held in Colorado, *The Denver Principles* were developed. This document, on the one hand, promotes the rights of those infected with HIV and, on the other hand, it emphasizes their responsibilities, especially as they relate to providing information about their HIV status to their partners.

Men who have sex with men (MSM) is one of the populations most affected by HIV infection, largely due to the multiple barriers that they face in the prevention of infection: reduced access to education and information, high levels of discrimination, lack of self-acceptance of their sexual orientation, and high levels of stress.

Sexual orientation and gender role may affect individuals' willingness to be tested for HIV. Research indicates that gay and bisexual men have delayed HIV testing because they feared a possible positive result and the stigma associated with their sexual orientation; many have symptoms suggestive of HIV infection when they present for testing. Heterosexual women are more likely to be tested for HIV due to their partners' sexual behavior rather than their own behavior. These findings suggest the need to incorporate discussions about sexual orientation and HIV testing in routine medical and mental health care.

HIV-infected persons may have additional psychological problems due to their labeling and stigmatization in the community and the perceived association between HIV and homosexuality, which may not be accepted in that particular community. HIV-infected African Americans are stigmatized because some members of the community believe that HIV infection can be contracted only by men having sex with men, and the church, which has an important role in the community, condemns homosexuality. Homophobia in the community leads to the silencing of HIV-infected persons with respect to their HIV status, and places additional psychological burden on them. A study of 98 HIV-infected African Americans from southern California HIV clinics, of whom 61 of the men were gay, found that the psychological discomfort caused by homophobia, the belief that HIV is transmitted only to men having sex with men, the fear of stigma, and the severity of depressive symptoms were more pronounced among HIV-infected heterosexual men than among gay men. In order to maintain silence about their condition, HIV-infected African American men delayed accessing health services, showed a reduced adherence to treatment and medical examinations, hid medication, and in many cases did not inform their partners about their HIV serostatus or adopt safer sexual practices.

Accordingly, it is critical that healthcare professionals talk openly with their patients about sexuality and safer sex practices, be informed about the sexuality of gay men and of HIV-infected persons, and be knowledgeable about the resources available in the community.

Related Topics: Adherence, Bisexuals and bisexuality, Gender identity, Stigma and stigmatization, Transgender, Transsexual.

Suggested Readings

American Psychiatric Association. (2000). *Diagnostic and statistical manual of mental disorders, fourth edition, text revision*. Washington, D.C.: Author.

Coleman, C. L., & Hummel, D. B. (2005). Sexual orientation a predictor of depressive symptoms among HIV-infected African American men: A descriptive correlational study. *Archives of Psychiatric Nursing, 19*(5), 236–241.

Goren, L. J., & Byne, W. (2009). Sexual orientation in men and women. In A. P. Arnold, A. M. Etgen, S. E. Fahrbach, R. T. Rubin, & D. W. Pfaff (Eds.), *Hormones, brain and behavior* (2nd ed., pp. 2429–2445). San Diego, CA: Elsevier Science.

Loue, S. (1999). *Gender, ethnicity and health research*. New York: Kluwer Academic/Plenum Publishers.

Loue, S., & Pike, E. C. (2007). *Case studies in ethics and HIV research*. New York: Springer.

Solomon, R. C., Nicholson, L. J., & Greene, J. K. (2003). Sexual identity. In S. Post (Ed.), *Encyclopedia of bioethics* (3rd ed., pp. 2434–2442). New York: Macmillan Library Reference.
Sanchez, F. J., Bocklandt, S., & Vilain, E. (2009). The biology of sexual orientation and gender identity. In A. P. Arnold, A. M. Etgen, S. E. Fahrbach, R. T. Rubin, & D. W. Pfaff (Eds.), *Hormones, brain and behavior* (2nd ed., pp. 1911–1924). San Diego, CA: Elsevier Science.
Siegel, K., Lekas, H. M., Olson, K., & VanDevanter, N. (2010). Gender, sexual orientation, and adolescent HIV testing: A qualitative analysis. *Journal of the Association of Nurses and AIDS Care, 21*(4), 314–326.

Sexually Transmitted Diseases

Laura Gheuca Solovastru, Dan Vata, and Diana Diaconu

A sexually transmitted disease (STD) is a disease that is transmitted by sexual contact. Once called "venereal diseases," STDs (also known as sexually transmitted infections or STIs), are among the most common infectious diseases today in the USA. Although prevention and education efforts have curbed the rise of certain STDs in the USA, the diseases continue to affect sexually active people in the USA as well as other countries.

There are more than 20 STDs, according to *Journal of the American Medical Association*. Major STDs that sexually active people must be aware of include HIV/AIDS, chlamydia, genital herpes, genital warts, gonorrhea, and syphilis. Other disorders that can be sexually transmitted include hepatitis B, scabies, pubic lice, trichomoniasis, and cytomegalovirus.

In today's era of widespread dissemination of these diseases, sexually active people definitely need a good understanding of STDs, how they are spread, their symptoms, and more. It is extremely important for people to know that many sexually transmitted diseases do not have symptoms at the outset, and sometimes—in fact, often—a partner may not even be aware that he or she has a disease. To complicate matters even more, safe sex (using a latex condom) is not a sure solution, because some STDs can be contracted even when condoms are used. This points to the obvious conclusion—that the only way a person can be sure of not contracting a sexually transmitted disease is to abstain from having sex and any sexual conduct, and that includes oral sex.

Millions of new sexually transmitted disease infections occur every year in the USA—as many as about 15 million—and this figure includes about four million cases of chlamydia, 800,000 cases of gonorrhea, 110,000+ cases of syphilis, several million cases of trichomonas vaginitis and nonspecific urethritis, 1–2 million cases of human papillomavirus, 200,000 to 1 million cases of hepatitis B, 200,000–500,000 cases of genital herpes, and 40,000–80,000 new HIV infections. Many of

L.G. Solovastru (✉) • D. Vata • D. Diaconu
Department of Dermatology, University of Medicine and Pharmacy "Gr. T. Popa", Iasi, Romania
e-mail: lsolovastru13@yahoo.com

S. Loue (ed.), *Mental Health Practitioner's Guide to HIV/AIDS*,
DOI 10.1007/978-1-4614-5283-6_80, © Springer Science+Business Media New York 2013

these, however, are not reported to the Centers for Disease Control and Prevention (CDC). Estimates suggest that in the USA, there are about one million Americans infected with human immunodeficiency virus, 31–50 million infected with herpes simplex virus, 24 million infected with human papillomavirus, and more than one million chronic hepatitis B carriers. Of the 15 million new cases of STDs in Americans each year, about 25% will be in the age group 15–19 years old. Although two-thirds of those who have STDs are younger than 25, it is not unusual for older people to contract these diseases, especially considering the trend toward multiple sex partners, which increases one's risk of getting an STD. To prevent an STD, a person can avoid all forms of sexual activity (abstinence) or practice safe sex to reduce the likelihood of contracting an STD.

A study of 3,500 visitors to an STD clinic in Atlanta, Georgia, revealed that although many people have no idea how to protect themselves from STDs, counseling does make a difference. What most surprised investigators were the many basic misconceptions about the kinds of behavior that prevent infection. Upon initial interviews, about one-half of respondents said they thought douching protected them from STDs. About 20% believed that the use of birth control pills protected them from STDs. Some thought that washing and urinating after sex were both protective measures. Three months after their visit to the clinic, one-half of those who previously believed myths were found to be better informed in a retrospective survey.

Ignorance of risk factors, denial of risk, and deliberate deception are three significant factors in the spread of STDs. In particular, the sharp rise of STDs in the teenage population reflects the perennial tendency of young people to perceive themselves as invulnerable. The startling news is that, according to the CDC, about three in five Americans living with HIV were infected as teens. Also, studies underscore that when HIV-positive people have other sexually transmitted diseases, they are more likely to have HIV present in their genital secretions, meaning that they are more infectious. Men infected with both gonorrhea and HIV are more than twice as likely to shed HIV in genital secretions as those who have HIV alone. The median concentration of HIV in semen can be ten times higher in men who have both HIV and gonorrhea than in men who are only HIV-infected. Thus, it is clear that STD treatment can help to reduce a person's ability to transmit HIV and also reduces the spread of HIV in communities.

It has been seen that continuous interventions to improve access to treatment are more effective in reducing HIV transmission than interventions that are intermittent, such as periodic mass treatments. Second, STD treatment is most effective in reducing HIV transmission where STD rates are high and the heterosexual HIV epidemic is young.

Third, treatment of symptomatic STDs appears to be especially important. The CDC emphasizes that a great deal of scientific evidence suggests that the presence of sexually transmitted disease(s) in an individual enhances his or her likelihood of both transmitting and getting HIV. For example, scientists are seeing much greater risk for HIV infection in women who have genital ulcers. Studies show a clear link between sexually transmitted diseases and the risk of sexual HIV transmission.

First, STDs probably increase a person's susceptibility to HIV infection in two ways: genital ulcers (syphilis, herpes, chancroid) cause breaks in the genital tract lining or skin, which can create portals of entry for HIV. Second, nonulcerative STDs (chlamydia, gonorrhea, and trichomoniasis) increase the concentration of cells in genital secretions that can serve as HIV targets (CD4+ cells). The upshot of this is that strong and comprehensive efforts to prevent, test, and treat STDs can go a long way toward preventing the spread of HIV sexually. Also, STD trends provide researchers with insights so that they can determine where the HIV epidemic may grow and try to address this trend with appropriate interventions.

Certainly, every proactive health consumer should arm himself or herself with information on STD symptoms and treatments. Those in the realm of health care should exercise increased vigilance; the discovery that a patient has a sexually transmitted disease should prompt physicians to check for other STDs, because occurrence of multiple concurrent infections is common. The truth is, however, that one reason so many STDs are undiagnosed and untreated is that many non-STDs health care workers are reluctant to ask about exposure to sexually transmitted diseases. One factor that complicates all forms of reporting demographics and statistics on sexually transmitted diseases is the private nature of sex—the means of transmission. Americans (and often even their doctors) do not like talking about STDs, and their reluctance makes tracking difficult.

There are a number of mental health issues that are associated with sexually transmitted diseases. Doctors note that some people are so devastated by hearing the news of a sexually transmitted disease diagnosis that they require counseling, whereas others seem to accept it relatively well. Much depends on the basic temperament of the individual, his or her medical history up to that point, and the particular disease. Naturally, those that are incurable affect the individual more drastically.

Depression and anxiety are common problems of those dealing with an STD diagnosis. An important factor for such individuals is finding help and support in treating the psychosocial and psychiatric complications that can go hand in hand with having an STD. Even psychiatric complications of AIDS, such as delirium, mania, psychosis, organic brain disease, depression, and panic disorder can be treated. Often, as someone becomes more ill with HIV/AIDS, he or she is more likely to experience a form of psychiatric distress, which can stem from central nervous system disease, complications from medications, and/or spiritual and emotional dysfunction. A particular mental health problem is seen in certain HIV-negative people with high-risk lifestyles, who become obsessed with whether their next HIV test will have a positive result.

Considering the physical and emotional devastation of all different STDs, it is impossible to overestimate their impact on individuals, couples, and families. For example, high levels of anxiety are related to HPV infections. Patients need to be educated about HPV, and their concerns should be answered. On initial diagnosis, a patient may be extremely upset by fears about health and sexual future. Patients usually want to know how they contracted this disease and how likely they are to spread it to a partner. Pain and disfigurement are also worries. The uncertainty makes some patients entertain the idea of rejecting treatment and maintaining denial. Some patients who have genital warts experience sleep problems, irritability, crying jags, anger outbursts, weight swings, and relationship difficulties. During treatment, new problems can arise from fear of the pain of treatment. Some tried-and-true methods are used when treatment occurs for HPV. Doctors like patient distraction, which may involve the nurse's chatting with the patient while colposcopy is done. One study found that entertaining adolescents with music videos reduced anxiety. Anxiety may be a particular issue among individuals diagnosed with human papillomavirus (HPV). Some estimate that about 30% of sexually active young women have HPV in the lower genital tract. Most HPV infections occur through sexual contact, but the virus can be dormant for years, so there is actually no way to pinpoint when and where a person got the infection. Intrapartum transmission from mother to baby, from nonsexual/casual contact between children and caregivers, between children, and through families possibly occurs, although these are thought to account for a small minority of cases in adults. Most HPV infection is time-limited, although it has been thought that all HPV is forever—a presumption that new evidence calls into question. Risk of serious consequences to the male partner, other than warts, is low. Yet, undiagnosed human papillomavirus may, in some women, lead to cervical cancer.

Psychological distress among those infected is also an enormously devastating result of herpes. In personal relationships, having herpes can feel like having leprosy, and, unfortunately, once it is contracted, there is little one can do other than try to suppress the symptoms and frequency of bouts and take an honest approach with prospective sexual partners. Decreased sense of self-worth is a huge problem with herpes, in that many people, after recovering from the initial feeling of betrayal and shock when they realize they have contracted the disease, move into a state of malaise and inaction. During this time, a redefinition of self can take place, as the individual assigns herself or himself the stigma of being "undesirable." A belief that repeated rejections will occur because of this diagnosis can prove to be an immense burden for a person to carry during youth. Emotional difficulties can cause mood swings and destructive thoughts, as the herpes sufferer experiences relationship rebuffs over months and years after the disease is contracted. To combat the feeling of helplessness that often accompanies this disease, the person with herpes needs to be fortified with knowledge. Knowing how this is spread and how it can be treated can go a long way toward easing the load of self-recrimination and low self-image.

One of the major difficulties occurs in learning how to broach the subject of herpes with a new sex partner, and some should be encouraged to seek counseling with a mental health professional on how to address this subject. In many people with herpes, the fear of rejection as a result of disclosure of herpes is mixed with chagrin and anxiety. Counseling, family support, and preventive measures can help patients cope successfully with this disease. A person who has contracted herpes needs to understand that this disease does recur, and that episodes can vary in severity. In some individuals, episodes tend to become less severe after a year or so; in others, herpes is treacherous to handle indefinitely. Because this disease has asymptomatic shedding, it is extremely important for the infected person to understand that sexual transmission can occur at times when he or she is not aware that the disease is resurfacing. During counseling, a doctor is likely to caution that it is imperative to refrain from sexual intercourse during times when there are prodromal symptoms or lesions. Consistent use of condoms during sexual activity with new or uninfected partners should be a rule of thumb for those with genital herpes. People who have HSV-2 infections are more likely than those with HSV-1 to have viral shedding minus symptoms.

Another key fact that should be shared in counseling is the risk of neonatal infection. Some women are reluctant to disclose that they have herpes when their doctors ask for their gynecologic history, and it is very important that the doctor who is delivering the baby be aware of the herpes. A pregnant woman living with active herpes may require a cesarean section to prevent infection of her baby.

In a study reported in 1998 researchers sought to identify the psychological factors that accompanied chronic recurrent vaginal candidiasis. A group of women with recurring candidiasis were compared with women with no history of this disease. Although the groups were similar in demographic characteristics and most sexual health issues, the ones with recurrent disease were much more likely to suffer from clinical depression and stress, to have low self-esteem, and to report decreased life satisfaction. They also believed that their candidiasis interfered greatly with their relationships, both sexual and emotional. Thus, the study underscored the need for psychological treatment for such patients.

A woman who is diagnosed with chlamydia often is very concerned about her ability to have children—a situation the woman must live with because treating the disease may not prevent its causing infertility. Thus, doctors cannot reassure women about their future reproductive ability. Researchers report that when women find out they have chlamydia, they have several reactions: they are shocked to discover they have a sexually transmitted disease, they feel anxiety about their future fertility, and they often experience difficulty in disclosing the infection to partners. Women report feelings ranging from self-disgust to distress. A group of women who were surveyed in the UK said that they felt isolated, reluctant to confide in friends, and disturbed because they had previously believed that STDs primarily affected only women who were promiscuous.

A person with syphilis can suffer blindness, paralysis, heart damage, mental illness, and death. In some people, hepatitis B leads to liver failure or liver cancer, and thus death. Gonorrhea can lead to pelvic inflammatory disease. HIV leads to AIDS, a terminal illness. Suicide attempts are not unusual among those who have just received HIV-positive test results.

Furthermore, people with sexually transmitted diseases are often ostracized because of prejudice or ignorance. For example, some people still think they can contract HIV by hugging or touching people with this disease. Ostracism can have a devastating effect on the mental health of those who suffer from STDs, and that is one of the reasons why the high incidence of depression in those who have HIV, AIDS, herpes, and other sexually transmitted diseases is not surprising. The USA has federal laws that preclude discrimination against those with disabilities, but there are still cases of workplace and schoolhouse discrimination against those with HIV and AIDS. There are laws designed to protect those afflicted with disabilities from job loss, but courts continue to see cases in which people are harassed and fired. Other legal and social issues that cause difficulties for those with sexually transmitted diseases, especially HIV/AIDS, are home health care, managed care, care for the indigent, and care for those who are rendered incapable of employment as a result of illness.

Related Topics: Discrimination, legal issues for the HIV-infected client, prevention strategies, stigma and stigmatization.

Suggested Reading

Lawrence, S., Walzman, M., Sheppard, S., & Natin, D. (2009). The psychological impact caused by genital warts: Has the Department of Health's choice of vaccination missed the opportunity to prevent such morbidity? *International Journal of STDs and AIDS, 20*(10), 696–700.

Suggested Resources

Centers for Disease Control and Prevention. (2012). *Chlamydia—CDC fact sheet.* Retrieved April 24, 2012 from http://www.cdc.gov/std/chlamydia/stdfact-chlamydia.htm

Centers for Disease Control and Prevention. (2012). *Genital herpes—CDC fact sheet.* Retrieved April 24, 2012 from http://www.cdc.gov/std/Herpes/STDFact-Herpes.htm

Centers for Disease Control and Prevention. (2012). *Human papillomavirus.* Retrieved April 24, 2012 from http://www.cdc.gov/std/hpv/default.htm

Centers for Disease Control and Prevention. (2010). *Syphilis—CDC fact sheet.* Retrieved April 24, 2012 from http://www.cdc.gov/std/syphilis/STDFact-Syphilis.htm

Social Support

Eric Rice, Hailey Winetrobe, and Heather Wollin

Effective social support can dramatically improve the lives of persons living with HIV/AIDS. Enhanced social support networks have been shown to improve: mental health outcomes, HIV medication treatment adherence, self-esteem, perceived quality of life, physical health outcomes, productivity at work, self-care behaviors and outcomes for pregnant women living with HIV. Social support can also reduce stress and fear associated with being HIV positive.

In this entry we: (1) provide a brief introduction to the types and sources of social support that can help persons living with HIV/AIDS, (2) examine issues specific to the lives of men who have sex with men, racial/ethnic minorities, women, and youth, (3) make specific recommendations for practitioners on how to help these populations obtain effective social support, and (4) discuss how online support networks may positively impact the lives of people living with HIV/AIDS. We recognize that race/ethnicity, gender, sexuality, and age are all important categories that define people's experiences with HIV/AIDS. However, we also recognize that people's lives cut across these categories, can impact how they live with the disease, and can compound the stressors they undergo. It is important to remember the potential effects of intersectionality between these categories when working with any individual.

Practitioners, clinicians, social service providers, and health care providers comprise the type of support referred to as *formal support*, whereas *informal support* is defined as the person's family, friends, and community organizations. Social support tends to have three major foci: emotions, information, and tangible resources. For persons living with HIV/AIDS, emotional support can involve feeling loved and cared for, receiving sympathy and pick-me-ups, and displays of physical affection. Informational support relates to assistance with medications, treatment options, health-promoting behaviors, resources, and social services.

E. Rice (✉) • H. Winetrobe • H. Wollin
School of Social Work, University of Southern California, Los Angeles, CA, USA
e-mail: ericr@usc.edu

S. Loue (ed.), *Mental Health Practitioner's Guide to HIV/AIDS*, DOI 10.1007/978-1-4614-5283-6_81, © Springer Science+Business Media New York 2013

Tangible or instrumental support includes help with appointment reminders, caretaking when ill, babysitting, chores, transportation, and money.

Men who have sex with men (MSM) rely heavily on sources of informal social support from partners, friends, family, and communities to cope with a diagnosis of HIV. MSM perceive that they receive less support from family and more support from friends, likely due to the extended friendship networks that exist within the lesbian, gay, bisexual, transgender (LGBT) communities. HIV-positive individuals can help newly diagnosed individuals manage their anxiety around diagnosis. Since there is a high percentage of MSM with HIV, gay community members or friends living with HIV may serve as an added source of support. MSM of a racial/ethnic minority are also faced with compounded stigma and discrimination directed at racial/ethnic minority and gay communities. To overcome this, African American MSM use multiple coping strategies, such as spiritual, passive problem solving, and positive action.

MSM seeking formal networks of social support may be faced with discrimination and homophobia from service providers. It is crucial that clinicians take steps to educate themselves about the unique needs of the LGBT community in order to provide comprehensive and caring services. Clinicians need to first address their own internalized homophobia to effectively work with this population. Clinicians also want to ensure they keep an open and non-judgmental attitude toward their clients' sexual behaviors. It is important for providers to acknowledge the potential for familial discrimination for some MSM and to understand that friends or other LGBT community members may serve as a better source of informal social support.

Relative to gay and bisexual men, women report higher sources of social support from family members. Supportive families of HIV-positive women can enhance their ability to adhere to HIV treatment and improve pregnancy outcomes. Clinicians should encourage women living with HIV to reach out to their family, particularly other female family members, as a major source of support. African American women identify perceived social support from friends and family as an important factor in their medication and treatment adherence. African American women may have lowered emotional support from their husbands, especially if their husbands are also HIV-positive, for they may spend more time taking care of their HIV-positive husbands, and miss out on their own health care needs. Of note, children and grandchildren can serve as a vital means of social support to African American women in sustaining medication adherence and providing emotional and tangible support.

HIV-positive adolescents and young adults rely heavily on family social support. Youth tend to identify family members, close friends, and friends who are aware of their HIV status as those in their support networks. Furthermore, youth who are perinatally infected report more social support than those who became infected through sexual risk or injection drug using behaviors. LBGT youth may experience less family social support and worse mental health symptoms, including depression. Mental health care professionals working with youth, especially for non-heterosexual youth and those who were infected behaviorally, should address social support so the youth may overcome HIV-related stigma and homophobia.

Clinicians should help youth to identify familial support, while understanding that LGBT youth may prefer to receive support from outside of the family. Furthermore, youth who acquired HIV behaviorally may need additional help in identifying positive sources of social support.

Many HIV-positive persons are now turning to the internet for social support. This provides easy access to a seemingly safe place with reduced stigma. Online social support websites, such as message boards, allow users to share personal experiences, provide encouragement and validation, and share resources with their fellow online community members. One study found that frequent users are those who may need the most support—persons recently diagnosed with HIV, persons experiencing great HIV-related symptoms, and persons with AIDS. Users were found to have greater active coping, planning, and emotional and tangible support. Online resources may be especially helpful for persons who live in rural communities and/or communities where HIV is highly stigmatized. Online social support is a useful tool that can be integrated into or combined with in-person formal and informal support.

In working with HIV-positive individuals, clinicians should take into consideration the following points:

1. Ask about the individual's needs related to his/her HIV diagnosis. Then determine how those needs may best be met by formal and/or informal social support through friends and/or family.
2. Assist the individual in identifying who specifically he/she can turn to for social support (formal and informal). This should be multiple people, with some persons serving different roles than others, while attempting to achieve all of the types of social support (i.e., emotional, informational, and tangible).
3. Demonstrate cultural competency. In addition to the aforementioned points, clinicians and providers must be aware of what is (and is not) appropriate for all cultures: women, MSM, racial/ethnic minorities, and youth. This includes avoiding stereotypes, assumptions, and judgments.

Related Topics: AIDS service organizations, coping, faith community, Internet, religion and spirituality.

Suggested Reading

Abramowitz, S., Koenig, L. J., Chandwani, S., Orban, L., Stein, R., Lagrange, R., et al. (2009). Characterizing social support: Global and specific social support experiences of HIV-infected youth. *AIDS Patient Care and STDs, 23*(5), 323–330.

Brashers, D. E., Neidig, J. L., & Goldsmith, D. J. (2004). Social support and the management of uncertainty for people living with HIV or AIDS. *Health Communication, 16*(3), 305–331.

Coursaris, C. K., & Liu, M. (2009). An analysis of social support exchanges in online HIV/AIDS self-help groups. *Computers in Human Behavior, 25*(4), 911–918.

Edwards, L. V. (2006). Perceived social support and HIV/AIDS medication adherence among African American women. *Qualitative Health Research, 16*(5), 679–691.

George, S., Garth, B., Wohl, A. R., Galvan, F. H., Garland, W., & Myers, H. F. (2009). Sources and types of social support that influences engagement in HIV care among Latinos and African Americans. *Journal of Health Care for the Poor and Underserved, 20*(4), 1012–1035.

Mo, P. K. H., & Coulson, N. S. (2008). Exploring the communication of social support within virtual communities: A content analysis of messages posted to an online HIV/AIDS support group. *CyberPsychology & Behavior, 11*(3), 371–374.

Poindexter, C. C. (2010). *Handbook of HIV and social work: Principles, practice, and populations*. Hoboken, NJ: Wiley.

Tate, D., Van Den Berg, J., Hansen, N. B., Kochman, A., & Sikkema, K. J. (2006). Race, social support, and coping strategies among HIV-positive gay and bisexual men. *Culture, Health and Sexuality, 8*(3), 235–249.

Standard of Care

Nicole M. Deming

Standard of care refers to those practices, procedures and quality of treatments that a patient should be accorded and a health care provider is obligated to make available. The phrase "standard of care" also refers to the evaluation of a provider's actions compared to what should have been done in a given situation. As medicine evolves, our knowledge increases and we modify our recommendations and treatment offerings to incorporate and improve our care of patients. As a result, the standard of care is not fixed, but instead, can change rapidly. Health care providers are obligated to stay current and continue to educate themselves on these changing standards. This obligation is often expressed in terms of continued education requirements, certifications, and practice guidelines.

Sometimes the standard of care is clearly defined in professional guidelines or hospital policies. However, these written standards are static and can be outdated if referencing a specific practice rather than general principles. Since the standard of care is a moving target, determining whether a particular action complied with what was required at the time is often determined retrospectively. For example, if a patient claims that a physician did not exercise the sufficient level of care, the standard can be determined by calling in expert witnesses to give testimony to a jury to decide whether the physician's actions reflect what a "reasonable person" would have done in that situation. If the answer is "no" then the physician has violated his or her duty and has been negligent. Several problems exist with defining the standard of care in court including: the variation among juries, the reactionary (rather than proactive) nature of the determination, and the utility of these decisions to health care professionals in practice. However, the standard of care should be viewed as a level of care below which providers cannot go rather than an aspirational ceiling or level of care to reach. This concept plays an important role in the context of research.

N.M. Deming (✉)
Department of Bioethics, Case Western Reserve University, Cleveland, OH, USA
e-mail: Nicole.Deming@case.edu

S. Loue (ed.), *Mental Health Practitioner's Guide to HIV/AIDS*,
DOI 10.1007/978-1-4614-5283-6_82, © Springer Science+Business Media New York 2013

In the USA, an Institutional Review Board (IRB) must evaluate the potential risks and benefits of new interventions in relation to the existing standard of care. The committee needs to know the current standard of care for the disease or condition in question, its relative effectiveness, and whether there is genuine uncertainty regarding which of the proposed treatments in the study will be more effective. The genuine uncertainty regarding the best treatment in a trial is referred to as clinical equipoise and is another source of debate within medicine.

For mental health practitioners, these concepts are important to understand because as the standard of care advances, the ethical permissibility of research and treatment changes accordingly. What further complicates the situation is that standard of care often varies due to location and resource availability. While some professionals and academics claim that standard of care is universal, there are real resource limitations and differences among hospitals, states and countries. As an example, there was a great deal of controversy regarding the use of placebo in HIV clinical trials abroad due to their use of a placebo in lieu of the standard of care as a comparison against the experimental treatment; such a study could not have been approved in the USA because of an established standard of care for treating HIV. These issues represent true ethical dilemmas: even after several decades of debate, reasonable minds can disagree on how standard of care should be defined when comparing different systems of health care.

A standard of care exists to help communicate effective practices in the care of patients. The challenge is to stay current as medicine advances and provide all patients with quality care. In the context of mental health practice, providers must be aware of and remain current with the standard of care in their field generally and in the subspecialty or specialty specifically. This can be achieved through participation in courses for continuing education credit; by seeking supervision, especially in situations involving complex clinical or ethical issues; and by reading the current literature. A failure to do so may place the client at risk of harm, such as through prescription of an inappropriate medication or dose or reliance on an inappropriate psychotherapeutic approach. It may also increase the likelihood that the mental health care provider will face malpractice and/or licensing issues.

Related Topics: Declaration of Helsinki, mental health comorbidity and HIV/AIDS.

Suggested Reading

Freedman, B. (1987). Equipoise and the ethics of clinical research. *New England Journal of Medicine, 317*(3), 141–145.

Lurie, P., & Wolfe, S. M. (1997). Unethical trials of interventions to reduce perinatal transmission of the human immunodeficiency virus in developing countries. *New England Journal of Medicine, 337*(12), 853–856.

Suggested Resources

Council for International Organizations of Medical Sciences c/o World Health Organization (CIOMS). Last accessed April 25, 2012 at http://www.cioms.ch/about/frame_about.htm
Hill, G., & Hill, K. (2012). Standard of care. *The people's law dictionary*. Retrieved April 27, 2012 from http://dictionary.law.com/Default.aspx?selected=2002
United States Department of Health and Human Services. Last accessed April 25, 2012 from http://www.hhs.gov/ohrp/index.html
World Health Organization. (2011). *HIV/AIDS fact sheet*. Retrieved April 27, 2012 from http://www.who.int/mediacentre/factsheets/fs360/en/index.html

Stigma and Stigmatization

Ezer Kang

As Weiss and Ramakrishna noted in 2006, stigma is "a social process or personal experience characterized by exclusion, rejection, blame or devaluation that results from experience or reasonable anticipation of an adverse social judgment about a person or group." In HIV-related stigma, this judgment is conferred by one's HIV-seropositive status. Framed as an individually constructed trait, early research on HIV stigma has focused on stereotype formation and its behavioral and emotional consequences. Studies have identified two categories of stigmatization—enacted and felt stigma, distinguished by experiences of actual discrimination (enacted stigma) and one's perceived fear of encountering stigmatizing practices (felt stigma). Both forms of HIV-related stigma are intertwined with the illness course and uniquely sustained or mitigated by the responses of broader society, friends, and families. Moreover, there are multiple layers of stigma particularly among women and ethnic and sexual minorities living with HIV. Perceptions of marginalization and social rejection, for example, could be perpetuated by virtue of one's serostatus, risk behaviors associated with HIV transmission, undocumented immigration status, gender, or sexual orientation. The immediate consequence of enacted HIV-related stigma is a loss or diminution of individual status. People living with HIV (PLHIV) who experience status loss often report poor mental health outcomes (depression, negative self-worth, social isolation), delayed access to and inconsistent utilization of HIV care, poor medical treatment adherence, and avoidance of serostatus disclosure, particularly among racial and ethnic minorities in the USA and groups that contend with inequalities that predate learning about their HIV serostatus.

Following an experience of actual discrimination, many PLHIVs develop a heightened "stigma consciousness" which informs their world view and behavior. Specifically, they vigilantly avoid situations that would place them at risk for repeated discrimination on account of their HIV-serostatus. They maintain their

E. Kang (✉)
Department of Psychology, Wheaton College, Wheaton, IL, USA
e-mail: Ezer.Kang@wheaton.edu

S. Loue (ed.), *Mental Health Practitioner's Guide to HIV/AIDS*,
DOI 10.1007/978-1-4614-5283-6_83,

illness a secret within public and personal social networks—a task that becomes a consuming priority. The emotional demand of sustaining this heightened sense of vigilance or awareness of social devaluation often has *more* deleterious effects than the immediate consequences of a discriminatory event.

The social setting in which stigma is perceived and experienced influences the degree of psychological damage exerted on PLHIVs. Stigmatizing encounters experienced within one's family and peer networks, as well as institutional settings including employment, healthcare, or recreation have varying affects on PLHIVs depending on the significance placed in these specific settings. Experiencing avoidance from family members or awkward social interactions in healthcare settings, for example, impacts adults with HIV more adversely than experiencing such avoidance or awkwardness in other social settings. Not all PLHIVs experience diminished well-being or negative emotional consequences from HIV-stigma. Responses to stigma-related events vary depending on the timing of the occurrence, one's repertoire of self-protective strategies, and the extent to which stigmatizing traits can be concealed.

Few studies have found that stigmatizing beliefs against PLHIVs are significantly correlated with lower HIV knowledge and beliefs, suggesting the importance of both correcting misinformation about HIV and mitigating the influences of stigma. Addressing HIV knowledge and stigma is particularly critical given the relationship between stigma and high risk sexual behavior. Studies, for example, have also found that stigmatizing perceptions of persons with HIV are associated with increased sexual risk behavior (multiple partners), less frequent use of condoms, and voluntary HIV testing in two major cities in China.

Although overt expressions of HIV-related stigmatization in the USA have declined since the 1990s, many people continue to have misinformed fears of HIV transmission by casual social contact, and punitive and negative attitudes towards persons living with HIV. Moreover, historic associations between HIV and marginalized groups such as gay men and injecting drug users continue to inform public attitudes towards PLHIVs.

Similarly in rural regions of East Asia, illness stigma is based largely on misconception of casual HIV transmission coupled with cultural proscriptions against high-risk groups. Recent scholarship, for example, has reconceptualized HIV stigma in China as a "moral process" that undermines one's social and familial obligation to preserve "face"—both moral (*lian*) and social (*mianzi*)—which governs inner social networks of family and kinship ties, and outer networks (e.g., friends, neighbors). Another dimension of HIV stigma to consider is pubic fear of HIV contagion—one that is shaped and reinforced by ingrained misconceptions of HIV transmission or unfamiliarity with the epidemic. Stigma in rural China is largely enacted by excluding and isolating PLHIVs out of fear of infection and not necessarily motivated by socio-moral condemnation of HIV risk behavior. In some regions, the inclination to avoid social contact with PLHIVs may reflect more instinctual self-preservation rather than a malicious intent to discredit another. In a study of HIV- and drug abuse-related stigma among the Dai community in the Dehong prefecture of Yunnan, HIV illness did not reinforce stigma against drug abusers per se; rather, the illness solicited a compassionate response, largely motivated by a desire to earn merits and ensure happiness and prosperity in the next life.

Recent scholarship has conceptually reframed HIV-related stigma as a social rather than individual process that perpetuates and sustains relations of power that exclude and devalue people and groups. This approach shifts the focus from how individuals act towards one another to consider how culture and history construct social hierarchies and breed intergroup difference and domination that underlie HIV and AIDS-related stigma. As such, researchers have challenged conventional individual-level interventions (e.g., cognitive-behavioral approaches) and argued for structural interventions aimed at shifting community paradigms about HIV and its intersection with other causes of inequity. This approach, for example, has recently informed studies that examine the unique roles of African American and Chinese ethnic churches in reshaping cultural scripts on HIV prevention in their respective communities.

Related Topics: Discrimination, faith community, gender identity, hate crimes, risk behaviors, risk groups.

Suggested Reading

Alonzo, A. A., & Reynolds, N. R. (1995). Stigma, HIV and AIDS: An explorations and elaboration of a stigma trajectory. *Social Science and Medicine, 14*(3), 303–315.

Link, B. G., & Phelan, J. (2001). Conceptualizing stigma. *Annual Review of Sociology, 27*, 363.

Major, B., & O'Brien, L. T. (2005). The social psychology of stigma. *Annual Review of Psychology, 56*, 393–421.

Parker, R., & Aggleton, P. (2003). HIV and AIDS-related stigma and discrimination: A conceptual framework and implications for action. *Social Science and Medicine, 57*(2003), 13.

Stutterheim, S. E., Pryor, J. B., Bor, A. E. R., Hogendijk, R., Muris, P., & Schaalma, H. P. (2009). HIV-related stigma and psychological distress: The harmful effects of specific stigma manifestations in various social settings. *AIDS, 23*, 2353–2357.

Weiss, M. G., & Ramak, J. (2006). Stigma interventions and research for international health. *Lancet, 367*, 536.

Yang, L. S., Kleinman, A., Link, B. G., Phelan, J. C., Lee, S., & Good, B. (2007). Culture and stigma: Adding moral experiences to stigma theory. *Social Science and Medicine, 64*, 1524–1535.

Substance Use

Beatrice Gabriela Ioan

Introduction

Substance use refers to the use of both legal (e.g., alcohol) and illegal drugs (e.g., cocaine). Substance use and HIV infection are considered to be "twin epidemics," often affecting the same individuals. Substance use has been found to be associated with HIV transmission and complicates the management of this disease. Because substance use often co-occurs with mental illness, it is critical that mental health care providers be aware of the HIV-related risks that are associated with substance use.

The United Nations Office on Drugs and Crime (UNDOC) estimates that approximately 16 million people around the world inject themselves with illicit substances, mainly opioids, and of these, three million are HIV-infected. In a cross-sectional survey in the USA, the prevalence of HIV infection was similar: 12–17% among heroin and cocaine users, regardless of the mechanism of administration. It has been estimated that of approximately 10% of the estimated six million users of illegal substances in the USA, about 10% inject drugs and about 40–45% of them are HIV infected. In contrast, it is estimated that 25–30% of substance users who do not inject are HIV-infected. However, the risk of HIV associated with substance use varies across substances.

HIV Transmission in Substance Users

Injection drug users face the highest risk of HIV infection. It is estimated that from the moment when HIV makes its way inside a community of substance users by injection, it takes less than 2 years for the infection to reach 90% prevalence.

B.G. Ioan (✉)
Legal Medicine, Medical Deontology and Bioethics Department, University of Medicine and Pharmacy "Gr. T. Popa", Iasi, Romania
e-mail: ioanbml@yahoo.com

S. Loue (ed.), *Mental Health Practitioner's Guide to HIV/AIDS*,
DOI 10.1007/978-1-4614-5283-6_84, © Springer Science+Business Media New York 2013

According to a survey of the Centers for Disease Control and Prevention (CDC) conducted in 33 US states between 2001 and 2004, 21% of the females and 21% of the males of adult and teen age who were newly diagnosed with HIV/AIDS were injecting drugs.

HIV transmission in injecting drug users is primarily due to high risk injecting techniques, such as injection in a shooting gallery, needle sharing, and the sharing of other injection paraphernalia such as cotton for filtering the heroin or cocaine solution. In the latter situation the blood containing the virus from the used syringe is deposited on the cotton wad. It is then "washed" in the filtered drug solution and the virus is transmitted to the next user by injecting this solution. Individuals who utilize this technique might consider themselves safe because they are not sharing the same needle with others. As a consequence, they are often unaware of their HIV-positive status and may unknowingly transmit the virus to others through unprotected sexual intercourse.

Individuals acting under the influence of a substance may become infected with HIV and/or transmit the virus to others as a result of engaging in risky sexual behaviors. A study conducted in San Francisco in 1999 with injecting cocaine users indicated that, in addition to sharing needles, they also displayed risky sexual behavior, in that they failed to use condoms or engaged in sexual intercourse in exchange for illegal substances. The recognition of the connection between injection drug use and HIV transmission led to the establishment of needle exchange programs as one approach to harm reduction. These programs provide injection drug users with clean needles and syringes in exchange for the used ones as a method of harm reduction. These programs can prevent HIV transmission, but they do not seem to be reducing the level of injection drug use.

Non-injection drug use is significantly more common than injection drug use. Non-injection drug use is characterized by heterogeneity of use patterns, the substances used, and the motivations underlying consumption. Non-injection substance use may indirectly increase the risk of HIV transmission through associated risky sexual behavior. Nevertheless, the risk of HIV transmission associated with non-injection drug use is lower compared to that associated with injection drug use. As a result, non-injecting substance users might falsely consider themselves protected from HIV transmission, unaware that the virus may be transmitted through risky sexual behavior, thus facilitating the spread of infection.

Specific Substances and HIV

Studies have found a statistically significant association between risky sexual behavior and non-injection substance use, especially in the case of amphetamines, methamphetamines, cocaine, and alcohol, and nitrates ("poppers"). Treatment for drug use leads to an important decrease in HIV transmission.

Alcohol consumption increases the risk of HIV transmission behavior by reducing inhibition and reason, impairing cognition and perception (also known as "alcohol myopia"), and causing a surge in sexual arousal. The association between alcohol consumption and unprotected sexual intercourse has been observed among both men who have sex with women and men who have sex with men (MSM). Studies have shown that consuming alcohol leads to a reduced use of condoms, but not in the case of new partners or newly established couples. HIV transmission is linked to alcohol consumption before intercourse and alcohol and drug abuse among men who have sex with men (MSM) both before and during sexual intercourse is linked to a high HIV incidence.

Amphetamines and methamphetamines increase sexual confidence, libido, sexual function, and pain endurance; prolong sexual encounters and increase their number during intoxication; dehydrate genital and rectal mucosal surfaces; and alter the mental state of the consumer. These substances also adversely affect individuals' ability to reason and make decisions. Hypersexuality is one of the main effects of amphetamine and methamphetamine use; consumers often report high sexual activity while using these drugs. Amphetamine and methamphetamine use are highly associated with HIV transmission. This association may be due to low use of condoms during anal or vaginal intercourse, participation in unprotected sexual activity in exchange for drugs or money, and effects of these substances on the immune system. Behavioral interventions for treating amphetamine and methamphetamine addiction have been found to reduce the frequency of unprotected sex as well as substance use.

The use of Ecstasy (methilenedioximethamphetamine—MDMA) by teenagers has been found to lead to low condom use. In the case of MSM, it favors unprotected anal sex and HIV seroconversion.

Cocaine, a central nervous system stimulant, is consumed annually by approximately 14 million people around the world. According to statistics provided by the Substance Abuse and Mental Health Services Administration in 2006, the cocaine consumption during the preceding year was more frequent amongst MSM (37%) than among the general population (1%). Cocaine consumption raises self-confidence, sexual appetite and libido, and alters mental state. Cocaine use before or during sexual intercourse induces high risk sexual behaviors such as unprotected anal sex with an HIV-infected partner or a partner with undetermined HIV status, reduced condom use, and the exchange of sex for money.

Nitrates (popper) increase sexual appetite, produce vasodilation, and relaxation of the anal sphincter, thus facilitating anal sexual intercourse. The frequency of anal sexual intercourse in the case of MSM and HIV seroconversion depend upon the level of nitrate consumption.

According to the United Nations, marijuana is consumed by approximately 160 million people around the world; it is the most consumed substance after alcohol. It alters mental state and intensifies sexual pleasure. Some studies have shown that using marijuana before sexual intercourse in the case of MSM favors unprotected passive anal intercourse and anal sexual intercourse with serodiscordant partners or with an unknown HIV status. In the case of self-identified heterosexuals, marijuana favors unprotected sexual intercourse.

Consumption of multiple substances, e.g., more than one substance at once, is more frequent among cocaine and amphetamine users. The simultaneous use of several substances and the order in which they are consumed may modify the quantities of used substances. For example, in a study conducted with college students, it was observed that alcohol consumption was higher when associated with cocaine consumption. There are some specific combinations of drugs, such as methamphetamines and erectile dysfunction drugs (e.g., Viagra) that increase the probability of engaging in risky sexual behavior, thereby increasing the risk of HIV transmission. Multidrug consumption among MSM has been found to increase the probability of unprotected anal sexual practice and the frequency of sex club and bathhouse visits. Teenagers tend to reduce the use of condoms and are more likely to consider exchanging sexual intercourse for money or drugs.

Specific Populations

Women who consume illicit substances are often victims of partner physical and sexual abuse. Because they are fearful of abuse, they may not approach their partners about condom use. As a result, they may be at increased risk of HIV transmission due to their partners' risky behaviors. If they are HIV-positive, they may also refrain from disclosing their serostatus due to fear of abuse.

Substance-using homeless individuals may be at increased risk of HIV infection due to the existence of psychiatric comorbidities and other serious health issues, participation in survival sex (engaging sex for money, drugs, shelter or food).

Prison inmates are prone to psychiatric disorders, suicide, self-mutilation, a high level of stress, sexual harassment, and physical and psychological abuse. In addition, there is frequent contact with others who are using illicit substances. This contact may create a high risk of substance use, which may be initiated or continued in prison. Studies reveal a strong connection between incarceration and blood-borne infectious diseases, including HIV.

The rate of illicit substance use among juvenile delinquents is higher than in the general teen population, a situation that leads to greater risk of transmitting HIV infection as well as other STDs. Juvenile delinquency is frequently associated with substance use during sexual intercourse, a high incidence of STDs and pregnancy, early start of sexual activity, multiple sexual partners, unprotected sex, and a high rate of mental disorders, each of which is associated with increased HIV risk.

The risk of HIV infection among mentally ill persons is significantly higher in comparison with the general population. Research studies report that mentally ill individuals have high rates of HIV risk behavior such as unprotected sexual intercourse, multiple partners, the exchange of sex for money, and injection drug use. The severity of the mental illness is predictive of the HIV infection risk. Research has found that those who suffer from mood swings are more likely to be sexually active than those suffering from psychotic disturbances. Individuals with bipolar disorder who are manic may experience euphoria, a highly energetic mood, hypersexuality, impulsiveness, and altered judgment that can lead to risky behavior. Studies show that the association between a recent manic episode and the intense use of substances increases the risk of HIV infection. Of all illicit substances, cocaine is most likely to induce risky sexual behavior and HIV transmission when associated with mania.

Treatment for HIV-Infected Substance Users

Substance users may be reluctant to undergo HIV testing because of denial, fear, and/or the belief that nothing can be done in case the result is positive. Since an early diagnosis offers an opportunity for an early treatment, treatment programs for substance use should encourage testing for HIV. Treatment interventions for substance use should also seek to decrease risky sexual behavior, encourage condom use, and access HIV treatment. That said, substance addiction and HIV infection are chronic conditions of varying evolution, including remissions and exacerbations.

Methadone treatment of injecting opiate users leads to a reduction of risky behavior by lessening drug- and sex-related risk behavior. Nevertheless, studies indicate that treatment for HIV infection and opiate addiction may be complicated by interactions between methadone and antiretroviral medicine. For other drugs, such as cocaine, behavioral therapies may be used to reduce or eliminate usage.

HIV-infected individuals with a history of substance use, particularly those who have been dependent on opiates such as heroin, frequently have a lower pain threshold compared to those who have not used these drugs. Pain may persist despite the opiate use, most likely due to particular neuropsychological issues. Opiate pseudoaddiction may occur due to the inadequate or partial treatment of pain. Medical staff may be concerned about prescribing and administering opiates due to an individual's abuse of or dependence on these substances. However, if pain is not controlled adequately, individuals may again resort to illegally using opiates, which may lead to the adoption of risky sexual behaviors. It is important that care providers treating individuals who have abused or are abusing opiates counsel them with respect to HIV prevention strategies.

There are a number of barriers to the provision of medical care to HIV-infected substance users, including poverty, malnutrition, an inadequate and stressful lifestyle, and self-neglect. Stress factors and the effects of illicit substances may throw consumers into a state of denial regarding medical care and even make them abandon treatment. Due to self-neglect, a precarious financial state, a lack of medical insurance, a low number of treatment facilities, and a lack of empathy from the medical system, substance users may find themselves in an advanced state of illness when they seek medical care. Also, due to financial issues they may not always be able to stay on the diets prescribed to them. Some HIV-infected substance users may refuse treatment because they have no confidence in the medical staff and others because they fear their HIV-positive status might be revealed.

The treatment of HIV-infected substance users calls for a multidisciplinary and multi-dimensional approach in order to tackle all medical, psychological and social issues that the clients are facing. The sensitivity and cultural competence of the medical staff are key points for convincing the HIV-infected substance user to join and stay with the programs. The medical team must provide services that are acceptable from the patients' point of view and cultural background. Thus, they must understand the way patients define and consider their own sexual orientation (e.g., they must be aware of the pressure gays, lesbians and bisexuals are under within their community or at the work place). Moreover, clients' families need to be taken into account (what exactly the concept of family is to them), as well as their community, gender, and spirituality (religious leaders, church members, and spiritual support may help attract and keep patients on treatment). Involving successfully recovering substance users in treatment programs for substance-dependent individuals may ensure cultural compatibility and lead to success.

Individuals with co-occurring substance use and HIV infection may be reluctant to participate in clinical trials to test antiretroviral medicine, either because they do not want to be on any kind of medication or because such an experience with untested medicine would remind them of illicit substance use. However, individuals who lack adequate health insurance coverage may be unable to obtain the care necessary to maintain their health. Too, active substance users with co-occurring substance use disorders may be excluded from clinical trials due to a belief that they will be unable or unwilling to adhere to the study protocol. This may not only result in a lack of access to the most innovative treatments, but also raises important ethical issues.

Related Topics: Access to care, harm reduction, housing and homelessness, mental health comorbidity and HIV/AIDS, prevention strategies, risk behaviors, stigma and stigmatization, syringe exchange.

Suggested Reading

American Psychiatric Association. (2000). *Diagnostic and statistical manual of mental disorders, fourth edition, text revision*. Washington, DC: Author.

Dookeran, N. M., Burgess, J. F., Bowman, C. C., Goetz, M. B., Asch, S. M., & Gifford, A. L. (2009). HIV screening among substance-abusing veterans in care. *Journal of Substance Abuse Treatment, 37*, 286–291.

Drumright, N. L., & Colfax, N. G. (2009). HIV risk and prevention for non-injection substance users. In K. H. Mayer & H. F. Pizer (Eds.), *HIV prevention. A comprehensive approach* (pp. 340–375). London: Academic/Elsevier.

Ghiza, U. E., Epstein, D. H., & Preston, K. L. (2008). Contingency management reduces injection-related HIV risk behaviors in heroin and cocaine using outpatients. *Addictive Behaviors, 33*, 593–604.

Gonzales-Guarda, R. M., Peragallo, N., Urrutia, M. T., Vasquez, E. P., & Mitrani, V. B. (2008). HIV risks, substance abuse, and intimate partner violence among Hispanic women and their intimate partners. *Journal of the Association of Nurses in AIDS Care, 19*(4), 252–266.

Mackesy-Amiti, M. E., Fendrich, M., & Johnson, T. P. (2009). Substance-related problems and treatment among men who have sex with men in comparison to another men in Chicago. *Journal of Substance Abuse Treatment, 36*, 227–233.
Meade, C. S., Graff, F. S., Griffin, M. L., & Weiss, R. D. (2008). HIV risk behavior among patients with co-ocurring bipolar and substance use disorders: Associations with mania and drug abuse. *Drug and Alcohol Dependence, 92*, 296–300.
Reback, C. J., Kamien, J. B., & Amass, L. (2007). Characteristics and HIV risk behaviors of homeless, substance-using men who have sex with men. *Addictive Behaviors, 32*, 647–654.
Tolou-Shams, M., Brown, L. K., Gordon, G., & Fernandez, I. (2007). Arrest history as an indicator of asolescent/young adult substance use and HIV risk. *Drug and Alcohol Dependence, 88*, 87–90.
Tsao, J. C. I., Stein, J. A., & Dobalian, A. (2007). Pain, problem drug use history, and aberrant analgesic use behaviors in persons living with HIV. *Pain, 133*, 128–137.

Suggested Resources

Centers for Disease Control and Prevention. *HIV testing*. Retrieved January 15, 2012 from http://www.cdc.gov/hiv/topics/testing/
Center for Substance Abuse Treatment. (1993). *SAMHSA/CSAT treatment improvement protocols*. Rockville, MD: Author. Retrieved January 15, 2012 from http://www.ncbi.nlm.nih.gov/books/NBK82999/
United Nations AIDS (UNAIDS). (2010). *UNAIDS report onthe global AIDS epidemic 2010*. Retrieved February 12, 2012 from http://www.unaids.org/globalreport/default.htm
United Nations Office on Drugs and Crime, & UNAIDS. (n.d.). *Protocol on assessing drug use and HIV in prison settings*. Retrieved February 12, 2012 from http://www.unodc.org/documents/hiv-aids/publications/UNODC_MENA_2009_Protocol_on_assessing_drug_use_and_HIV_in_prison_settings_-EN.pdf
World Health Organization. *Management of substance abuse: Facts and figures*. Retrieved February 12, 2012 from http://www.who.int/substance_abuse/facts/en/

Suicide and HIV

Kristen G. Shirey

Suicidal ideation, attempts, and completions are common among people living with HIV/AIDS (PLWHA). Recent cohort studies have found that the rate of suicide completion among PLWHA in Switzerland is three times that of the general population, and, in the USA, one in five HIV positive patients report having had suicidal ideation in the previous week. Many factors contribute to this phenomenon, including highly prevalent comorbid depression, substance use disorders, social isolation, stigma, and chronic pain and fatigue associated with the disease. During the early years of the HIV epidemic, suicide rates in the USA and Western Europe were extremely high, particularly among men. With the advent of combination antiretroviral therapy (cART), and resultant prolonged life expectancy, suicide rates have declined and are now similar to those of other populations living with chronic medical illnesses such as amyotrophic lateral sclerosis, end-stage renal disease, and spinal cord injury. However, even with the decline in suicide rates since the 1990s, suicidal ideation and behaviors remain alarmingly high among PLWHA, and it is urgent for providers caring for this population to evaluate and address suicide risk in routine clinical practice.

Though life expectancy for HIV positive patients has improved dramatically with cART, it remains lower than that of the general population. Further, cART is often accompanied by a number of adverse side effects and toxicities that markedly impair quality of life. Certain antiretroviral drugs, notably the non-nucleoside reverse transcriptase inhibitor efavirenz, directly cause neuropsychiatric side effects including depression and worsening suicidal ideation. Some characteristics of those who complete suicide have changed since the pre-cART era; now suicide completers more commonly have an underlying diagnosis of mental illness and are

K.G. Shirey (✉)
Department of Psychiatry and Behavioral Sciences, Duke University Medical Center, Durham, NC, USA

Department of Medicine, Duke University Medical Center, Durham, NC, USA
e-mail: kristen.shirey@duke.edu

S. Loue (ed.), *Mental Health Practitioner's Guide to HIV/AIDS*,
DOI 10.1007/978-1-4614-5283-6_85,

likely to have received some treatment for mental illness. In the 1980s and 1990s, pre-cART, suicide completion appeared to be influenced more by HIV disease progression than by psychiatric comorbidities. The associations between mental illnesses, particularly depression, and HIV are complex. People with baseline mental illness and substance use disorders are at elevated risk for contracting HIV due to increased risk behaviors. Once infected, people with mental illness or substance use disorders are at increased risk of transmitting the virus to others. Such comorbidities are associated with suicidal ideation and behaviors in those without HIV, so adding this stressor compounds risk in an already vulnerable population.

While the risk of suicide in PLWHA is elevated throughout the lifespan, there are points during the disease course during which individuals are at particularly high risk. These points include time of HIV diagnosis, signs of disease progression such as first opportunistic infection or diagnosis of AIDS, changes in medication regimen, and stressful live events related to bereavement or disease-related stigma. In contrast to pre-cART era suicide rates that did increase with disease progression, there is no longer a clear relationship between suicide attempt and duration of HIV infection. In fact, some studies suggest that HIV positive individuals develop effective coping strategies over the course of the illness that lead to reduced suicide risk over time. Apart from the stress of having a chronic disease compiled with other stressors and comorbidities in the lives of PLWHA, the HIV virus itself may increase suicide risk in that individuals with HIV associated dementia complex can experience mood lability, impulsivity, and impaired judgment that heighten suicide risk.

Almost all studies of suicidal ideation, attempts, and completions have taken place in the developed world, where only 15 % of suicides occur. In the developing world, where 85 % of suicides occur, and where the burden of the HIV epidemic lies, the relationship between suicide and HIV status is not as well characterized. In North America and Western Europe, suicide has traditionally been associated with mental illnesses, particularly depression and alcohol abuse. However, studies in Asian countries suggest that different risk factors play a greater role in suicide, including impulsiveness, financial stress, and interpersonal conflict.

The issues of suicidal ideation and attempts among PLWHA are challenging indeed, related to complex relationships between psychosocial stressors, comorbid mental illness and substance use disorders, and the HIV virus itself through a combination of direct effects of the virus on mediating symptoms such as fatigue and cognitive changes, adverse side effects and impaired quality of life from cART, and the stigma and social isolation associated with HIV. While this is a complicated problem and the challenges are many, it is clear that suicidal ideation and attempts are a major source of suffering and mortality and need to be addressed. Clinicians should routinely screen HIV positive patients, no matter what stage of disease, for suicidal ideation and for comorbid psychiatric illness and should treat and refer accordingly. Individual and group psychotherapy may greatly benefit in providing support and bolstering coping skills. Psychotropic medications, including antidepressants, are generally well tolerated even in combination with cART and effectively treat comorbid depression that so frequently contributes to suicide in

PLWHA. Further, in collaboration with prescribers of cART, regimens can be tailored to avoid medications such as efavirenz that may escalate risk in at-risk individuals.

Related Topics: Cognitive impairment, HIV-associated dementia, mental health comorbidity and HIV/AIDS, stigma and stigmatization, substance use.

Suggested Reading

Baidee, J., Moore, D. J., Atkinson, J. H., Vaida, F., Gerard, M., Duarte, N. A., et al. (2011). Lifetime suicidal ideation and attempt are common among HIV+ individuals. *Journal of Affective Disorders*. doi:10.1016/j.jad.2011.06.044 (epub ahead of print).

Carrico, A. W., Johnson, M. O., Morin, S. F., Remien, R. H., Charlebois, E. D., Steward, W. T., et al. (2007). Correlates of suicidal ideation among HIV-positive persons. *AIDS, 21*, 1199–1203.

Clifford, D. B., Evans, S., Yang, Y., Acosta, E. P., Goodkin, K., Tashima, K., et al. (2005). Impact of efavirenz on neuropsychological performance and symptoms in HIV-infected individuals. *Annals of Internal Medicine, 143*, 714–721.

Keiser, O., Spoerri, A., Brinkhof, M. W. G., Hasse, B., Gayet-Ageron, A., Tissot, F., et al. (2010). Suicide in HIV-infected individuals and the general population in Switzerland, 1998–2008. *American Journal of Psychiatry, 167*, 143–150.

Robertson, K., Parsons, T. D., Van der Horst, C., & Hall, C. (2006). Thoughts of death and suicidal ideation in nonpsychiatric human immunodeficiency virus seropositive individuals. *Death Studies, 30*(5), 455–469.

Survival Sex

Vanessa A. Forro

Survival sex has been used to describe a transactional relationship in exchange for money, sex, drugs, food, shelter, or any other daily means of survival. It encompasses sex as work as well as other forms of small scale, money-making, in informal sectors such as selling homemade goods, brewing illicit beer or liquor, petty trade and other crimes. The term "survival sex" originated among researchers and sex workers in Durban, South Africa. Many women and men engage in some type of these activities at some point in their lives, which is primarily due to increasing unemployment, lack of options for financial support, war and conflict, and basic daily survival. Survival sex is about getting by in a world of poverty, prejudice, and disempowerment. As one woman put it, "This is how we survive" (Preston-Whyte, Varga, Oosthuizen, Robert, & Blose, 2000).

Like HIV/AIDS, sex for money or other survival needs are both the center of debate over the nature and limits of sexual relationships. The danger that lies in sex work is not necessarily the "work" itself, but rather the contexts and geographical areas in which it is practiced. Transactional sex need not be a one-time interaction, and some individuals who have long-standing sexual relationships for survival needs often do not consider themselves as sex workers. The paradox of "survival" sex in the heightened exposure to HIV/AIDS is achieved only at the expense of long-term illness or death.

Gender inequality has also been a pervasive factor in HIV/AIDS risk. Women are at risk for HIV because poverty is the primary determining condition of their lives. Women's vulnerability in the HIV epidemic in most developing countries is determined by their social, political, and economic subordination as well as poverty-driven survival sex.

In conflict-driven nations women and girls are particularly vulnerable to participate in survival sex activities, increasing their acquisition of HIV/AIDS. The United Nations Development Fund for Women (UNIFEM) reports that about

V.A. Forro (✉)
Neurological Outcomes Center, Case Western Reserve University, Cleveland, OH, USA
e-mail: Vanessa.Forro@case.edu

S. Loue (ed.), *Mental Health Practitioner's Guide to HIV/AIDS*,

DOI 10.1007/978-1-4614-5283-6_86,

75% of the more than 35 million displaced persons worldwide are women and children. Women make up over half of the HIV/AIDS infections in sub-Saharan Africa. The breakdown of family, community, and social networks, lack of access to health care, stigma and discrimination fuels the imbalances between women and men. This destitute environment heightens the reliance of women on men for physical and emotional security. In a report from sub-Saharan Africa, it was revealed that refugee women and girls are propositioned and forced to have sex with soldiers, police, or peace-keeping officers in exchange for food, shelter, and protection. In these situations, women are trying to provide for themselves, their husbands, children, and even orphans. Young, orphaned girls are forced to fend for themselves and often their siblings. The prevalence of HIV among military and police officials in these areas can range above 50%, leaving women and girls at a disproportionate risk.

Commercial sex worker's vulnerability to HIV/AIDS varies and is multidimensional. One dimension relates to the law, where sex work is legal, has degrees of legality, or illegal. Discrimination compounds the vulnerability of commercial sex workers to HIV/AIDS, and unprotected sex is a serious issue among this group. Clients often refuse to use a condom, sometimes to the point of being violent. Due to their illegal status, many commercial sex workers are often unable to report this violence for fear of being prosecuted. In addition, the cost of a pack of condoms is often far greater than what commercial sex workers receive for sex. Poverty-induced exploitation of commercial sex workers increases the difficulty of negotiating safer sex practices and work environments.

Women who engage in survival sex are significantly more likely to have experienced trauma in their lives, and are more likely to fall victim to assault and episodes of violence as adults. In one study looking at the HIV/AIDS knowledge and behavior of women engaged in sex for survival in Durban, South Africa, researchers discovered that although most of the individuals were well-informed about HIV/AIDS, their attitude was that they have more pressing issues to consider. Thus, having sex without a condom pays more and is often the decision they are willing to make in order to survive. The structural relationship of poverty and risk is clear, but HIV has made this risk a matter of not only survival, but of death.

A study from sexually transmitted infections (STIs) clinics in Seattle attempted to identify the concurrent factors related to sexual behavior and STIs. They found that women who reported engaging in survival sex often had a main sexual partner or many short-term partners. Their transactions were either for money or drugs, and the survival sex was generally with the non-main partner. The researchers also found that women who engaged in survival sex for money were more likely to use a condom than those reporting having sex for drugs, where negotiation is compromised.

Street youth are another HIV/AIDS at-risk group that has been identified as participating in survival sex. Several studies have shown that street youth are particularly vulnerable due to increased criminalization and violence, risk-enhanced environments, and high HIV prevalence in social networks. Street youth are at 25–40% increased risk for participating in survival sex, and this activity is equally common among males and females. A multisite US study found that approximately one quarter of street and homeless or runway youth reported ever participating in survival sex. The prevalence of survival sex among this population is linked to individual circumstances and duration of homelessness. Additionally, street youth are at increased risk of other adverse health outcomes such as depression, suicidality, and victimization. Sexual minority street youth are significantly more likely to report engaging in survival sex, report significantly greater numbers of clients, and are more likely to report inconsistent condom use.

The medical and social services communities recognize the social, cultural, and legal vulnerabilities of survival sex interactions. The development of vaginal microbicides is one preventive measure that is being developed particularly for individuals who lack the power or resources to negotiate condom use. These products will place some control back into the hands of women who engage in survival sex. Other measures to educate and provide resources to commercial sex workers and street youth include peer-education programs, street-based outreach, and drop-in centers that provide HIV and STI testing, counseling, and other health-related referrals. The dynamics of survival sex are varied and the risk of HIV acquisition is great, yet the roots of these issues include a much larger picture than the activity of sex for survival itself.

Related Topics: Housing and homelessness, sexually transmitted infections, women.

Suggested Reading

Gorbach, P. M., Stoner, B. P., Aral, S. O., Whittington, W. L. H., & Holmes, K. K. (2002). Understanding concurrent sexual partnerships in Seattle, Washington. *Sexually Transmitted Diseases, 29*(8), 453–462.

Green, J. M., Ennett, S. T., & Ringwalt, C. L. (1999). Prevalence and correlates of survival sex among runaway and homeless youth. *American Journal of Public Health, 89*(9), 1406–1409.

Marshall, B. D. L., Shannon, K., Kerr, T., Zhang, R., & Wood, E. (2010). Survival sex work and increased HIV risk among sexual minority street-involved youth. *Journal of AIDS, 53*(5), 661–664.

Preston-Whyte, E., Varga, C., Oosthuizen, H., Robert, R., & Blose, F. (2000). Survival sex and HIV/AIDS in an African city. In R. Parker, R. M. Barbosa, & P. Aggleton (Eds.), *Framing the sexual subject: The politics of gender, sexuality, and power* (pp. 165–190). Berkeley and Los Angeles, CA: University of California Press.

Renzaho, A. M. N., & Pallotta-Chiarolli, M. (2009). Commercial sex work, survival sex, sexual violence and HIV/AIDS prevention in Arumeru District, Arusha Region of Tanzania. *The Open Tropical Medicine Journal, 2*, 27–38.

Suggested Resources

National Alliance to End Homelessness. (2009, October 30). *Homeless youth and sexual exploitation: Research findings and practice implications*. Retrieved from http://www.endhomelessness.org/content/general/detail/2559

Otsuki, J. *Refugee women, girls in sub-Saharan Africa among hardest hit by HIV/AIDS crisis*. Retrieved from http://www.ypwc.org/beta/files/pdf/hiv-aids/Otsuki.pdf

Syringe Exchange

Bettina Rausa

Syringe exchange programs (SEPs) are designed to provide a way for individuals who inject drugs intravenously to exchange their used syringes for new, sterile ones. They also provide safe disposal of used syringes. Because syringes are not always easy to obtain (i.e., a prescription may be required in some states), the practice of sharing needles and syringes among injection drug users (IDUs) is common, and the sharing of syringes greatly increases the chances of contracting and transmitting HIV. In fact, injection drug use and HIV are explicitly connected and injection drug use is considered one of the highest risk activities contributing to the spread of HIV.

SEPs are part of a public health approach to addressing community health problems and concerns referred to as harm reduction. Harm reduction programs are designed to meet clients "where they are at" by creating safe, non-threatening and non-judgmental options for individuals who engage in high-risk health behaviors. The goal of a SEP is to discourage the sharing of syringes among IDUs, therefore lowering the risk of disease. In 1997, a series of studies conducted in 81 cities around the world with SEPs found that HIV infection rates decreased by 6% in 29 cities that provided this service, whereas infection rates increased by 6% in 52 cities that did not have a SEP.

In addition to providing clean syringes, SEPs provide a variety of care and prevention services that are fundamental to helping IDUs reduce their risks of acquiring HIV and other diseases. These services include: HIV/AIDS education, counseling, on-site HIV testing, and crisis intervention; condom distribution; referrals to substance abuse treatment, medical and social services; distribution of sterilizing equipment such as alcohol and cotton swabs to help prevent sores and wound infections; screening for diseases such as tuberculosis (TB) and hepatitis C and B; and the provision of primary healthcare services. SEPs operate in various settings including storefronts, drop-in centers, mobile vans, other street outreach

B. Rausa (✉)
Salk Institute for Biological Studies, La Jolla, CA, USA
e-mail: brausa@cox.net

S. Loue (ed.), *Mental Health Practitioner's Guide to HIV/AIDS*,
DOI 10.1007/978-1-4614-5283-6_87, © Springer Science+Business Media New York 2013

activities, 24-h vending machines, health clinics, pharmacies, and in places were IDUs gather.

According to the Centers for Disease Control and Prevention (CDC), in 2008, there were at least 184 SEPs in 36 states in the USA that exchanged 29.1 million syringes. This figure is an underestimate because at least one third of the SEPs surveyed that year did not respond to the CDC questionnaire. SEPs are also cost effective. In 2005, the CDC estimated that the medical cost of treating a person infected with HIV was $190,000. It is safe to assume that in the last several years, this cost has risen. In sharp contrast, the cost of a syringe is less than $1.00.

SEPs are not without controversy which is expressed in many public arenas. Some people feel that SEPs encourage drug use because they provide the tools needed to consume drugs like heroin and methamphetamine. Moral and legal perspectives are often the drivers when drug use is discussed publically, especially by elected officials and candidates for elected office. The controversy exists even at the highest levels of global decision making. Notably, although harm reduction, which includes SEPs, is supported by many organizations within the United Nations (UN) including UNAIDS, the UN Office on Drugs and Crime and the World Health Organization, it is not even considered by global organizations that influence and guide drug policies internationally. For example, the UN Commission on Narcotic Drugs' 2009 outline of international cooperation on drug strategy for a ten-year period does not refer to SEPs at all, which was encouraged by the USA, Russia, Sweden, Italy, Japan, and the Vatican, among others.

Advocates of SEPs however point to the scientific evidence that SEPs actually reduce HIV infection rates and do not promote drug use. Findings from four groups of IDUs who have been followed over time show the number of new cases of HIV (HIV incidence) declined significantly from 5.5 cases per 100 person-years in 1988–1989 to 0 cases per 100 person-years in 1998, and remained at 0 cases in 2005–2008. The authors state that the "large-scale expansion of [needle exchange programs] and opiate substitution treatment programs appear to have reduced HIV transmission among IDUs." The scientific evidence shows that the benefits of a SEP go beyond the drug user to the general society because they support education and recovery, reduce deaths, crime, and HIV infection. Accordingly, mental health care providers may wish to refer their clients who continue to inject drugs to syringe exchange programs, in an effort to reduce the clients' risk of contracting HIV or other blood-borne diseases, such as hepatitis B and C, and the risk of bacterial infections.

Related Topics: Harm reduction, mental health comorbidity and HIV/AIDS, prevention strategies.

Suggested Reading

Centers for Disease Control and Prevention (CDC). (2007). Syringe exchange programs—United States, 2005. *Morbidity and Mortality Weekly Report*, 56(44), 1164–1167. Retrieved February 26, 2012 http://www.cdc.gov/mmwr/preview/mmwrhtml/mm5945a4.htm?s_cid=mm5945a4_e

Centers for Disease Control and Prevention (CDC). (2010). Syringe exchange programs—United States, 2008. *Morbidity and Mortality Weekly Report*, 59(45), 1488–1491. Retrieved February 27, 2012 from http://www.cdc.gov/mmwr/preview/mmwrhtml/mm5945a4.htm?s_cid=mm5945a4_e

Drucker, E., Lurie, P., Wodak, A., & Alcabes, P. (1998). *Measuring harm reduction: The effects of needle and syringe exchange program and methadone maintenance on the ecology of HIV*. AIDS, 12(Suppl A), S217–S230.

Mehta, S. H., Astemborski, J., Kirk, G. D., Strathdee, S. A., Nelson, K. E., et al. (2011). Changes in blood-borne infection risk among injection drug users. *Journal of Infectious Diseases, 203*(5), 587–594. Retrieved on March 17, 2012 from http://www.hivandhepatitis.com/hep_c/news/2011/0211_2011_a.html.

Okie, S. (2007). Sex, drugs, prisons, and HIV. *New England Journal of Medicine*, *356*, 105–108. Retrieved on March 3, 2012 from http://www.nejm.org/doi/full/10.1056/NEJMp068277

Suggested Resources

AVERT: Averting HIV and AIDS. *Needle exchange and harm reduction/needle exchange and HIV*. Retrieved February 13, 2012 from http://www.avert.org/needle-exchange.htm

Centers for Disease Control and Prevention (CDC). (2005). *Syringe exchange program (factsheet)*. Retrieved February 25, 2012 from http://www.cdc.gov/idu/facts/AED_IDU_SYR.pdf

Kaiser Family Foundation/statehealthfacts.org. (2011). *Sterile syringe exchange programs, 2011*. Retrieved February 23, 2012 from http://www.statehealthfacts.org/comparetable.jsp?ind=566&cat=11

Transgender

Ana-Gabriela Benghiac

Transgender is a term that defines individuals whose gender identity, expression or behavior differs from their birth sex. There are no national surveillance data regarding the number of transgender persons in USA and the local data and literature estimates suggest high differences regarding HIV/AIDS infection in the transgender population. However, it is known that this community is one of the highest risk groups for HIV/AIDS. According to the Centers for Disease Control and Prevention (CDC), up to 69% of transgender persons are HIV-infected, the highest prevalence being registered among male-to-female transgender sex workers. It is believed that African American transgender persons are at even higher risk of HIV infection due to the stigma associated with being transgender and a minority.

Several prevention measures can be implemented in order to better control the transmission of HIV infection among the transgender communities. A better understanding of the definition of transgender individuals must be attained. However, identifying individuals with specificity is difficult due to the diversity of sexual orientations. Many transgender individuals have multiple partners and practice unprotected sex, some of which may be related to commercial sex work. The consumption of alcohol and drugs can impact individuals' capacity and judgment, leading to decisions and actions that can increase infection risk. Efforts should be made to develop tailored interventions that encourage the reduction of sexual partners, the use of protective measures for sex, and the diminution or elimination of alcohol intake and substance use. Contextual factors that lead to the manifestation of such risk behaviors must also be addressed, such as the exchange of sex for housing, food, money, or drugs (survival sex) and the shared use of needles for silicone injections and hormones.

Due to discrimination and stigma, most transgender individuals have a lower income compared to other HIV risk groups, often lacking high school or advanced

A.-G. Benghiac (✉)
Department of Bioethics, Case Western Reserve University, Cleveland, OH, USA
e-mail: dr.gabriela_benghiac@yahoo.com

S. Loue (ed.), *Mental Health Practitioner's Guide to HIV/AIDS*,
DOI 10.1007/978-1-4614-5283-6_88,

education, health insurance, permanent housing or jobs. Even those who have health insurance may be underinsured. Mental health problems are frequent and are influenced by social instability and risk behaviors. The prevalence of depression, isolation, anxiety, loneliness, lower self-esteem, and suicidal ideation is considered to be high in this population. A history of sexual harassment, trauma and cross-sex hormonal therapy are other issues that have to be addressed; patients should benefit from support in order to cope with events that impact their daily life.

Attitudes of healthcare providers towards transgender individuals have often been less than helpful, leading to individuals' reluctance to seek advice, medical care and social services. There is a tendency among transgender people to distrust the healthcare providers due to barriers created over time. There is a clear need to offer practical advice to healthcare providers involved in activities with transgender individuals in order to improve communication skills, increase their patients' well-being, and avoid health care inequities. Screening for mental health illnesses, substance abuse, sexually transmitted diseases, and HIV testing must be promoted in these communities and people should be referred to institutions that offer prevention and treatment programs. These programs should address other important problems in the community such as education for employment, the promotion of a healthy life style, psychological support, and appropriate access to medical care. The World Professional Association for Transgender Health (WPATH) publishes on its website the *Standards of Care for Health of Transsexual, Transgender and Gender Nonconforming People*. These standards are provided for healthcare providers as a means of guiding them in their profession and to institutions and individuals interested in promoting optimal health in transgender communities. These guidelines are important for healthcare providers as they offer a good image of the general and medical issues that transgender individuals have. Mental health professionals can play an important role in addressing several problems reported by the transgender population such as difficulties in finding specialized professionals; refusal of counseling, treatment and referral services; and misconceptions and judgmental attitudes.

Studies show that many transgender individuals access health care services seeking hormone therapy. Thus, the attitude of healthcare providers who interact with transgender individuals is crucial. Patients should benefit not only from hormone treatment but also from preventive measures and counseling regarding STDs, HIV/AIDS, mental health issues and substance abuse. Support groups should be implemented and transgender individuals should be referred to other professionals that could offer them immediate and real solutions for their problems.

Since identity issues are life-time processes that affect this population, a positive attitude manifested by society, educators and healthcare providers towards this vulnerable group will contribute to an increased quality of life, societal integration and acceptance, disease prevention, and treatment adherence.

Related Topics: Gender identity, gender role, transsexuality.

Suggested Reading

Garofalo, R., Deleon, J., Osmer, E., Doll, M., & Harper, G. W. (2006). Overlooked, misunderstood and at-risk: Exploring the lives and HIV risk of ethnic minority male-to-female transgender youth. *Journal of Adolescent Health, 38*, 230–236.

Moriarty, H. J., Thiagalingam, A., & Hill, P. D. (1998). Audit of service to a minority client group: Male to female transsexuals. *International Journal of STD and AIDS, 9*, 238–240.

Valenta, L. J., Elias, A. N., & Domurat, E. S. (1992). Hormone pattern in pharmacologically feminized male transsexuals in the California State prison system. *Journal of the National Medical Association, 84*, 241–250.

White, J. C., & Townsend, M. H. (1998). Transgender medicine: Issues and definitions. *Journal of the Gay and Lesbian Medical Association, 2*, 1–3.

Suggested Resources

Centers for Disease Control and Prevention. *HIV/AIDS and transgender persons*. Retrieved March 7, 2012 from http://www.cdc.gov/lgbthealth/pdf/fs-transgender-06192007.pdf

The World Professional Association for Transgender Health. (2011). *Standards of care for health of transsexual, transgender and gender nonconforming people, 7th version*. Retrieved March 7, 2012 from http://www.wpath.org/documents/Standards%20of%20Care%20V7%20-%202011%20WPATH.pdf

Transsexuality

Lisa R. Norman

Transsexuals have been defined as individuals with a cross-sexual identity. Although a transsexual individual is transgender, not all transgender individuals are transsexual. The distinction may be more clearly understood by thinking of transsexuals as wishing to change or attempting to change their sex from that at birth and transgender individuals as those who blur the boundaries between genders, e.g., the societally accepted representation for masculinity/femininity or male/female roles. An individual may be transsexual even if he or she has not undergone sexual reassignment surgery to change his or her biological sex. It has been estimated that approximately 1 out of every 11,900 men (male to female) and approximately 1 out of every 30,400 women (female to male) are transsexuals. Estimates of the sex ratio have varied widely, from 2.5 men to 1 woman in the Netherlands to 5.5 women to 1 man in Poland.

Transsexual persons may identify as heterosexual, homosexual, bisexual, or none of the above in terms of their sexual orientation. Because of the small reported number of transsexual persons in the USA and elsewhere, little effort has been made to create a new demographic category for the purpose of epidemiology, e.g., tracking health conditions, including HIV, in different populations. The general lack of inclusion of gender variance variables in health surveys makes collecting true estimates of the transsexual population and transsexual HIV population that much more difficult. However, it appears that transsexual persons often face a myriad of challenges that place them at increased risk of HIV infection. Precarious economic status, substance use, low self-esteem, social vulnerability, and a lack of social support are common barriers to adopting and maintaining safer behaviors that can prevent the acquisition of HIV or transmission of HIV.

With respect to mental health issues, social marginalization is one that is experienced by many transsexual persons due to rejection by their peers and families, and a lack of connection to the lesbian, gay, and bisexual community,

L.R. Norman (✉)
Ponce School of Medicine, Ponce, Puerto Rico
e-mail: lnorman@psm.edu

S. Loue (ed.), *Mental Health Practitioner's Guide to HIV/AIDS*,
DOI 10.1007/978-1-4614-5283-6_89,

intensifying the risk of HIV transmission and disease progression. Rejection from family and peers may lead to alienation and feelings of hopelessness, and may increase psychological and social vulnerability, which may in turn, increase HIV risk.

Many transsexual persons have an increased risk of depression, substance abuse, and a history of forced sex, gender-based discrimination, and gender-based victimization, which are all associated with attempting suicide. As such, a complete psychological history should be taken and any necessary mental health treatment should be started before hormone therapy, to ensure the best possible outcomes. The health care needs of transsexual individuals are complex and may intimidate health care providers; due to the lack of culturally competent medical settings, transsexual individuals may struggle to find appropriate medical care. Other barriers to care include fear of exposure or disclosure, geographic isolation, and a dearth of transsexual-specific clinical research and medical literature.

Overall, the transsexual population is severely underserved and carries a disproportionate burden of HIV and mental health problems. By adopting culturally appropriate steps, health care provides can take significant steps toward relieving some of the health disparities experienced by transgendered persons.

Related Topics: Access to care, transgender, stigma and stigmatization.

Suggested Reading

Bolin, A. (1992). Coming of age among transsexuals. In T. L. Whitehead & B. V. Reid (Eds.), *Gender constructs and social issues* (pp. 13–39). Chicago, IL: University of Chicago Press.

Bolin, A. (1994). Transcending and transgendering: Male-to-female transsexuals, dichotomy and diversity. In G. Herdt (Ed.), *Third sex, third gender: Beyond sexual dimorphism in culture and history* (pp. 447–485). New York, NY: Zone Books.

Coleman, E. J. (2001). *Transgender and HIV: Risks, prevention, and care*. Binghamton, NY: The Hawthorne Press.

Israel, G. E. (2002). *Transgender care, recommended guidelines, practical information, and personal accounts*. Philadelphia, PA: Temple University Press.

Suggested Resources

Center of Excellence for Transgender HIV Prevention. Retrieved February 29, 2012 from www.transhealth.org

National Center for Transgender Equality. Retrieved February 29, 2012 from www.nctequality.org

The World Professional for Transgender Health (WPATH). Retrieved February 29, 2012 from www.wpath.org

Tuskegee Syphilis Study

Brittany Daugherty-Brownrigg

The field of medicine has benefited tremendously from human research and experimentation. Yet, these advances have come at a cost. There have been many incidences in which individuals used in research studies were treated unfairly and harmed. One historically relevant incident was called the Tuskegee Syphilis Study. This federally funded study was initiated in 1932 in Macon County, Alabama by the US Public Health Service to address the epidemic of syphilis.

Syphilis is a sexually transmitted disease caused by the bacterium *Treponema pallidum*. Its symptoms often mimic other diseases making it hard to diagnose without a specific blood test. It can be passed from person to person through unprotected sexual relations and blood. The infection often goes unnoticed because symptoms can be dormant. Although syphilis is easily curable, the infection can cause significant problems if it remains untreated. There are three stages to the infection: primary, secondary, and late or latent stages. The primary stage is triggered by the presence of chancre sores. The secondary stage is reached when there is the presence of mild skin rashes and lesions on mucous membranes.

The latent stage begins after the cessation of primary and secondary stage symptoms. In some individuals, the latent stage never ends. However, approximately 15 % of individuals with untreated syphilis will go onto develop late stage syphilis, which will bring additional health problems and may even be fatal. Problems may occur within the lymph glands, vital organs, bone structure or central nervous system.

Untreated syphilis in its late stage can cause neurosyphilis, an infection of the central nervous system. Neurosyphilis can lead to symptoms such as blindness, confusion, numbness, paralysis, dementia and difficulties coordination muscle movements. Blood tests can be preformed to detect the bacterium that causes syphilis. However, testing of the spinal fluid is a prime indicator of neurosyphilis.

B. Daugherty-Brownrigg (✉)
John Carroll University, South Euclid, OH, USA
e-mail: bdaugherty10@jcu.edu

S. Loue (ed.), *Mental Health Practitioner's Guide to HIV/AIDS*,
DOI 10.1007/978-1-4614-5283-6_90,

The only treatment for syphilis is penicillin or other antibiotics for individuals allergic to penicillin. Follow-up blood tests and lumbar punctures may be performed to monitor the progression of the infection and the effectiveness of the treatment.

All of the study subjects in the Tuskegee Syphilis Study were poor Black sharecroppers. They were not told that they were the subjects in a natural history study of syphilis or that they were infected with syphilis. Instead, they were informed that they were to be treated for "bad blood," a euphemism that referred to a variety of maladies including anemia, syphilis and others. The standard of care for syphilis at the time the study began, 1932, consisted of injections of arsenic and mercury for a period of 1 year. Later, following the discovery of penicillin, the infection was treatable with this antibiotic. Nevertheless, the men were not provided with the standard of care that prevailed for syphilis during the course of the study and were actively prevented in some cases from obtaining treatment for the infection from providers outside of the study. The incentives for continuing to present for the ostensible treatment included free physical examinations, free transportation to and from clinics, hot meals and a guaranteed burial stipend. However, there was no official protocol for the experiment and the men were simply being tested for the complications of the disease instead of being treated.

During this time racial tension was prevalent in the South. This set a dramatic tone for the way this cohort of Black men was treated. Scientists and physicians emphasized differences between Whites and Blacks in their facial features, skin color, cranium and brain size as a means to both explain and justify their portrayal of Blacks. African American subjects were portrayed as inferior on many different levels. Black sexuality was equated to what was perceived as Blacks' innate sexual promiscuity a character flaw that was inherently problematic.

During the 1960s, questions began to be raised regarding the ethics of the Tuskegee Syphilis Study. An investigation of the study ultimately led to its cessation in 1972. No longer can researchers use human beings as merely a means to an end in the conduct of research. Since the Tuskegee Syphilis Study, laws have been promulgated to protect participants from harm. Prospective study participants must be provided with adequate information about the study objectives as well as the risks and benefits associated with participation; this information constitutes elements of what is known as informed consent. Additionally, their consent to participate must be voluntary, unlike that of the men in the Tuskegee Syphilis Study, who faced the possible loss of their employment if they refused to participate.

Many institutions that conduct research have established committees to review the ethical aspects of a study prior to its approval and conduct. These are known in the USA as Institutional Review Boards (IRBs) and in many other countries as Research Ethics Committees (RECs). These committees review the risks and benefits of proposed research to ensure that the protocol complies with international and national standards for the conduct of research with human beings. In the USA, the federal agency of the Office of Human Protections, established by the US

Department of Health and Human Services, focuses on the protection of human research participants.

This study exemplifies the exploitation of Blacks by researchers and medical professionals; the study led to injury to the men's bodies and displayed utter disregard of their rights as patients seeking care. Importantly, the study has led to the distrust of medical "establishments," which helps to explain not only the reduced involvement of African Americans in clinical trials, but also their greater reluctance to seek HIV testing and to seek out and utilize medical and behavioral health services if HIV positive. In a widely cited 1991 analysis, Thomas and Quinn suggested that the enduring power of intra-community memory of the infamous Tuskegee Syphilis Study within the African American community has significant impact on trust of medical institutions and, therefore, the effectiveness of HIV prevention programs designed and delivered by those institutions. Bogart and Thorburn (2005) found significant endorsement of conspiracy theories about the origin of HIV/AIDS among African Americans, and a strong association between the acceptance of conspiracy theories and a distrust of and reduced use of condoms among men. In an abstract presented at the 2004 AmFAR National Update Conference, Nessel and Primm of the Addiction Research and Treatment Corporation reported having found high levels of distrust of medical institutions among individuals from groups who were surveyed about the origins of HIV.

Related Topics: African Americans, cognitive impairment, conspiracy theories, denialism, discrimination, informed consent, sexually transmitted infections.

Suggested Reading

Bogart, L. M., & Thorburn, S. (2005). Are HIV/AIDS conspiracy beliefs a barrier to prevention among African Americans? *Journal of Acquired Immune Deficiency Syndromes, 38*(2), 213–218.

Foster, C. (2001). *The ethics of medical research on humans*. New York, NY: Cambridge University Press.

Jones, J. H. (1981). *Bad blood: The Tuskegee syphilis experiment*. New York, NY: The Free Press.

Thomas, S. B., & Quinn, S. C. (1991). The Tuskegee Syphilis Study, 1932–1972: Implications for HIV education and AIDS risk reduction programs in the black community. *American Journal of Public Health, 8*(11), 1498–1504.

Washington, H. A. (2006). *Medical apartheid: The dark history of medical experimentation on black Americans from colonial times to the present*. New York, NY: Doubleday.

Suggested Resources

Centers for Disease Control and Prevention. (2010, September 16). *Sexually transmitted diseases: Syphilis–CDC fact sheet*. Retrieved January 30, 2012 from http://www.cdc.gov/std/syphilis/stdfact-syphilis.htm

Centers for Disease Control and Prevention. (2011, June 15). *U.S. Public Health Service Syphilis Study at Tuskegee*. Retrieved January 30, 2012 from http://www.cdc.gov/tuskegee/timeline.htm

Office of Human Research Protections. U.S. Department of Health & Human Services. http://www.hhs.gov/ohrp/index.html

PubMed Health. (2010, September 15). *Neurosyphilis*. Retrieved January 30, 2012 from http://www.ncbi.nlm.nih.gov/pubmedhealth/PMH0001722/

United Nations

Beatrice Gabriela Ioan

The United Nations is an international organization, founded in 1945 by 51 countries around the world. Currently, this organization consists of 193 countries.

The ultimate goal of the United Nations is to harmonize the efforts of the nations to maintain peace and security in the world, to promote friendly relations among peoples and nations of the world helping them to achieve better living standards and respect for human rights and freedoms. Through its activities that seek to create a safer world, the United Nations virtually reaches all over the corners of the world and covers various areas such as: sustainable development, environmental protection, problems of refugees, disarmament, promoting democracy, human rights, gender equality, health, etc.

United Nations activities for the prevention and combating HIV infection worldwide are coordinated by the *Joint Nations Programme on HIV/AIDS* (*UNAIDS*). This program is co-sponsored by ten other United Nations agencies: the United National High Commissioner for Refugees (UNHCR), the United Nations Children's Fund (UNICEF), the United Nations World Food Programme (WFP), the United Nations Development Programme (UNDP), the United Nations Population Fund (UNFPA), the United Nations Office on Drugs and Crime (UNDOC), the International Labor Organization (ILO), UNESCO, the World Health Organization (WHO), and the World Bank.

In 2000 the General Assembly's Millennium Summit set specific goals for halting and reducing the spread of HIV epidemic in the world. The following year, during a special session of the General Assembly, these purposes were extended through the development of a reference document entitled *Declaration of Commitment on HIV/AIDS*, in which were set national targets and actions to reduce global HIV epidemic. In 2002, The Global Fund to Fight AIDS, Tuberculosis and Malaria was created.

B.G. Ioan (✉)
Legal Medicine, Medical Deontology and Bioethics Department, University of Medicine and Pharmacy "Gr. T. Popa", Iasi, Romania
e-mail: ioanbml@yahoo.com

S. Loue (ed.), *Mental Health Practitioner's Guide to HIV/AIDS*,
DOI 10.1007/978-1-4614-5283-6_91,

In 2006 the General Assembly adopted an important document, entitled *Political Declaration on HIV/AIDS*, which aimed at ensuring, by 2010, universal access to prevention programs, treatment, care and support services for people infected with HIV. It also created a system for the United Nations Member States to report annually their results and to monitor their actions against HIV/AIDS.

In 2011, based on the fact that the deadline for achieving the goals agreed by the member countries through the *2001 Declaration of Commitment on HIV/AIDS* and *the 2006 Political Declaration on HIV/AIDS* passed, and many countries have not succeeded in fulfilling their commitments, the UN General Assembly adopted the *Political Declaration on HIV/AIDS: Intensifying our Efforts to Eliminate HIV/AIDS (A/RES/65/277)*. This document outlines the strategy of the United Nations and its member countries and is aimed at ensuring that by 2015, universal access to prevention programs, treatment, care and support for persons suffering from HIV/AIDS will exist. The Declaration indicates that while the issue of HIV/AIDS is not resolved, as a result of sustained efforts at national, regional and international levels, the rate of new HIV infections has been reduced by over 25% in 30 countries, and antiretroviral treatment is available for more than six million people infected with HIV, which has reduced AIDS deaths by 20% in the last 5 years.

However, despite international efforts, HIV epidemics continue to be alarming, especially affecting the population in sub-Saharan African countries, followed by Caribbean countries. At the same time, the number of HIV infections is increasing in countries from Eastern Europe, Central Asia, North Africa, the Middle East and parts of Asia and the Pacific. The Declaration points to the main characteristics of the present HIV epidemics to envisage the main directions of intervention directed to fulfill its goals.

The HIV epidemic affects mainly agrarian economies, leading to an increase in poverty in these countries. Poor diet favors premature deaths caused by AIDS, due to immune deficiency and inadequate response of the body to opportunistic infections or other diseases. Moreover, the maximum benefit of antiretroviral therapy can be achieved only if individuals are able to maintain an appropriate diet.

Girls and women continue to be the most affected by the epidemic due to their reduced ability to protect themselves from HIV infection as the result of physiological factors, gender inequalities, and inadequate access to medical services. They also have an increased risk of sexual violence and exploitation. In these circumstances the UN has an important role in combating HIV through promoting gender equality, which may reduce the vulnerability of women and girls to HIV infection.

Young persons, aged between 15 and 24 years, account for more than a third of all new HIV infections, and many young people have limited access to programs for sexual and reproductive health. The increased incidence of HIV infection among those who inject drugs and use drugs continues to be a real threat to public health and welfare of humanity, especially affecting young people. Another concern is the vertical transmission of HIV infection from mother to child, even in high-income countries that have made significant progress to eradicate this mechanism of transmission. Also, people with disabilities are not sufficiently included in programs to prevent, treat, care and support cases of HIV/AIDS.

According to the Declaration, programs to fight against HIV/AIDS should be customized in each country according to the epidemiological and cultural characteristics. In the global response to HIV/AIDS, prevention must be the key element, achieved through various actions such as: public information and education campaigns; the reduction of risk behaviors, including the promotion of responsible sexual behavior; the implementation of harm reduction programs among drug users; provision of sterile injection equipment; the elimination of gender inequalities, including that involving men and boys; and the increased access of pregnant women to prevention and treatment programs.

Targets set out in the Declaration for 2015 include the reduction by 50% of sexual transmission of HIV and of transmission among drug injecting users, the elimination of HIV transmission from mother to child and a substantial decrease of maternal deaths due to AIDS. In terms of treatment, the Declaration sets out the goal to ensure access to antiretroviral treatment to 15 million HIV-infected people by 2015. It also requires the elimination of barriers to access to antiretroviral treatment in low and middle-income countries.

The Declaration also stipulates the need to intensify national efforts to reduce stigma, discrimination and violence associated with HIV. To this end, HIV-infected persons should have equal access to education, employment, health and social services. Special attention should be given to people who are vulnerable to HIV infection, such as migrants who should have access to prevention programs, treatment, care and support.

In order to ensure the necessary funds to fight HIV/AIDS, the Declaration emphasizes the need to increase the funds allocated by each country. Many developed countries, for example, have proposed an allocation of up to 0.7% of their GDP for actions to reduce HIV/AIDS. In addition, the Global Fund to Fight AIDS, Tuberculosis and Malaria plays a key role in financing the global response to HIV/AIDS.

The declaration recommends strengthening national health systems, particularly primary health systems, with the inclusion of measures designed to combat HIV/AIDS. This document also emphasizes the importance of basic research in accelerating the development of sustainable and affordable treatments for HIV and TB, and the development of a safe, affordable, and effective HIV vaccine.

To achieve the goal of universal access to prevention programs, treatment, care and support for those affected by HIV/AIDS, UNAIDS has developed a strategy for 2011–2015, entitled *Getting to Zero*. The document proposes three strategic directions to respond to HIV infection: the prevention of transmission of infection; the introduction of new methods of treatment and support that are both simple and accessible; and the promotion of human rights and gender equality.

In June 2011 the Resolution 1983 (2011) of the UN Security Council was adopted. It starts from the first resolution of the UN Security Council on HIV/AIDS (Resolution 1308/2000) which was limited to only the risk placed on the UN representatives in the peacekeeping missions in areas affected by the HIV/AIDS pandemic. Resolution 1308/2000, adopted at the initiative of the USA, encourages Member States to cooperate for the prevention, voluntary testing, confidentiality, counseling and treatment of the staff of the peacekeeping missions. Resolution 1983/2011 has a broader approach and it starts from the impact of the HIV/AIDS on the process of maintaining peace and security in armed conflict and post-conflict areas. By its terms, this Resolution encourages the incorporation of prevention programs, treatment, care and support for cases of HIV/AIDS in the mandates of UN peacekeeping missions, adopting the most appropriate measures to protect civilians, particularly girls and women against sexual violence, human trafficking, sexual exploitation in conflict and post-conflict areas. At the heart of the 2011 Resolution are vulnerable persons, particularly girls and women, who are the most frequent victims of sexual violence and trafficking. These measures are based on the fact that rape is a weapon in many areas of armed conflict and post-conflict and violence and instability in these areas may favor expansion of HIV through sexual violence and population movements.

Related Topics: Human rights, human trafficking, prevention strategies, World Health Organization.

Suggested Reading

United Nations General Assembly. *Political declaration on HIV/AIDS: Intensifying our efforts to eliminate HIV/AIDS*. Retrieved October 25, 2011 from http://www.unaids.org/en/media/unaids/contentassets/documents/document/2011/06/20110610_UN_A-RES-65-277_en.pdf

United Nations General Assembly Special Session on HIV/AIDS (2001, June 25–27). *Declaration of Commitment on HIV/AIDS*. Retrieved October 25, 2011 from http://www.unaids.org/en/media/unaids/contentassets/dataimport/publications/irc-pub03/aidsdeclaration_en.pdf

UNAIDS. (2011–2015). *Strategy. Getting to zero*. Retrieved October 25, 2011 from http://www.unaids.org/en/media/unaids/contentassets/documents/unaidspublication/2010/JC2034_UNAIDS_Strategy_en.pdf

Suggested Resources

http://www.un.org/en/aboutun/index.shtml. Last accessed October 25, 2011.

http://www.un.org/en/globalissues/aids/index.shtml. Last accessed October 25, 2011.

http://www.un.org/News/Press/docs/2011/sc10272.doc.htm. Last accessed October 25, 2011.

Universalism

Nicole M. Deming

Universalism is a branch of ethics that states that there are principles of ethics (such as rules of right and wrong) that apply to all humans regardless of situation, location or even time. One example of universalism in practice is The Universal Declaration of Human Rights. Adopted in December 1948, this document states that all humans have inalienable rights including life, liberty, and security of person regardless of race, sex, language, religion, political opinions, nationality, or any other status. In healthcare, we adopt similar universal rules and rights such as the Patient Bill of Rights and Responsibilities.

There are many different theories of ethics that fall under Universalism; three of the most well-known are utilitarian theories (consequentialism), deontological theories and virtue ethics. Utilitarians hold that whether an action is right or wrong depends solely on the consequences that result from that action. For a utilitarian, the right action is the action that produces the most good, regardless of how this might affect an individual personally. In contrast, deontology looks not to consequences but to an individual's duty to determine what is right and wrong. Immanuel Kant is one of the most recognizable deontologists. Kant wrote about the "Categorial Imperative" which holds that to determine what is right, an individual must be able to make the action into a universal law. Kant also held that it was important to treat all human beings with respect, as an "end" in themselves rather than just a means to an end. Aristotelian virtue ethics is discussed in terms of good and bad traits referred to as virtues and vices. Under this theory, a moral person does not act based on consequences or a sense of duty, but because it is the right action. A virtuous individual possessing all the virtues can achieve practical wisdom (*phronesis*) and ultimately live a happy or flourishing life (*eudaimonia*).

Like all theories, there are problems with the application of universalism in the real world. Utilitarians are faced with the problem of predicting the consequences. Deontologists are faced with the problem of conflicting duties or an inability to

N.M. Deming (✉)
Department of Bioethics, Case Western Reserve University, Cleveland, OH, USA
e-mail: Nicole.Deming@case.edu

S. Loue (ed.), *Mental Health Practitioner's Guide to HIV/AIDS*,

DOI 10.1007/978-1-4614-5283-6_92,

create a rule that could be applied universally. Critics of virtue ethics point to the difficulty in teaching character development rather than actions and rules. Despite these various problems with universalism, most health professionals are familiar with and rely upon universal rules in daily life. We are comfortable incorporating rules of law, religion, hospital policy, and standards of professionalism when deciding what is the right course of action.

As health care professionals, we must be aware that all patients have a right to care. While it is a reality that not all patients are treated equally, universalism challenges us to examine why patients are treated differently and determine if there is a morally justifiable rationale (i.e., could we justify treating all patients in this manner?). However, even when universal rules or principles exist, mental health care providers must question whether they are the true or correct rule. Looking back at history, we can see many examples of behaviors and laws that are unethical by today's standard. Like all policies, the rules and guiding principles we use in practice must be evaluated over time to ensure that they are in fact ethical and not just a product of tradition.

Ethical theories can be useful tools to analyze a difficult situation when the "right thing to do" is not obvious. By asking questions about the consequences, responsibilities, rules and what a wise mentor would do, we create a framework to examine a dilemma and decide upon a course of action in a thoughtful manner.

Related Topics: Declaration of Helsinki, human rights.

Suggested Reading

Alexander, L., & Moore, M. (2008). Deontological ethics. In E. N. Zalta (Ed.), *The Stanford encyclopedia of philosophy*. Retrieved April 2, 2012 from http://plato.stanford.edu/archives/fall2008/entries/ethics-deontological/

Driver, J. (2009). The history of utilitarianism. In E. N. Zalta (Ed.), *The Stanford encyclopedia of philosophy*. Retrieved April 2, 2012 from http://plato.stanford.edu/archives/sum2009/entries/utilitarianism-history/

Hursthouse, R. (2012). Virtue ethics. In E. N. Zalta (Ed.), *The Stanford encyclopedia of philosophy*. Retrieved April 2, 2012 from http://plato.stanford.edu/archives/spr2012/entries/ethics-virtue/

Oakley, J. (2007). Virtue theory. In R. Ashcroft et al. (Eds.), *Principles of health care ethics* (2nd ed.). West Sussex: Wiley.

Sinnott-Armstrong, W. (2011). Consequentialism. In E. N. Zalta (Ed.), *The Stanford encyclopedia of philosophy*. Retrieved April 2, 2012 from http://plato.stanford.edu/archives/win2011/entries/consequentialism/

Suggested Resources

The Universal Declaration of Human Rights. http://www.un.org/en/documents/udhr/

Women

Sana Loue

Incidence and Prevalence of HIV Among Women

Worldwide, approximately one-half of all individuals infected with HIV are women. It has been estimated that 1 out of every 139 women in the USA will be diagnosed with HIV during their lifetimes. However, Black and Latina women are at increased risk; one out of every 32 Black women and 1 out of every 106 Latina women will be diagnosed with HIV. Native Hawaiian, Pacific Islander, American Indian, and Alaskan Native women are at less risk. Non-Hispanic White women and Asian women have the least risk; it is estimated that 1 out of every 526 will be diagnosed with HIV infection.

In 2009, approximately 11,200 women in the USA became newly infected with HIV. This accounted for almost one-quarter of new infections that year. That same year, the rate of new HIV infections among Black women was approximately 15 times the rate among non-Hispanic White women and three times the rate among Latina women. In 2008, approximately one-quarter of all adults and individuals living with HIV were female.

Risk Factors for HIV Transmission to Women

The majority of women who become HIV-infected contract the infection through unprotected sex with a HIV-infected male partner. Many times, the woman may not know that her partner is HIV-infected. Even when she suspects that her partner is HIV-infected or is having sexual relations with other women or men, she may be

S. Loue (✉)
Department of Epidemiology and Biostatistics, Case Western Reserve University, Cleveland, OH, USA
e-mail: sana.loue@case.edu

S. Loue (ed.), *Mental Health Practitioner's Guide to HIV/AIDS*,
DOI 10.1007/978-1-4614-5283-6_93,

reluctant to insist on condom use because of the possibility of partner violence. Also, unprotected anal sex increases the risk of HIV transmission compared to vaginal sex due to a greater likelihood of ruptures.

The second most common means of becoming infected is through injection drug use, using contaminated injection equipment. The use of alcohol and drugs may also affect risk indirectly, by making it more likely that a woman will engage in unprotected sex while under the influence of the alcohol or drug.

The extent to which women who have sex with women (WSW) are at risk for 18 HIV infection remains unclear, due in large part to the way that risk behaviors are 19 reported. As an example, although some studies suggest that a large number of 20 female injection drug users areWSW, their risk if they are found to be HIV positive 21 is classified as that of injection drug use. Women who self-identify as WSW may 22 report having had sexual relations with a gay or bisexual man and, as a result, are 23 often classified as having heterosexual transmission risk.

Women who have been victims of abuse may experience increased risk as well. They may find it more difficult to refuse unwanted sexual overtures or may use drugs or alcohol as a means of coping with the abuse. The alcohol or drug use may, as indicated above, lead to increased HIV risk, directly or indirectly.

Women with severe mental illness may be at even greater risk of HIV infection in comparison with women who do not have a diagnosis of a severe mental illness. Researchers have found that women with severe mental illness who reported having sexual activity outside of an exclusive relationship or with high-risk partners are at increased risk of contracting HIV in comparison to men by virtue of *being female*. This may result from several factors. First, women with mental illness may experience difficulties in processing information, so that they are less able to identify and avoid situations that are risky. Second, they may be less competent socially because of their mental illness. As a result, they may not be able to form lasting relationships, refuse unreasonable requests, solve problems effectively, or negotiate risky situations. Third, women with a severe mental illness may be at increased risk of partner violence, which may place them at increased risk of HIV infection. Fourth, HIV may not rank as a high priority in relation to the women's daily struggle with poverty and unemployment. Finally, the various anatomical and hormonal characteristics of women render them more vulnerable to HIV transmission in comparison with men.

Additional factors may increase the risk of HIV among women. Infection with a sexually transmitted disease may increase the risk by facilitating HIV transmission. Poverty may also lead to increased risk, forcing some women, particularly those who are homeless, to exchange sex for shelter, food, or safety.

Other Implications of HIV for Women

Maternal-Infant Transmission

HIV infection can be transmitted vertically from mother to child during pregnancy, during labor and delivery, and through breast milk. UNAIDS has estimated that worldwide, at the end of 2009, approximately 2.5 million children under the age of 15 were HIV-infected and that the vast majority had contracted the infection from their mothers. In the USA, mother-to-child transmission has become less frequent with the administration of AZT before, during, and following delivery.

Women who are HIV-positive should be sure to consult with their doctor about their medications during pregnancy and even before becoming pregnant if at all possible. The type and/or dosage of medication may need to be adjusted depending upon the woman's CD4 count, the woman's weight, the stage of pregnancy, what is known about a drug's effects on the fetus, and what seems to be best for the mother's health. For women who are mentally ill and utilizing medications for their mental illness, it is particularly important that care be coordinated between the gynecologist and a physician specializing in HIV care in order to be alert to possible drug interactions and possible drug contraindications.

Caregiving

Women are also more likely to be caregivers to someone who is HIV-infected than are men. This may be particularly difficult for women with a serious mental illness due to the need to maintain the HIV-infected individual on a specific medication regimen, make sure that the individual's dietary needs are adequately addressed, and calendar and facilitate the individual's visits to his or her physicians. It is important that women in this situation receive emotional support themselves through available community resources.

Suggestions for Mental Health Care Providers

Due to the increased risk of HIV transmission that mentally ill women face, it is important that mental health care providers conduct a sexual history to determine if a particular client is at increased risk of HIV due to poverty, homelessness, substance use, violence, or other factors. This assessment likely needs to be conducted periodically as clients' circumstances can change. Safer sex practices, e.g., condom use, and safer needle-sharing practices, e.g., the use of a needle exchange service if available, should be discussed with clients for whom these issues are relevant. Providers will also want to be aware of HIV-related services that are available in the community, such as venues for HIV testing, needle exchange, HIV-related information, and support groups for HIV-infected women and for women who are caregivers of HIV-infected persons.

Related Topics: Caregivers and caregiving, mental health comorbidity and HIV/AIDS, partner violence, prevention strategies, risk behaviors.

Suggested Reading

Brabin, L. (2001). Hormonal markers of susceptibility to sexually transmitted infections: Are we taking them seriously? *British Medical Journal, 323*, 394–395.

Dworkin, S. L. (2005). Who is epidemiologically fathomable in the HIV. AIDS epidemic? Gender, sexuality, and intersectionality in public health. *Culture, Health & Sexuality, 7*(6), 6150623.

Gearon, J. S., & Bellack, A. S. (1999). Women with schizophrenia and co-occurring substance use disorders: An increased risk for violent victimization and HIV. *Community Mental Health, 35*, 401–419.

Hatters-Friedman, S., & Loue, S. (2007). Incidence and prevalence of intimate partner violence by and against women with severe mental illness. *Journal of Women's Health, 16*(4), 471–480.

Katz, R. C., Watts, C., & Santman, J. (1994). AIDS knowledge and high risk behaviors in the chronically mentally ill. *Community Mental Health Journal, 30*, 395–402.

Nicolosi, A., Leite, M. L. C., Musicco, M., Arici, C., Gavazzeni, G., & Lazzarin, A. (1994). The efficiency of male-to-female and female-to-male sexual transmission of the human immunodeficiency virus: A study of 730 stable couples. *Epidemiology, 5*(6), 570–575.

Padian, N. S., Shiboski, S. C., Glass, S. O., & Vittinghoff, E. (1997). Heterosexual transmission of human immunodeficiency virus (HIV) in northern California: Results from a ten-year study. *American Journal of Epidemiology, 146*(4), 350–357.

Weinhardt, L. S., Carey, M. P., & Carey, K. B. (1998). HIV-risk behavior and the public health context of HIV/AIDS among women living with a severe and persistent mental illness. *Journal of Nervous and Mental Disease, 186*, 276–282.

Suggested Resources

AVERT. (n.d.). *Women, HIV, and AIDS*. Retrieved December 23, 2011 from http://www.avert.org/women-hiv-aids.htm

Centers for Disease Control and Prevention. (2011, August). *HIV among women*. Retrieved December 23, 2011 from http://www.cdc.gov/hiv/topics/women/

World Health Organization

Anton Knieling

The World Health Organization (WHO) is a specialized agency of the United Nations (UN) that is concerned with international public health. It was established on April 7, 1948, with headquarters in Geneva, Switzerland and is a member of the UN Development Group. The membership of the WHP includes 193 countries and 2 associate members. Six regional committees, located in the Americas, Europe, the Eastern Mediterranean, South-East Asia, the Western Pacific, and Africa, focus on regional health concerns.

The WHO's constitution states that its objective "is the attainment by all people of the highest possible level of health". Apart from coordinating international efforts to control outbreaks of infectious disease, such as SARS, malaria, tuberculosis, influenza, and HIV/AIDS, the WHO also sponsors programs to prevent and treat such diseases. The WHO supports the development and distribution of safe and effective vaccines, pharmaceutical diagnostics, and drugs, such as through the Expanded Program on Immunization.

The WHO Disease Staging System for HIV Infection and Disease was first produced in 1990 by the WHO and was updated in September 2005. It can be used in resource-limited settings, is widely used in Africa and Asia, and has been used in research focusing on progression to symptomatic HIV disease. Most of these conditions are opportunistic infections that can be easily treated in healthy people. The staging system is different for adults and adolescents and children.

The WHO published an interim policy on collaborative TB/HIV activities to assist countries in need of immediate guidance to decrease the dual burden of tuberculosis (TB) and human immunodeficiency virus (HIV). The term interim was used because the evidence was incomplete at that time. Since then, additional evidence has been obtained from randomized controlled trials, observational studies, operational research, and the identification of best practices from programmatic implementation of the collaborative TB/HIV activities recommended by the policy.

A. Knieling (✉)
University of Medicine and Pharmacy Gr. T. Popa, Iasi, Romania
e-mail: tony_knieling@yahoo.com

S. Loue (ed.), *Mental Health Practitioner's Guide to HIV/AIDS*,
DOI 10.1007/978-1-4614-5283-6_94,

A number of TB and HIV guidelines and policy recommendations have been developed by WHO's Stop TB and HIV/AIDS departments.

Access to evidence-informed HIV prevention, testing and counseling, treatment and care services in low- and middle-income countries has increased and the global incidence of HIV infection is declining in many countries with generalized epidemics. The number of people receiving antiretroviral therapy continues to increase. The WHO Global Health Sector Strategy on HIV/AIDS: Getting to Zero, and the UNICEF's strategic and programmatic focus on equity will emphasize the need to tailor national HIV responses to the local epidemics, to decentralize programs, and to integrate with other health and community services to achieve the greatest impact.

UNAIDS and WHO have established several new targets: zero new infections, zero discrimination and zero AIDS-related deaths. The Global Health Sector Strategy on HIV/AIDS, endorsed by all WHO Member States in May 2011, guides national HIV responses in the health sector and outlines the role of WHO and other partners in achieving targets. The strategy focuses on four strategic directions: optimizing HIV prevention, diagnosis treatment and care; leveraging broader health outcomes through HIV responses; building strong and sustainable health and community systems; and reducing vulnerability and removing structural barriers that impede access to needed services. The prevention of mother-to-child HIV transmission through increased access to antiretroviral therapy and prophylaxis has energized the efforts of UN members to eliminate new infections among children and improve maternal health.

Related Topics: Standard of care, United Nations.

Suggested Resource

World Health Organization. (2007). *Working for health: An introduction to the World Health Organization*. Geneva, Switzerland: Author. Retrieved April 17, 2012 from http://www.who.int/about/brochure_en.pdf

World Health Organization. (2011). *Global health sector strategy on HIV/AIDS 2011–2015*. Geneva, Switzerland: Author. Retrieved April 17, 2012 from http://whqlibdoc.who.int/publications/2011/9789241501651_eng.pdf

World Trade Organization

Domniţa Oana Bădărău

Established in 1994 following the Uruguay Round, The World Trade Organization (WTO) is the result of multilateral trade negotiations; it seeks to promote and intensify commercial activities between its members. The rules to which the States agreed represent their declared effort to support an international trading system created through free markets policies. In the same year, The General Agreement on Tariffs and Trade (GATT) was adopted and added to the GATT 1947 provisions. Through GATT, the WTO established the most-favored-nation treatment stating that upon signing the agreement, member States must apply to the signing parties, without delay or under any conditions, the same circumstances that they already offered to suppliers from other countries. The main document regulates areas such as agriculture, rules of origin, subsidies and countervailing measures, safeguards and customs valuation; the additional protocols include agreements on trade services and information technology. Among the provisions which regulate drug commercialization and thus impact access to medication and treatments is the Trade-Related Aspects of Intellectual Property Rights (TRIPS).

In combating HIV/AIDS, significant progress has been made since the 1990s; this includes the development of antiretroviral drugs (ARVs). The positive results following antiretroviral treatment (ART) in HIV-infected patients were recognized by the World Health Organization (WHO) and were followed by the WHO's recommendation to make it available for larger populations in need, especially in developing countries. However, this goal appears harder to achieve given the intellectual property rights regulations in trade relations agreed upon by the WTO.

Beginning with 2005, developing countries had to adhere to Annex 1C of the GATT 1994 agreements on Trade-Related Aspects of Intellectual Property Rights (TRIPS). The TRIPS agreement aims to reduce barriers and imbalances in international legitimate trade, while guaranteeing that intellectual property rights are respected. In setting an international framework for member countries operating

D.O. Bădărău (✉)
Institute for Biomedical Ethics, University of Basel, Basel, Switzerland
e-mail: domnita14@gmail.com

S. Loue (ed.), *Mental Health Practitioner's Guide to HIV/AIDS*,
DOI 10.1007/978-1-4614-5283-6_95, © Springer Science+Business Media New York 2013

within the global trade, the Agreement stipulates that intellectual property rights must be recognized as private rights and protected by national laws, even when these differ between countries. Signatory States are responsible for creating laws and amending them, consistent with the Agreement's provisions. Exceptions or limitations from these provisions will be exclusively allowed in regard to particular cases and as long as they will not result in an infringement upon holder's rights. In addition, States agree to offer national treatment to all other Members, thus adopting a unitary standard for the recognition of intellectual rights protections. On the other hand, under the most-favored-nation treatment, it is guaranteed that any privilege offered by a signatory State to any other national or foreign agent shall apply to all parties in the Agreement. To explain it another way, there are two concepts here. National treatment means that a State gives to a country or number of countries the same privileges that the State gives to its own national agents. Most-favored-nation treatment refers to a situation in which a country signs an agreement with several other countries and is required to provide those countries or their national agents with at least the same preferential treatment that was agreed upon with a third country, which is not a signatory to this agreement.

Regarding ART, TRIPS seems to operate in a way that restricts competition with generics, which represents the key determinant to the reduction of the first-line medical therapy's prices starting with 2000. Developing countries such as India and Thailand produce the generic antiretroviral drugs which successfully competed with the multinational pharmaceutical companies' brand-name drugs. As a result, prices were reduced for brand-name drugs under "preferential prices" agreements, while generic drugs were available at even more reduced prices, thus leading to increased access to ART for the developing countries. However, the newer ART lines of treatment are patented by large pharmaceutical corporations. These patents, which require that intellectual property rights be respected, can be extended even longer under specific conditions. During the period of time in which the patent is held, TRIPS signatory countries are prohibited from producing generic versions of these pharmaceutical products. Under these circumstances, developing countries unable to afford the newer ART lines, priced at high levels due to the brand-name and latest technology, would continue to provide older, less effective and therefore cheaper drug medication.

The highest prevalence of HIV/AIDS occurs in some of the most impoverished populations, in developing countries, mainly sub-Saharan Africa, for which access to new medication at low prices is essential. Anuproar followed the TRIPS agreement on the commercialization and availability of ART for these populations. Subsequently, the Doha Declaration was signed, amending the Agreement on Trade-Related Aspects of Intellectual Property Rights and recognizing the value of public health needs. Under this Act, the member States facing difficulties in procuring the medication for a population severely affected by a disease, such as HIV, can interpret the patent regulations and apply them in a manner designed to best serve the public health issue.

Despite these concessions, access to HIV treatment is not completely without difficulties and is affected by economic and political factors. Fears exist that the growing number of people in need of medication and newer therapies, and the increasing costs of developing new drugs and adding patent regulations, will only exacerbate the problem. New antiretroviral medications continue to be patented in developed countries at higher and higher prices and the legal framework seems to limit the production of reverse engineered drugs in developing countries. A negative contributing factor to these limitations is represented by the so called "pay for delay" settlements between major pharmaceutical companies and generic producers. Under these settlements, generic manufacturers interested in producing newer therapies would agree to stop legal procedures to invalidate the brand-name producer's patent, the time ownership of the patent or to abandon procedures to patent the generic as a version that does respect the original patent. Financial payments are offered to the generic producer by the brand-name producer and patent holder, which ensures that generics of newer therapies will not reach the market. As these practices are becoming more and more common, HIV treatment will become restricted and higher prices for newer drugs will be maintained.

Related Topics: Antiretroviral therapy, economic impact.

Suggested Reading

Hoen, E., Berger, J., Calmy, A., & Moon, S. (2011). Driving a decade of change: HIV/AIDS, patents and access to medicines for all. *Journal of the International AIDS Society, 14*, 15. doi:10.1186/1758-2652-14-15.

Kesselheim, A. S., Murtagh, L., & Mello, M. M. (2011). "Pay for delay" settlements of disputes over pharmaceutical patents. *New England Journal of Medicine, 365*(15), 1439–1445. doi:10.1056/NEJMhle1102235.

Meiners, C., Sagaon-Teyssier, L., Hasenclever, L., & Moatti, J. P. (2011). Modeling HIV/AIDS drug price determinants in Brazil: Is generic competition a myth? *PLoS One, 6*(8), e23478. doi:10.1371/journal.pone.0023478.

Orsi, F., & d'almeida, C. (2010). Soaring antiretroviral prices, TRIPS and TRIPS flexibilities: A burning issue for antiretroviral treatment scale-up in developing countries. *Current Opinion in HIV and AIDS, 5*(3), 237–241. doi:10.1097/COH.0b013e32833860ba.

Van Puymbroeck, R. V. (2010). Basic survival needs and access to medicines—coming to grips with TRIPS: Conversion + calculation. *Journal of Law, Medicine and Ethics, 38*(3), 520–549. doi:10.1111/j.1748-720X.2010.00510.x.

Waning, B., Diedrichsen, E., & Moon, S. (2010). A lifeline to treatment: The role of Indian generic manufacturers in supplying antiretroviral medicines to developing countries. *Journal of the International AIDS Society, 13*, 35. doi:10.1186/1758-2652-13-35.

Index

S. Loue (ed.), *Mental Health Practitioner's Guide to HIV/AIDS*,
DOI 10.1007/978-1-4614-5283-6,

MIX
Papier aus verantwortungsvollen Quellen
Paper from responsible sources
FSC® C105338

If you have any concerns about our products,
you can contact us on
ProductSafety@springernature.com

In case Publisher is established outside the EU,
the EU authorized representative is:
Springer Nature Customer Service Center GmbH
Europaplatz 3, 69115 Heidelberg, Germany

Printed by Libri Plureos GmbH
in Hamburg, Germany